The Pathogenesis of
Infectious Disease

The Pathogenesis of Infectious Disease

Third Edition

CEDRIC A. MIMS

*Department of Microbiology,
Guy's Hospital Medical School, UMDS,
London Bridge, London SE1*

ACADEMIC PRESS

Harcourt Brace Jovanovich, Publishers
London   San Diego   New York
Boston   Sydney   Tokyo   Toronto

ACADEMIC PRESS LIMITED
24/28 Oval Road
London NW1 7DX

United States Edition published by
ACADEMIC PRESS, INC.
San Diego, CA92101

British Library Cataloguing in Publication Data is available

ISBN 0-12-498260-3
ISBN 0-12-498261-1 Pbk

This book is printed on acid-free paper

Photoset by Paston Press, Loddon, Norfolk
Printed by The Alden Press, Oxford, London, Northampton

Preface to the Third Edition

I have once again updated the text, but the general layout of the book still seems appropriate and has not been altered. I continue to look at things from the point of view of the infectious agent, which is perhaps becoming a more respectable thing to do.

The first edition was written in 1975–6 and the last line in the text contained my ultimate justification for the study of pathogenesis. It refers to the need for greater knowledge of disease processes and pathogenicity because it helps with "our ability to deal with any strange new pestilences that arise and threaten us", and it is still included on page 322. The emergence of AIDS has provided an immense stimulus to pathogenesis studies, particularly those dealing with the interaction of viruses with the immune system.

Studies of microbial pathogenesis are flourishing these days, and the final analysis of virulence at the molecular level has begun. Molecular biology, pathology and immunology will come together to explain just how a given gene product contributes to disease, giving not only intellectual satisfaction to scientists but also a rich fallout for human and veterinary medicine.

December, 1986   C. A. Mims

Preface to the Second Edition

I have brought things up to date, especially in the fast moving fields of phagocytes and immunology. Important subjects such as diarrhoea and persistent infections are given greater attention, and there is a brief look at infectious agents in human diseases of unknown aetiology, a confusing area for which an overview seemed timely. Otherwise the general layout of the book is unaltered, and it is still quite short. There are more references, but not too many, and they remain at the end of the chapters so as not to weigh down the text or inhibit the generalizations!

At times I have been taken to task for calling viruses "microorganisms". I do so because there is no collective term embracing viruses, chlamydias, rickettsias, mycoplasmas, bacteria, fungi and protozoa other than "infectious agents", and for this there is no equivalent adjective. I prefer to take this particular liberty with microbiological language rather than stay tied to definitions (which can end up with tautologies such as "viruses are viruses".)

March, 1982   C. A. Mims

Preface to the First Edition

For the physician or veterinarian of course, the important thing about microorganisms is that they infect and cause diseases. Most textbooks of medical microbiology deal with the subject either microbe by microbe, or disease by disease. There are usually a few general chapters on the properties of microorganisms, natural and acquired resistance to infection etc., and then the student reads separately about each microbe and each infectious disease. It is my conviction that the centrally significant aspect of the subject is the mechanism of microbial infection and pathogenicity, and that the principles are the same, whatever the infectious agent. When we consider the entry of microorganisms into the body, their spread through tissues, the role of immune responses, toxins and phagocytes, the general features are the same for viruses, rickettsiae, bacteria, fungi and protozoa. This book deals with infection and pathogenicity from this point of view. All microorganisms are considered together as each part of the subject is dealt with. There are no systematic accounts of individual diseases, their diagnosis or their treatment, but the principal microorganisms and diseases are included in a series of tables and a figure at the end of the book.

Just as the virologist has needed to study not only the virus itself but also the cell and its responses to infection, so the student of infectious diseases must understand the body's response to infection as well as the properties of the infecting microorganism. It is hoped that this approach will give the reader an attitude towards infection and pathogenicity that will be relevant whatever the nature of the infectious agent and whatever the type of infectious disease. Most of the examples concern infections of man, but because the principles apply to all infections, the book may also prove of value for the student of veterinary or general science.

C. A. Mims

For creatures your size I offer
   a free choice of habitat,
so settle yourselves in the zone
   that suits you best, in the pools
of my pores or the tropical
   forests of arm-pit and crotch,
in the deserts of my fore-arms,
   or the cool woods of my scalp

Build colonies: I will supply
   adequate warmth and moisture,
the sebum and lipids you need,
   on condition you never
do me annoy with your presence,
   but behave as good guests should
not rioting into acne
   or athlete's-foot or a boil.

From: "A New Year Greeting" by W. H. Auden. (Epistle to a Godson and other poems. Published by Faber and Faber (UK) and Random House, Inc. (USA).)

Contents

1

General Principles

In general biological terms, the type of association between two different organisms can be classified as parasitic, where one benefits at the expense of the other, or symbiotic (mutualistic), where both benefit. There is an intermediate category called commensalism, where only one organism derives benefit, living near the other organism or on its surface without doing any damage. It is often difficult to use this category with confidence, because an apparently commensal association often proves on closer examination to be really parasitic or symbiotic, or it may at times become parasitic or symbiotic.

The same classification can be applied to the association between microorganisms and vertebrates. Generalized infections such as measles, tuberculosis or typhoid are clearly examples of parasitism. On the other hand, the microflora inhabiting the rumen of cows or the caecum of rabbits, enjoying food and shelter and at the same time supplying the host with food derived from the utilization of cellulose, are clearly symbiotic. Symbiotic associations perhaps also occur between man and his microbes, but they are less obvious. For instance, the bacteria that inhabit the human intestinal tract might theoretically be useful by supplying certain vitamins, but there is no evidence that they are important under normal circumstances. In malnourished individuals, however, vitamins derived from intestinal bacteria may be significant, and it has been recorded that in individuals with subclinical vitamin B_1 (thiamine) deficiency, clinical beri-beri can be precipitated after treatment with oral antibiotics. Presumably the antibiotics act on the intestinal bacteria that synthesize thiamine.

The bacteria that live on human skin and are specifically adapted to this habitat might at first sight be considered as commensals. They enjoy shelter and food (sebum, sweat etc.) but are normally harmless. If the skin surface is examined by the scanning electron microscope, the bacteria, such as *Staphylococcus epidermidis* and *Propionibacterium acnes*, are seen in small colonies scattered over a moon-like landscape. The colonies contain several hundred individuals* and tend to get smeared over the surface. Skin bacteria adhere to the epithelial squames that form the cornified skin surface, and extend between the squames and down the mouths of the hair follicles and glands opening onto the skin surface. They can be reduced in numbers, but never eliminated, by scrubbing and washing, and are most numerous in moister regions such as the armpit, groin and perineum. The dryness of the stratum corneum makes the skin an unsuitable environment for most bacteria, and merely occluding and thus hydrating an area with polythene sheeting leads to a large increase in the number of bacteria. The secretions of apocrine sweat glands are metabolized by skin bacteria and odoriferous amines and other substances such as 16-androstene steroids are produced, giving the body a smell that modern man, at least, finds offensive.† Deodorants, containing aluminium salts to inhibit sweating, and often antiseptics to inhibit bacterial growth, are therefore applied to the apocrine gland areas in the axillae. But for other mammals, and perhaps primitive man, body smells have been of great significance in social and sexual life. Not all body smells are produced by bacteria, and skin glands may secrete substances that are themselves odoriferous. Skin bacteria nevertheless contribute to body smells and could for this reason be classified as symbiotic rather than parasitic. There is also evidence that the harmless skin bacteria, by their very presence, inhibit the growth of more pathogenic bacteria, again indicating benefit to the host and a symbiotic classification for these bacteria.

A microbe's ability to multiply is obviously of paramount importance; indeed, we call a microbe dead or nonviable if it cannot replicate.‡ The ability to spread from host to host is of equal importance. Spread can be horizontal in a species, one individual infecting another by contact, via insect vectors and so on (Fig. 1). Alternatively spread can be "vertical" in a species, parents infecting offspring via sperm, ovum, the placenta, the milk, or by contact. Clearly if a microbe does not spread from individual to individual it will die with the individual, and cannot persist in nature. The crucial significance of the ability of a microbe to spread can be illustrated by

---

* The average size of these colonies is determined by counting the total number of bacteria recovered by scrubbing and comparing this with the number of foci of bacterial growth obtained from velvet pad replicas. The sterile pad is applied firmly to the skin, then removed and applied to the bacterial growth plate.

† The smell of feet encased in shoes and socks is characteristic, and in many European languages it is referred to as cheese-like. Between the toes lives *Brevibacterium epidermidis*, which converts L-methionine to methane thiol, a gas that contributes to the smell. A very similar bacterium is added to cheeses such as Brie to enhance odour and flavour.

‡ Sterilization is the killing of all forms of microbial life, and appropriately the word means making barren, or devoid of offspring.

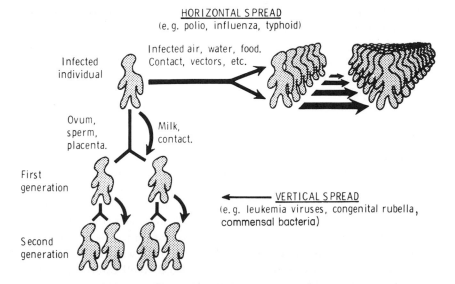

Fig. 1. Vertical and horizontal transmission of infection.

comparing the horizontal spread of respiratory and venereal infections. An infected individual can transmit influenza or the common cold to a score of others in the course of an innocent hour in a crowded room. A venereal infection also, must spread progressively from person to person if it is to maintain itself in nature, but even the most energetic lover could not transmit a venereal infection on such a scale. A chain of horizontal infection in this case, however, requires a chain of venery (sexual relations) between individuals. If those infected at a given time never had sexual relations with more than one member of the opposite sex, the total incidence could double in a lifetime, and when the infected people died the causative microbe would be eliminated. In other words, venereal infections must be transmitted to more than one member of the opposite sex if they are to persist and flourish. The greater the degree of sexual promiscuity, the greater the number of sex partners, the more successful such infections can be. Further discussion of sexually transmitted infection is included in the next chapter.

Only a small proportion of the microorganisms associated with man give rise to pathological changes or cause disease. Vast numbers of bacteria live harmlessly in his mouth and intestines, on his teeth and skin, and most of the 150 or so viruses that infect man cause no detectable illness in most infected individuals, in spite of cell and tissue invasion. This is to be expected because, from an evolutionary point of view, successful microbes must avoid extinction, persist in the world, multiply, and leave descendants. A successful parasitic microbe lives on or in the individual host, multiplies, spreads to fresh individuals, and thus maintains itself in nature.

A successful parasitic microbe, like all successful parasites, tends to get what it can from the infected host without causing too much damage. If an infection is too often crippling or lethal, there will be a reduction in numbers of the host species and thus in the numbers of the microorganism. Thus, although a few microorganisms cause disease in a majority of those infected, most are comparatively harmless, causing either no disease, or disease in only a small proportion of those infected. Polioviruses, for instance, are transmitted by the faecal–oral route, and cause a subclinical intestinal infection under normal circumstances. But in an occasional host the virus invades the central nervous system, and causes meningitis, sometimes paralysis, and very occasionally death. This particular site of multiplication is irrelevant from the virus point of view, because growth in the central nervous system is quite unnecessary for transmission to the next host. If it occurred too frequently, in fact, the host species would be reduced in numbers and the success of the virus jeopardized. Well-established infectious agents have therefore generally reached a state of balanced pathogenicity in the host, and cause the smallest amount of damage compatible with the need to enter, multiply and be discharged from the body.

The importance of balanced pathogenicity is strikingly illustrated in the case of the natural evolution of myxomatosis in the Australian rabbit. After the first successful introduction of the virus in 1950 more than 99% of infected rabbits died, but subsequently new strains of virus appeared that were less lethal. Fewer infected rabbits died, so that the host species was less severely depleted. Also, because even those that died now survived longer, there were greater opportunities for the transmission of virus to uninfected individuals. The less lethal strains of virus were therefore selected out during the evolution of the virus in the rabbit population, and replaced the original highly lethal strains because they were more successful parasites. The rabbit population also changed its character, because those that were genetically more susceptible to the infection were eliminated. Cholera in man appears to be evolving in rather similar fashion towards a more balanced pathogenicity, as discussed in Ch. 10. Rabies, a virus infection of the central nervous system, seems to contradict, but in fact exemplifies, this principle. Infection is classically acquired from the bite of a rabid animal and the disease in man is almost always fatal, but the virus has shown no signs of becoming less virulent. Man, however, is an unnatural host for rabies virus, and it is maintained in a less pathogenic fashion in animals such as vampire bats and skunks. In these animals there is a relatively harmless infection and virus is shed for long periods in the saliva, which is the vehicle of transmission from individual to individual. Rabies is thus maintained in the natural host species without serious consequences. But bites can infect the individuals of other species, "accidentally" from the virus point of view, and the infection is a serious and lethal one in these unnatural hosts.

Although successful parasites cannot afford to become too pathogenic, some degree of tissue damage may be necessary for the effective shedding of microorganisms to the exterior, as for instance in the flow of infected fluids from the nose in the common cold or from the alimentary canal in infectious diarrhoea. Otherwise there is ideally very little tissue damage, a minimal inflammatory or immune response, and a few microbial parasites achieve the supreme success of causing zero damage and failing to be recognized as parasites by the host (see Ch. 7). Different microbes show varying degrees of attainment of this ideal state of parasitism.

The concept of balanced pathogenicity is helpful in understanding infectious diseases, but many infections have not yet had time to reach this ideal state. In the first place, as each microorganism evolves, occasional virulent variants emerge and cause extensive disease and death before disappearing after all susceptible individuals have been infected, or before settling down to a more balanced pathogenicity. Secondly, some of the microbes responsible for serious human diseases had appeared originally in one part of the world, where there had been a weeding out of genetically susceptible individuals and a move in the direction of a more balanced pathogenicity. Subsequent spread of the microorganism to a new continent has resulted in the infection of a different human population in whom the disease is much more severe because of greater genetic susceptibility. Examples include tuberculosis spreading from resistant Europeans to susceptible Africans or North American Indians, and yellow fever spreading from Africans to Europeans (see p. 276). Finally, there are a number of microorganisms that have not evolved towards a less pathogenic form in man because the human host is clearly irrelevant for the survival of the microorganism. Microorganisms of this sort, such as those causing rabies (see above), scrub typhus, plague, leptospirosis and psittacosis, have some other regular host species which is responsible, often together with an arthropod vector, for their maintenance in nature.* The pathogenicity for man is of no consequence to the microorganism. Several human infections that are spillovers from animals domesticated by man also come into this category, including brucellosis, Q fever and anthrax. As man colonizes every corner of the earth, he encounters an occasional microbe from an exotic animal that causes, quite "accidentally" from the point of view of the microorganism, a

---

*These infections are called *zoonoses* (see p. 34).

serious or lethal human disease. Examples include Lassa fever and Marburg disease from African rodents and monkeys respectively.*

On the other hand, a microorganism from one animal can adapt to a new species. Every infectious agent has an origin, and studies of nucleic acid sequence homologies are removing these things from the realm of speculation. Measles, which could not have existed and maintained itself in humans in the Palaeolithic era, probably arose at a later stage from the closely related rinderpest virus that infects cattle. New human influenza viruses continue to arise from birds, and the virus of AIDS, the modern pestilence (see p. 162), seems to have arisen from a very similar virus infecting monkeys in Africa.

Microorganisms multiply exceedingly rapidly in comparison with their vertebrate hosts. The generation time of an average bacterium is an hour or less, as compared with about 20 years for the human host. Consequently, microorganisms evolve with extraordinary speed in comparison with their vertebrate hosts. Vertebrates, throughout their hundreds of millions of years of evolution, have been continuously exposed to microbial infections. They have developed highly efficient recognition (early warning) systems for foreign invaders, and effective inflammatory and immune responses to restrain their growth and spread, and eliminate them from the body (see Ch. 9). If these responses were completely effective, microbial infections would be few in number and all would be terminated rapidly; microorganisms would not be allowed to persist in the body for long periods. But microorganisms, faced with the antimicrobial defences of the host species, have evolved and developed a variety of characteristics that enable them to bypass or overcome these defences. The defences are not infallible, and the rapid rate of evolution of microorganisms ensures that they are always many steps ahead. If there are possible ways round the established defences, microorganisms are likely to have discovered and taken advantage of them. Successful microorganisms, indeed, owe their success to this ability to adapt and evolve, exploiting weak points in the host defences. The ways in which the phagocytic and immune defences are overcome are described in Chs 4 and 7.

It is the virulence and pathogenicity of microorganisms, their ability to kill and damage the host, that makes them important to the physician or veterinarian. If none of the microorganisms associated with man did any

---

* Lassa fever is a sometimes lethal infection of man caused by an arenavirus (see Table 34). The virus is maintained in certain rodents in West Africa as a harmless persistent infection, and man is only occasionally infected. Another serious infectious disease occurred in 1967 in a small number of laboratory workers in Marburg, Germany, who had handled tissues from vervet monkeys recently imported from Africa. The Marburg agent is a virus and has since reappeared to cause fatal infections in Zaire and the Sudan, but nothing is known of its natural history. Monkeys are not natural hosts and are probably accidentally infected, like man.

damage, and none was notably beneficial, they would be interesting but relatively unimportant objects. In fact, they have been responsible for the great pestilences of history, have at times determined the course of history, and continue today, in spite of vaccines and antibiotics, as important causes of disease. Also, because of their rapid rate of evolution and the constantly changing circumstances of human life, they continue to present threats of future pestilences. It is the purpose of this book to describe and discuss the mechanisms of infection and the things that make microorganisms pathogenic. As will be seen, little is known about this aspect of microbiology, but it is the central significant core of microbiology as applied to medicine, and our understanding is now steadily increasing as molecular biological and immunological techniques are brought to bear on the problems.

References

Burnett, F. M. and White, D. O. (1972). "The Natural History of Infectious Disease", 4th edn. Cambridge University Press.

Christie, A. H. (1980). "Infectious Diseases, Epidemiology and Clinical Practice", 3rd edn. Churchill Livingstone, Edinburgh.

Fenner, F. (1959). Myxomatosis in Australian wild rabbits—evolutionary changes in an infectious disease. Harvey lectures 1957–8; 25–55.

Fenner, F. and Ratcliffe, F. N. (1965). "Myxomatosis". Cambridge University Press.

Mims, C. A. (1980). The emergence of new infectious diseases. *In* "Changing Disease Patterns and Human Behaviour" (N. F. Stanley and R. A. Joske, eds), pp. 231–250. Academic Press, London.

Noble, W. C. (1981). "Microbiology of the Human Skin". Lloyd-Luke, London.

Simpson. D. I. H. (1978). Viral hemorrhagic fevers of man. *Bull. W.H.O.* **56**, 819–832.

Smith, H. (1968). Biochemical challenge of microbial pathogenicity. *Bact. Rev.* **32**, 164.

Smith, H., Arbuthnot, J. P. and Mims, C. A. (Eds) (1983). The determinants of bacterial and viral pathogenicity. *Phil. Trans Roy. Soc. London, Series B* **303**, 63–227.

2

Entry of Microorganisms into the Body

Introduction

Figure 2 shows a simplified diagram of the mammalian host. In essence, the body is traversed by a tube, the alimentary canal, with the respiratory and urinogenital tracts as blind diverticula from the alimentary canal or from the region near the anus. The body surface is covered by skin, with a relatively impermeable dry, horny outer layer, and usually fur. This gives a degree of insulation from the outside world, and the structure of skin illustrates the compromise between the need to protect the body, yet at the same time maintain sensory communication with the outside world, give mechanical mobility, and, especially in man, act as an important thermoregulatory organ. It is the largest "organ" in the body, with a weight of 5 kg in humans.

The dry, protective skin cannot cover all body surfaces. At the site of the eye it must be replaced by a transparent layer of living cells, the conjunctiva. Food must be digested and the products of digestion absorbed, and in the alimentary canal therefore, where contact with the outside world must be facilitated, the lining consists of one or more layers of living cells. Also in the lungs the gaseous exchanges that take place require contact with the outside world across a layer of living cells. There must be yet another discontinuity in the insulating outer layer of skin in the urinogenital tract, where urine and sexual products are secreted and released to the exterior. The cells on all these surfaces are covered by a fluid film containing mucin, a complex

8

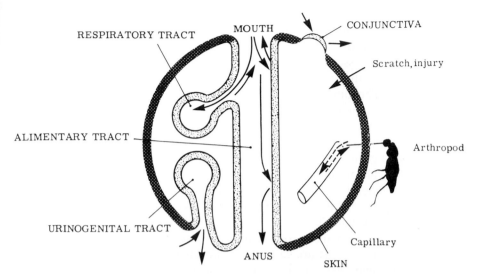

Fig. 2. Body surfaces as sites of microbial infection and shedding.

hydrated gel that waterproofs and lubricates. In the alimentary canal the lining cells are inevitably exposed to mechanical damage by food and they are continuously shed and replaced. Shedding and replacement is less pronounced in respiratory and urinogenital tracts, but it is an important phenomenon in the skin, the average person shedding about 5×10^8 skin squames per day.

The conjunctiva and the alimentary, respiratory and urinogenital tracts offer pathways for infection by microorganisms. Penetration of these surfaces is more easily accomplished than in the case of the intact outer skin. A number of antimicrobial devices have been developed in evolution to deal with this danger, and also special cleansing systems to keep the conjunctiva and respiratory tract clean enough to carry out their particular function. In order to colonize or penetrate these bodily surfaces, microorganisms must first become attached, and there are many examples of specific attachments that will be referred to (see Table 2). One striking feature of acute infectious illnesses all over the world is that most of them are either respiratory or dysentery-like in nature. They are not necessarily severe infections, but for sheer numbers they are the type that matter. In other words, infectious agents are for much of the time restricted to the respiratory and intestinal tracts.

It is of some interest to divide all infections into three groups. First, those in which the microorganisms have specific mechanisms for attaching to and sometimes penetrating the body surfaces of the normal, healthy host. This includes the infections listed in Table 2. In the second group, the micro-organism is introduced into the body of the normal healthy host by a biting arthropod, as with malaria, plague, typhus or yellow fever. Here the microorganism possesses specific mechanisms for infection of the arthropod, and depends on the arthropod for introduction into the body of the normal healthy host. The third group includes infections in which the microorganism is not by itself capable of infecting the normal healthy host. There must be some preliminary damage and impairment of defences at the body surface, such as a skin wound, damage to the respiratory tract initiated by a microbe from the first group, or an abnormality of the urinary tract interfering with the flushing, cleansing action of urine (see below). Alternatively, there could be a general defect in body defences. The opportunistic infections described later in this chapter come into this third group, and further examples are given in Ch. 11.

Although microorganisms only reach the tissues of the body by penetrat-ing body surfaces, some are capable of causing disease without doing this. Certain intestinal bacteria, for instance, secrete toxic substances that act locally to cause disease, as in the case of cholera. The bacteria exert their pathogenicity while remaining in the intestinal canal; inside the host in one sense, but outside in another (Fig. 2). The bacteria responsible for dental caries and periodontal disease act in a similar way (see pp. 20–1). Other bacteria remain on the body surface and release toxins that cause generalized disease after absorption, as in the case of diphtheria.

The Skin

The skin is a natural barrier to microorganisms and is penetrated at the site of breaks in its continuity, whether macroscopic or microscopic (Table 1).

Microorganisms other than commensals (residents) are soon inactivated, probably by fatty acids (skin pH is about 5.5) and other materials produced from sebum by the commensals. In the perianal region, for instance, where billions of faecal bacteria are not only deposited daily, but then, in man at least, rubbed into the area, there is evidently an astonishing resistance to infection. Faecal bacteria are rapidly inactivated here, but the exact mechanism, and the possible role of perianal gland secretions, is unknown.

Bacteria on the skin, as well as entering hair follicles and causing lesions (boils, styes), can also cause trouble after entering other orifices. Staphylococcal mastitis occurs in many mammals, but is of major importance in the dairying industry, and is thought to arise when the bacteria are carried up and past the teat canal of the cow as a result of vacuum fluctuations during milking.

Table 1. Microorganisms that infect the skin or enter the body via the skin

Microorganisms	Disease	Comments
Arthropod-borne viruses	Various fevers	150 distinct viruses, transmitted by infected arthropod bite
Rabies virus	Rabies	Bite from infected animals
Vaccinia virus	Skin lesion	Vaccination against smallpox
Wart viruses	Warts	Infection restricted to epidermis
Staphylococci	Boils etc.	Commonest skin invaders
Rickettsia	Typhus, spotted fevers	Infestation with infected arthropod
Leptospira	Leptospirosis	Contact with water containing infected animals' urine
Streptococci	Impetigo, erysipelas	
Bacillus anthracis	Cutaneous anthrax	Systemic disease following local lesion at inoculation site
Treponema pallidum and *pertenue*	Syphilis, yaws	Warm, moist skin is more susceptible
Yersinia pestis	Plague	Bite from infected rodent flea
Plasmodia	Malaria	Bite from infected mosquito
Trichophyton spp. and other fungi	Ringworm, athlete's foot	Infection restricted to skin, nails, hairs

Large or small breaks in the skin due to wounds are obvious routes for infection, and a small wound used to be produced artificially in the process of vaccination against smallpox. Live vaccinia virus entered the epidermis and dermis after damage by the vaccinator's needle. The virus of hepatitis B can be introduced into the body if the needle of the doctor, tattoist, drug-addict, acupuncturist or ear-piercer is contaminated with infected blood. Shaving upsets the antimicrobial defenses in the skin and can lead to staphylococcal infection of the shaved area in the male face (sycosis barbae) or female axilla. Pre-operative shaving, although a well-established ritual, seems to enhance rather than prevent infection in surgical wounds.

Bites are also important sites for the entry of microorganisms.

Small bites

Biting arthropods such as mosquitoes, mites, ticks, fleas and sandflies penetrate the skin during feeding and can thus introduce pathogenic agents into the body. Some infections are transmitted mechanically, the mouthparts of the arthropod being contaminated with the infectious agent, and there is no multiplication in the arthropod. This is what happens in the case of myxomatosis. Fleas or mosquitoes carry myxoma virus on their contaminated mouth-parts from one rabbit to another. When transmission is said to be biological, as in yellow fever or malaria, this means that the infectious agent multiplies in the arthropod, and, after an incubation period, appears in the saliva and is transmitted to the susceptible host during a blood feed. Mosquitoes or ticks, in the act of feeding, probe in the dermal tissues, emitting puffs of saliva as they do so. The mosquito proboscis may enter a blood capillary and is then threaded along the vessel, further injections of saliva occurring during the ingestion of blood. Infected saliva is thus introduced directly into the dermis and often into the vascular system, the counterpart of a minute intradermal or intravenous injection of micro-organisms. Other diseases transmitted biologically by arthropods include typhus and plague, and in these cases the microorganisms multiply in the alimentary canal of the arthropod. Plague bacteria from the infected flea are regurgitated into the skin during feeding, and the human body louse infected with typhus rickettsiae defaecates during feeding, the rickettsiae subsequently entering the body through the bite-wound.

Large bites

The classical infectious disease transmitted by a biting mammal is rabies. Virus is shed in the saliva of infected dogs, wolves, vampire bats etc. and thus introduced into bite wounds. Human bites are not common, most people having neither the temperament nor the teeth for it. When they do occur, human bites can cause troublesome sepsis because of the fusiform and spirochaetal bacteria normally present in the mouth that are introduced into the wound. Teeth often make an involuntary inoculation of bacteria into skin during fist fights. The hero's decisive punch can then bring him knuckle sepsis as well as victory.

Respiratory Tract

Air contains a variety of suspended particles, and the total quantity seems large if one says that there are more than 1000 millions tonnes of suspended particular matter in the earth's atmosphere. Most of this is smoke, soot and dust, but microorganisms are inevitably present. Inside buildings there are 400–900 microorganisms m^{-3}, nearly all of them nonpathogenic bacteria or moulds. Therefore with a ventilation rate of 6 litres min^{-1} at rest, the average man would inhale at least 8 microorganisms min^{-1} or about 10 000 day^{-1}. Efficient cleansing mechanisms remove inhaled particles and keep the

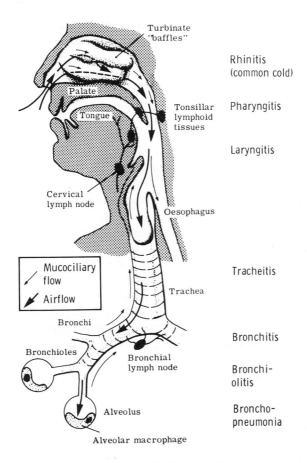

Fig. 3. Mechanisms of infection in the respiratory tract.

respiratory tract clean, and infection of the respiratory tract has to be thought of in relation to these mechanisms, which are designed to remove and dispose of inhaled particles, whatever their nature.

A mucociliary blanket covers most of the surface of the lower respiratory tract. It consists of ciliated cells together with single mucus-secreting cells (goblet cells) and subepithelial mucus-secreting glands. Foreign particles deposited on this surface are entrapped in mucus and born upwards from the lungs to the back of the throat by ciliary action (Fig. 3). This has been called the mucociliary escalator. The nasal cavity (upper respiratory tract) has a similar mucociliary lining, and particles deposited here are also carried to the back of the throat and swallowed.* The average person produces 10–100 ml mucus from the nasal cavity each day and a similar amount from the lung. The terminal portions of the lower respiratory tract are the alveoli, and these have no cilia or mucus but are lined by macrophages.

A great deal of experimental work has been carried out on the fate of inhaled particles, and particle size is of paramount importance. The larger the particle, the less likely it is to reach the terminal portions of the lung. All particles, whether viral, bacterial, fungal or inert, are dealt with in the same way. Larger visible particles are filtered off by the hairs lining the nostrils, and particles 10 μm or so in diameter tend to be deposited on the "baffle plates" in the nasal cavity, consisting of the turbinate bones covered by nasal mucosa. Smaller particles are likely to reach the lungs, those 5 μm or less in diameter reaching the alveoli. Nearly all observations have been made with animals but human subjects have been used on a few occasions. If a person inhales 5-μm particles of polystyrene tagged with ^{51}Cr and the fate of the particles is determined by external gamma measurements, about half of the labelled material is removed from the lungs within hours, after being deposited on the mucociliary escalator and carried up to the back of the throat. The rest is removed very slowly indeed, with a half-life of more than 150 days, having been phagocytosed by alveolar macrophages after settling on alveolar walls. The marker particles in this experiment are nondegradable, and nonpathogenic microorganisms for instance would have been disposed of more rapidly. Inhaled particles of soot are taken up by alveolar macrophages, some of which later migrate to the pulmonary lymph nodes. The town dweller can be recognized in the post-mortem room because of the grey colour of his pulmonary lymph nodes.†

If a microorganism is to initiate infection in the respiratory tract, the initial requirements are simple. First the microorganism must avoid being caught up in mucus, carried to the back of the throat and swallowed. Secondly, if it is deposited in alveoli it must either resist phagocytosis by the alveolar macrophage, or if it is phagocytosed it must survive or multiply rather than be digested and killed.

---

* If human serum albumin aggregates labelled with ^{131}I are introduced into the nose of a volunteer, their movement can be followed with a crystal scintillation detector. The speed of movement is variable, but averages 0.5–1.0 cm min^{-1}.

† There is also a movement of macrophages from the lower respiratory tract up to the back of the throat on the mucociliary escalator. At least 10^7 macrophages a day are recoverable in normal rats or cats, a similar quantity in normal people and more than this in patients with chronic bronchitis. This is a route to the exterior for macrophages laden with indigestible materials.

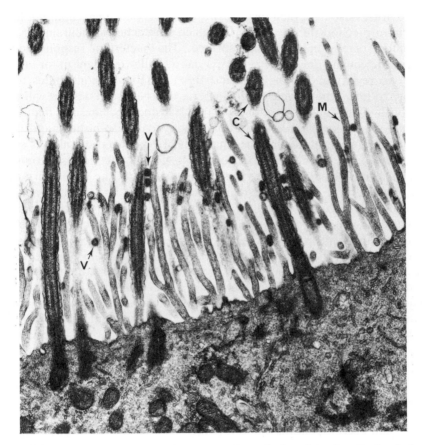

Fig. 4. Portion of ciliated epithelial cell from organ culture of guinea pig trachea after incubation with influenza virus for 1 h at 4°C. Electron micrograph of thin section showing virus particles (V) attached to cilia (C) and to microvilli (M). The fluid between the cilia is watery, the viscous mucoid layer lying above the cilia. (Electron micrograph very kindly supplied by Dr R. Dourmashkin.)

It would seem inevitable that a microorganism has little chance of avoiding the first fate unless the mucociliary mechanisms are defective, or unless it has some special device for attaching firmly if it is lucky enough to encounter an epithelial cell. The highly successful myxoviruses, for instance, of which influenza is an example, have a haemagglutinin on their surface which specifically reacts with receptor substance (sialic acid groupings on a glycoprotein) on the epithelial cells. A firm union is established (Fig. 4) and the virus now has an opportunity to infect the cell. The common cold rhinoviruses also have their own receptors.* *Mycoplasma pneumoniae* has a special projection on its surface by which it attaches to neuraminic acid receptors on the epithelial cell surface. The bacterium responsible for whooping cough (*Bordetella pertussis*) has a similar mechanism for attachment to respiratory epithelium, and this undoubtedly contributes to its ability to infect the normal lung. Bacteria that lack such devices will only establish infection when the mucociliary cleansing mechanism is damaged. *Streptococcus pneumoniae* has the opportunity to invade the lungs and cause pneumonia when mucociliary mechanisms are damaged or there is some other weakening of natural host defences. A virus infection is a common source of mucociliary damage. Destructive lesions of the respiratory tract are induced by viruses such as measles or influenza, and various bacteria, especially streptococci, then have the opportunity to grow in the lung and produce a secondary pneumonia. People with chronic bronchitis show disturbed mucociliary function, and this contributes to the low-grade bacterial infection in the lung which may be a semi-permanent feature of the disease. Also, there is suggestive evidence that cigarette smoking and atmospheric pollutants lead to temporary or permanent impairment of the mucociliary defences (see Ch. 11). Finally, there are many ways in which natural host defences are weakened in hospital patients. Patients with indwelling tracheal tubes, for instance, are particularly susceptible to respiratory infection because the air entering the tracheal tube has been neither filtered nor humidified in the nose. Dry air impairs ciliary activity and the indwelling tube causes further epithelial damage. General anaesthesia decreases lung resistance in a similar way, and in addition depresses the cough reflex.

Certain microorganisms that infect the respiratory tract directly depress ciliary activity, thus inhibiting their removal from the lung and promoting infection. *Bordetella pertussis* attaches to respiratory epithelial cells and in some way interferes with ciliary activity. *Haemophilus influenzae* produces a factor that could be important *in vivo*. The factor slows the ciliary beat, interferes with its coordination and finally causes loss of cilia. At least seven ciliostatic substances are produced by *Pseudomonas aeruginosa*, which causes a devastating respiratory infection in those with cystic fibrosis (see p. 35). Ciliary activity is also inhibited by *Mycoplasma pneumoniae*. The

---

*Although made use of by invading microorganisms, receptors are clearly not there for this purpose, and presumably serve other functions such as hormone binding, cell–cell recognition etc. Sometimes virus receptors are present only on certain types of cell, which can account for cell tropisms and other features of the disease. For instance, the receptor for EB virus is the C3d receptor on B cells, which are thus infected and undergo polyclonal activation (see p. 147), and the receptor for HIV (Human Immunodeficiency Virus, or HTLV3) is the T4 (CD4) receptor on T helper cells, whose infection and depletion contributes to the serious immune deficit in AIDS.

mycoplasma multiply while attached to the surface of respiratory epithelial cells, and the ciliostatic effect is possibly due to hydrogen peroxide produced locally by the mycoplasma. Cilia are defective in certain inherited conditions. In Kartagener's Syndrome, for instance, impaired ciliary movement leads to chronic infections in lung and sinuses. Spermatozoa are also affected and males with this condition are infertile.

The question of survival of airborne microorganisms after phagocytosis by alveolar macrophages is part of the general problem of microbial survival in phagocytic cells, and this is dealt with more fully in Ch. 4. Tubercle bacilli tend to survive in the alveolar macrophages of the susceptible host and respiratory tuberculosis is thought to be initiated in this way. The common cold viruses, in contrast, which are very commonly phagocytosed by these cells, fail to survive and multiply, and therefore cause no perceptible infection in the lower respiratory tract. Growth of many of these viruses is in any case restricted at 37°C, being optimal at about 33°C, the temperature of nasal mucosa. Under certain circumstances the antimicrobial activity of alveolar macrophages is depressed. This occurs, for instance, following the inhalation of toxic asbestos particles and their phagocytosis by alveolar macrophages. Patients with asbestosis have increased susceptibility to respiratory tuberculosis. Alveolar macrophages infected by respiratory viruses sometimes show decreased ability to deal with inhaled bacteria, even those that are normally nonpathogenic, and this can be a factor in secondary bacterial pneumonias (see Ch. 8).

Normally the lungs are almost sterile, because the microorganisms that are continually being inhaled are also continually being phagocytosed and destroyed or removed by mucociliary action.

Intestinal Tract

The intestinal tract must take what it is given during eating and drinking, and also various other swallowed materials originating from the mouth, nasopharynx and lungs. Apart from the general flow of intestinal contents, there are no particular cleansing mechanisms, unless diarrhoea and vomiting are included in this category. The lower intestinal tract is a seething cauldron of microbial activity, as can readily be appreciated from the microscopic examination of fresh faeces. Multiplication of bacteria is counter-balanced by their continuous passage to the exterior with the rest of the intestinal contents. A single *E. coli*, multiplying under favourable conditions, might well increase its numbers to about 10^8 within 12–18 h, the normal intestinal transit time. The faster the rate of flow of intestinal contents the less the opportunity for microbial growth, so that there is a much smaller total

Pathogenesis of Infectious Disease

number of bacteria in diarrhoea than in normal faeces. On the other hand, a reduced flow rate leads to increased growth of intestinal bacteria. This is not known to be harmful in individuals on a low-fibre diet, but is a more serious matter in the blind-loop syndrome. Here, surgical excision of a piece of intestine results in a blind length in which the flow rate is greatly reduced. The resulting bacterial overgrowth, especially in the small intestine, is associated with symptoms of malabsorption, because the excess bacteria metabolize bile acids needed for absorption of fats and also compete for vitamin B12 and other nutrients.

The commensal intestinal bacteria are often associated with the intestinal wall, either in the layers of mucus or attached to the epithelium itself. If a mouse's stomach or intestine is frozen with the contents intact and sections are then cut and stained, the various commensal bacteria can be seen in large numbers, intimately associated with the epithelial cells. This makes it easier for them to maintain themselves as permanent residents. Pathogenic intestinal bacteria must establish infection and increase in numbers, and they too often have mechanisms for attachment to the epithelial lining so that they can avoid being carried straight down the alimentary canal with the rest of the intestinal contents. Indeed, their pathogenicity is likely to depend on this capacity for attachment or penetration. The pathogenicity of cholera, for instance, depends on the adhesion of bacteria to specific receptors on the surface of intestinal epithelial cells, and other examples are included in Table 2. Clearly, the concentration and thus the adsorption of bacterial toxins will also be affected by the balance between production and removal of bacteria in the intestine. Certain protozoa cause intestinal infections without invading tissues, and they too depend on adherence to the epithelial surface. *Giardia lamblia* attaches to the upper small intestine of man by means of a sucking disc.

The likelihood of infection via the intestinal tract is certainly affected by the presence of mucus, acid, enzymes and bile. Mucus protects epithelial cells, perhaps acting as a mechanical barrier to infection, and contains secretory IgA antibodies that protect the immune individual against infection. Motile microorganisms (*Vibrio cholerae*, certain strains of *E. coli*) can propel themselves through the mucus layer and are thus more likely to reach epithelial cells to make specific attachments.* *Vibrio cholerae* also produces a mucinase that probably helps its passage through the mucus. Microorganisms infecting by the intestinal route are often capable of surviving in

---

*Nonmotile microorganisms, in contrast, rely on random and passive transport in the mucus layer. How important is mucus as a physical barrier? Gonococci and chlamydia are known to attach to spermatozoa, and they could be carried through the cervical mucus as "hitch-hikers" so that spermatozoa could help transmit gonorrhoea and nonspecific urethritis.

the presence of acid, proteolytic enzymes and bile. This also applies to microorganisms shed from the body by this route. The streptococci that are normal human intestinal inhabitants (*Streptococcus faecalis*) grow in the presence of bile, unlike other streptococci. This is also true of other normal (*E. coli, Proteus, Pseudomonas*) and pathogenic (*Salmonella, Shigella*) intestinal bacteria. It is noteworthy that the enteroviruses (hepatitis A, coxsackie-, echo- and polioviruses) are resistant to bile salts and to acid. The fact that tubercle bacilli resist acid conditions in the stomach favours the establishment of intestinal tuberculosis. Most bacteria, however, are acid sensitive and prefer slightly alkaline conditions.* Intestinal pathogens such as salmonella or *Vibrio cholerae* are more likely to establish infection when they are sheltered inside food particles or when acid production in the host is impaired (achlorhydria). Volunteers who drank different doses of *Vibrio cholerae* contained in 60 ml saline showed a 10^4-fold increase in susceptibility to cholera when 2 g of sodium bicarbonate were given with the bacteria. Classical strains of cholera were used, and the minimal disease-producing dose without bicarbonate was 10^8 bacteria. Similar experiments have been done in volunteers with *Salmonella typhi*. The minimal oral infectious dose was 10^3–10^4 bacteria, and this was significantly reduced by the ingestion of sodium bicarbonate.

The intestinal tract differs from the respiratory tract in that it is always in motion, with constantly changing surface contours. The surface is made up of villi, crypts and other irregularities, and the villi themselves contract and expand. Particles in the lumen are moved about a great deal and have good opportunities for encounters with living cells; this is what the alimentary canal is designed for, if food is to be mixed, digested and absorbed. Viruses, by definition, multiply only in living cells; thus enteric viruses must make the most of what are primarily chance encounters with epithelial cells. Polio-, coxsackie- and echoviruses and presumably the human diarrhoea viruses (rotaviruses, certain adenoviruses etc.) form firm unions with receptor substances on the surface of intestinal epithelial cells, thus giving time for the penetration of virus into the cell. On the other hand, enteric bacteria that enter the mucosa are able to increase their numbers by growth in the lumen before entry, but it is not surprising that there are also mechanisms for bacterial attachment to epithelial cells (Table 2). The adhesive components on bacteria mediating attachment to host cells have been called *adhesins* by J. P. Duguid. Penetration of viruses into cells is discussed at a later stage, but it can take place either by phagocytosis of the virus particle, or by fusion of the virus surface with the cell membrane so that the contents of the virus

---

* The standard Sabouraud's medium for the isolation of yeasts and moulds has an acid pH (5.4) in order that bacterial growth should be generally inhibited.

Table 2. Examples of specific attachments of microorganisms to host cell or body surface

Microorganism	Disease	Attachment site	Mechanism
Influenza virus	Influenza	Respiratory epithelial cell	Viral haemagglutin reacts with neuraminic acid receptor on cell
Poliovirus	Poliomyelitis	Susceptible tissue cell (e.g. neuron)	Viral capsid protein reacts with specific receptor on cell
Adenovirus	Conjunctivitis Pharyngitis Respiratory illness	Susceptible tissue cell	Viral capsid protein reacts with specific receptor on cell
Chlamydia	Conjunctivitis Urethritis	Conjunctival or urethral epithelium	Unknown (sialic acid-containing receptors on epithelial cell?)
Mycoplasma pneumoniae	Atypical pneumonia	Respiratory epithelial cell	"Foot" on Mycoplasma surface attaches to neuraminic acid receptor on cell
Neisseria meningitidis	Carrier state	Nasopharyngeal epithelium	Pili
Neisseria gonorrhoeae	Gonorrhoea	Urethral epithelium	Defined peptide fragment on bacterial pili attaches to carbohydrate polymer on cell
Vibrio cholerae	Cholera	Intestinal epithelium	Receptor is fucose and mannose
E. coli (certain strains)	Diarrhoea	Intestinal epithelium	Requires specific bacterial surface component on pili (e.g. K88 and K99 antigens in pig and calf diarrhoea) attaching to D-mannose receptor
	Urinary infection	Urinary tract epithelium	Pili adhere to D-mannose receptor
Salmonella typhi	Enteric fever	Intestinal epithelium	Bacterial adhesin attaches to mannose-like receptor on epithelial cell
Shigella flexneri	Dysentery	Colonic epithelium	Unknown (pili?)
Streptococcus mutans	Caries	Tooth	Bacteria bind to glycosyl-transferase, linked to glucan "glue" (bacterial product), and attached to teeth

Table 2. (*Contd.*)

Microorganism	Disease	Attachment site	Mechanism
Streptococcus pyogenes	Sore throat	Pharyngeal epithelium	Bacteria bind via lipoteichoic acid on pili
Streptococcus salivarius	Nil	Buccal epithelium and tongue	
Streptococcus agalactiae	Mastitis (cow)	Duct epithelium	Unknown
Corynebacterium diphtheriae	Diphtheria	Mucosal epithelium	Unknown (specific?)
Bordetella pertussis	Whooping cough	Respiratory epithelium	Unknown
Treponema pallidum	Syphilis	Protein (fibronectin) on host cell surface or in tissue	Peptide in outer envelope of bacterium binds to host cell
Haemophilus infleuenzae	Pneumonia	Respiratory epithelium	Unknown
Plasmodium vivax	Malaria	Erythrocyte of susceptible human	Malarial merozoite attaches to "Duffy" antigen on erythrocyte surface. Complement not necessary
Babesia	Babesiasis in cattle	Erythrocyte	Babesia binds complement and attaches to C3b receptor on erythrocyte
Giardia lamblia	Diarrhoea	Epithelium of duodenum, jejunum	Binding to mannose 6-phosphate on host cell, plus mechanical sucker
Entamoeba histolytica	Dysentery	Colonic epithelium	Amoebic adhesins bind to receptors (asialofetuin) on epithelial cell

particle enter the cell. These alternatives are not so distinct, because the virus particle in a phagocytic vacuole is still in a sense outside the cell and still has to penetrate the cell membrane for its contents to be released into the cytoplasm.

Most epithelial cells, whether epidermal, respiratory or intestinal, are capable of phagocytosis, but this is on a small scale compared with those specialist phagocytes, the macrophages and polymorphonuclear leucocytes (see Ch. 4). Certain pathogenic bacteria in the alimentary canal are taken into intestinal epithelial cells by a process that looks like phagocytosis. As seen by electron microscopy in experimental animals, *Salmonella typhimurium* or pathogenic strains of *E. coli* attach to microvilli forming the brush border of intestinal epithelial cells. The microvilli degenerate locally at the site of attachment, enabling the bacterium to enter the cell, and the breach in the cell surface is then repaired. A zone of degeneration precedes the bacterium as it advances into the apical cytoplasm. Commensal intestinal bacteria do not appear to be taken up when they are attached to intestinal epithelium, but the factors that promote or prevent uptake are not known. After penetration of the epithelium, final pathogenicity depends on bacterial multiplication and spread (see Ch. 3), on toxin production, cell damage and inflammatory responses (see Ch. 8).

Microbial toxins, endotoxins and proteins can certainly be absorbed from the intestine on a small scale, and immune responses may be induced. Antibodies to materials such as milk, eggs and black beans can be detected when they form a significant part of the diet, and insulin is absorbed after ingestion as shown by the occurrence of hypoglycaemia. Diarrhoea promotes the uptake of proteins, and absorption of protein also takes place more readily in the infant, especially in species such as the pig or horse that need to absorb maternal antibodies from milk. As well as large molecules, particles the size of viruses can be taken up from the intestinal lumen,* and recent work suggests that Peyers patches are the sites at which this occurs. Peyers patches are isolated collections of lymphoid tissue lying immediately below the intestinal epithelium. The epithelial cells here are highly specialized (so-called M cells) and take up particles and foreign proteins, delivering them to underlying immune cells with which they are intimately associated by means of cytoplasmic processes. When large amounts of a reovirus for instance (see Table 34) are introduced into the intestine of a mouse the uptake of virus particles by M cells and delivery to immune cells, from whence they reach local lymph nodes, can be followed by electron microscopy. It seems appropriate that microorganisms in the intestine are sometimes "focused" into immune defence strongholds.

---

* When rats drink water containing very large amounts of bacteriophage T7 (diameter 30 nm), intact infectious phages are recoverable from thoracic duct lymph within 20 minutes.

The normal intestinal microorganisms of man are specifically adapted to life in this situation, and most of them are anaerobes of the *Bacteroides* group, although *E. coli*, enterococci, lactobacilli and diphtheroids are common. The total numbers increase as the intestinal contents move from the small to the large intestine, and there are about 10^8–10^{10} bacteria g^{-1} in the terminal ileum, increasing to 10^{11} g^{-1} in the colon and rectum. Bacteria normally comprise about a quarter of the total faecal mass. The normal flora are in a balanced state, and tend to resist colonization with other bacteria.* Possible mechanisms include killing other bacteria by bacteriocins (see Glossary), competition for food substances or attachment sites, and the production of bacterial inhibitors. For instance, in mice the resident coliforms and *Bacteroides* produce acetic and propionic acids which are inhibitory for shigella (dysentery) bacteria. Patients treated with broad-spectrum antibiotics show changes in normal intestinal flora and this may allow an abnormal overgrowth of antibiotic-resistant microorganisms, such as the fungus, *Candida albicans*. In breast-fed infants, the predominant bacteria in the large bowel are lactobacili and their metabolic activity produces acid and other factors that inhibit other microorganisms. As a result of this, and perhaps also because of antibacterial components present in human milk, breast-fed infants resist colonization with other bacteria, such as the pathogenic strains of *E. coli*. Bottle-fed infants, on the other hand, lacking the protective lactobacilli, are susceptible to pathogenic strains of *E. coli*, and these may cause serious gastroenteritis.

Intestinal microorganisms that utilize ingested cellulose serve as important sources of food in herbivorous animals. In the rabbit, for instance, volatile fatty acids produced by microorganisms in the caecum yield 20% of the daily energy requirements of the animal. The rumen of a 500-kg cow is a complex fermentation chamber whose contents amount to 70 litres. In this vast vat 17 species of bacteria multiply continuously, utilizing cellulose and other plant materials, and protozoa (seven genera) live on the bacteria. As the microbial mass increases the surplus passes into the intestine to be killed, digested and absorbed. Large volumes of CO_2 and methane are formed and expelled from both ends of the cow. The passage of methane represents a loss of about 10% of the total energy derived from food. In man, intestinal bacteria do not normally have a nutritive function; they break down and recycle the components of desquamated epithelial cells, and perhaps synthesize vitamins, but this is unimportant under normal circumstances.

---

* For instance, lactobacilli are normally present on the nonsecretory epithelium of the mouse stomach, and are attached to keratinized squamous cells. If penicillin is added to the drinking water the lactobacilli disappear, and their place is taken by yeasts that normally inhabit only the secretory surfaces of the stomach. The natural distribution is restored when the penicillin treatment ceases.

Oropharynx

The throat (including tonsils, fauces etc.) is a common site of residence of microorganisms as well as of their entry into the body.

The microbial inhabitants of the normal mouth and throat are varied, exceedingly numerous, and are specifically adapted to life in this environment. Bacteria are the most numerous, but yeasts (*Candida albicans*) and protozoa (*Entamoeba gingivalis, Trichomonas tenax*) occur in may individuals. Oral bacteria include streptococci, micrococci and diphtheroids, together with *Actinomyces israeli* and other anaerobic bacteria. Some of these are able to make very firm attachments to mucosal surfaces, and others to teeth which provide a longterm, nondesquamating surface. *Streptococcus mutans*, for instance, uses the enzyme glycosyl transferase to synthesize glucan (a high molecular weight polysaccharide) from sucrose. The glucan forms an adhesive layer, attaching bacteria to the surface of teeth (Table 2). If there are no teeth, as in the very young or the very old, *Streptococcus mutans* has nothing to "hold on to" and cannot maintain itself in the mouth. The dextran-containing secretions constitute a matrix in which various other bacteria are present, many of them anaerobic. It forms a thin film attached to the surface of the tooth which is called dental plaque, and is visible as a red layer when a dye such as erythrosine is taken into the mouth. Dental plaque is a complex microbial mass containing about 10^9 bacteria g^{-1}. Certain areas of the tooth are readily colonized, especially surface fissures and pits, areas next to the gum, and contact points between neighbouring teeth. The film is largely removed by thorough brushing, but re-establishes itself within a few hours. When teeth are not cleaned for several days the plaque becomes quite thick, a tangled forest of microorganisms (Fig. 5). Dietary sugar is utilized by bacteria in the plaque and the acid that is formed decalcifies the tooth and is responsible for dental caries. The pH in an active caries lesion may be as low as 4.0. Unless the bacteria, the sugar (and the teeth) are present, dental caries does not develop. When monkeys are fed on a caries-producing diet, the extent of the disease can be greatly reduced by vaccination against *Streptococcus mutans*,[*] and vaccines are being developed for use against caries in man. Caries is already becoming less common, but if the vaccines are effective, caries (and many dentists) could one day be eliminated.

---

[*] Antibodies are presumably protective and it is noteworthy that in one study of 11 agammaglobulinaemic patients all were badly affected by caries, and four lost all their teeth quite rapidly between the age of 20 and 30 years. Secretory IgA antibodies would be expected to coat bacteria and prevent attachment to teeth and additional antimicrobial forces are present nearby in crevicular spaces. The crevicular space is a small fluid-filled cleft between the edge of the gum and the tooth, containing antibodies (IgG, IgM), complement and phagocytic cells derived from plasma.

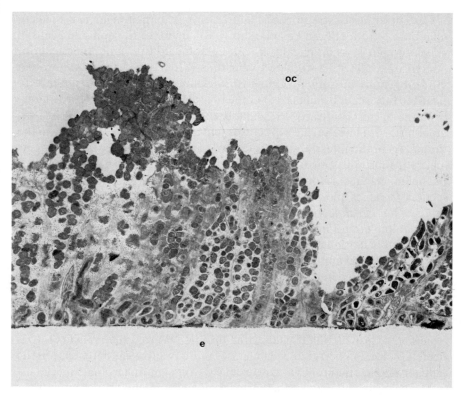

Fig. 5. Electron microscope section through dental plaque at gingival margin of a child's tooth, showing microcolonies of cocci. Thickness of plaque from enamel (e) to free border (oral cavity, oc) above is variable. Magnification ×4000. (Photograph kindly supplied by Dr H. N. Newman, Institute of Dental Surgery, Gray's Inn Road, London.)

Western man with his tightly packed, bacteria-coated teeth and his sugary, often fluoride-deficient diet, has been badly affected, and it is legitimate to regard dental caries as one of his most prevalent infectious diseases.

Periodontal disease is another important dental condition that affects nearly everyone (and most animals) to a greater or lesser extent. The space between the tooth and gum margin has no natural cleansing mechanism and it readily becomes infected. This results in inflammation, with accumulation of polymorphs and a serum exudate. The inflamed gum bleeds readily and later recedes, while the multiplying bacteria can cause halitosis. Eventually the structures that support the teeth are affected and teeth become loose as bone is resorbed and ligaments weakened. Bacteria such as *Actinomyces viscosis*, *Actinobacillus actinomycetemcomitans*, and *Bacteroides* spp. are commonly associated with periodontal disease.

Certain strains of streptococci adhere strongly to the tongue and cheek of man but not to teeth, and can be shown to adhere to the epithelial cells in cheek scrapings. Pharyngeal cells can be obtained by wiping the posterior pharyngeal wall with a wooden applicator stick, and experiments show that virulent strains of *Streptococcus pyogenes* make firm and specific attachments to these cells by means of lipoteichoic acid on threads (pili) protruding from the bacterial surface. Presumably the corynebacteria responsible for diphtheria also have surface structures that attach them to epithelium in the throat. As in the intestines, the presence of the regular microbial residents makes it more difficult for other microorganisms to become established. Possible mechanisms for this interference were mentioned in the preceding section. Changes in oral flora upset the balance. For instance, the yeast-like fungus *Candida albicans* is normally a harmless inhabitant of the mouth, but after prolonged administration of broad-spectrum antibiotics, changes in the normal bacteria flora enable the pseudomycelia of *Candida albicans* to penetrate the oral epithelium, grow and cause thrush.

Saliva is secreted in volumes of a litre or so a day, and has a flushing action in the mouth, mechanically removing microorganisms as well as providing antimicrobial materials such as lysozyme (see Glossary) and secretory antibodies. It contains leucocytes, desquamated mucosal cells and bacteria from sites of growth on the cheek, tongue, gingiva etc. When salivary flow is decreased for 3–4 h, as between meals,* there is a four-fold increase in the number of bacteria in saliva. Disturbances in oral antimicrobial and cleansing mechanisms may upset the normal balance. In dehydrated patients, or those ill with typhus, typhoid, pneumonia etc., the salivary flow is greatly reduced, and the mouth becomes foul as a result of microbial overgrowth, often with some tissue invasion. Vitamin C deficiency reduces mucosal resistance and allows the normal resident bacteria to cause gum infections. As on all bodily surfaces, there is a shifting boundary between harmless coexistence of the resident microbes and invasion of host tissues, according to changes in host resistance.

During mouth breathing the throat acts as a baffle on which larger inhaled particles can be deposited, and microorganisms in saliva and nasal secretions are born backwards to the pharynx. Microorganisms in the mouth and throat need to be attached to the squamous epithelial surface or find their way into crevices if they are to avoid being washed away and are to have an opportunity to establish infection. The efficiency of infection may be increased by the act of swallowing. As material from the nasal cavity, mouth and lung is brought to the pharynx, that great muscular organ the tongue pushes backwards with a vigorous thrust and firmly wipes this material

---

* Salivary flow continues between meals, the average person swallowing about 30 times an hour.

against the pharyngeal walls. One of the earliest and most regular symptoms of upper respiratory virus infections is a sore throat, suggesting early viral growth in this area, with an inflammatory response in the underlying tissues. It may also signify inflammation of submucosal lymphoid tissues in the tonsils, back of the tongue, and throat, which form a defensive ring guarding the entrance to alimentary and respiratory tracts.

Urinogenital Tract

Urine is normally sterile, and since the urinary tract is flushed with urine every hour or two, invading microorganisms have problems in gaining access and becoming established. The urethra in the male is sterile, except for the terminal third of its length, and microorganisms that progress above this point must first and foremost avoid being washed out during urination. That highly successful urethral parasite, the gonococcus, owes much of its success to its special ability to attach very firmly to the surface of urethral epithelial cells, partly by means of fine hairs (pili) projecting from its surface (Fig. 6.).* The bladder is not easily infected in the male; the urethra is 20 cm long and generally bacteria need to be introduced via an instrument such as a catheter to reach the bladder. The female urethra is much shorter, only about 5 cm long, and more readily traversed by microorganisms; it also suffers from a dangerous proximity to the anus, the source of intestinal bacteria. Urinary infections are about 14 times as common in women, and most women have urinary tract infections at some time. Bacteruria,† however, often occurs without frequency, dysuria, or other symptoms. Even the urethral deformations taking place during sexual intercourse may introduce infection into the female bladder.‡ Spread of infection to the kidney is promoted by the refluxing of urine from bladder to ureter that occurs in some young females.

---

*The gonococcus is soon killed in urines that are acid ($<$pH 5.5), and this helps explain why the bladder and kidney are not invaded. The prostate is at times affected and the gonococcus accordingly grows in the presence of spermine and zinc, materials that are present in prostatic secretions and that would inhibit many other bacteria.

† By the time it has been voided and tested in the lab, urine always contains bacteria. For routine purposes it is not regarded as significant unless there are more than 10^5 bacteria (ml urine)$^{-1}$. But many women have frequency and dysuria with smaller numbers of bacteria in urine and in some cases, perhaps, the infection has spread no further than the urethra.

‡ The importance of sexual activity is often assessed by comparing nuns or prostitutes with "ordinary" women. Bacteruria is 14 times commoner in ordinary women than in nuns, and in one study sexual intercourse was the commonest precipitating factor for dysuria and frequency in young women. On the other hand, an innocent bubble bath may facilitate spread of faecal organisms into the urethra.

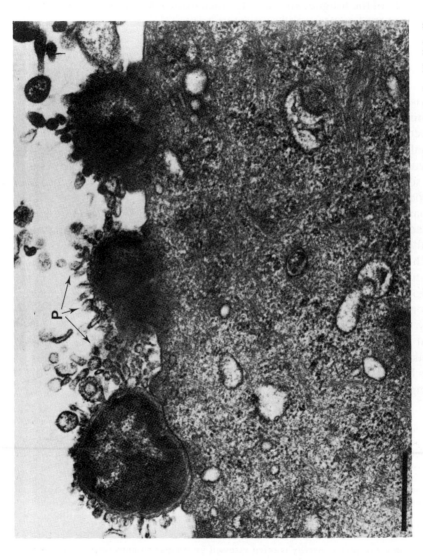

Fig. 6. Electron micrograph showing gonococci closely attached to the surface of a human urethral epithelial cell: 40–50 pili (P) project from the gonococcal surface. Adherence of *Neisseria gonorrhoeae* to urethral mucosal cells: An electron microscope study of human gonorrhoea. (Ward, M. E. and Watt, P. J. (1972). *J. Inf. Dis.* **126**, 601–604.)

Urine, as long as it is not too acid, provides a fine growth medium for many bacteria and the entire urinary tract is more prone to infections when there is interference with the free flow and flushing action of urine, or when a "sump" of urine remains in the bladder after urination. Urinary infections are thus associated with structural abnormalities of the bladder, ureter etc., with stones, or with an enlarged prostate that prevents complete emptying of the bladder. Incomplete emptying also leads to urinary infection in pregnant women, and this is partly due to the sluggish action of muscles in the bladder wall. But the bladder is more than an inert receptacle for infected urine, and responds with inflammation and secretory antibody production. The normal bladder wall, moreover, appears to have some intrinsic but poorly understood antibacterial activity.

The vagina has no particular cleansing mechanism and would appear to present an ideal site for colonization by commensal microorganisms. During reproductive life, however, from puberty until the menopause, the vaginal epithelium contains glycogen because of the action of circulating oestrogens. Döderlein's bacillus (a lactobacillus) colonizes the vagina, metabolizing the glycogen to produce lactic acid. The lactic acid gives a vaginal pH of about 5.0, and together with other products of metabolism inhibits colonization by all except Döderlein's bacillus and a select number of bacteria, including various nonpyogenic streptococci and diphtheroids. Normal vaginal secretions contain up to 10^8 bacteria ml^{-1}. Other microorganisms are unable to establish infections, except the specialized ones that are therefore responsible for venereal diseases. Oestrogens thus generate an antimicrobial defence mechanism just at the period of life when contaminated objects are being introduced into the vagina. Before puberty and after the menopause, the vaginal epithelium lacks glycogen, the secretion is alkaline, and bacteria from the vulva, including staphylococci and streptococci, can become established.

Conjunctiva

The conjunctiva is kept moist and healthy by the continuous flow of secretions from lacrymal and other glands. Every few seconds the lids pass over the conjunctival surface with a gentle but firm windscreen wiper action. Although the secretions (tears) contain lysozyme (see Glossary) and other antimicrobial substances, their principal protective action is the mechanical washing away of foreign particles. Microorganisms alighting on the conjunctiva are treated like inanimate particles of dirt or dust and swept away via the tear ducts into the nasal cavity. Clearly there is little or no opportunity for initiation of infection in the normal conjunctiva unless microorganisms have some special ability to attach to the conjunctival surface. The conjunctiva, however, suffers minor injuries whenever we get "something in the eye", and these give opportunities for infection, as would defects in the cleansing mechanisms due to lacrymal gland or lid disease. The chlamydia responsible for inclusion conjunctivitis and for that greatest eye infection in history, trachoma, are masters in the art of conjunctival infection. They probably attach to receptors on the cell surfaces, doubtless also taking advantage of breaches in the defence mechanisms. The conjunctiva is also infected from the "inside" during the course of measles, when the virus spreads via the circulation and is somehow seeded out to conjunctival blood vessels (see p. 115).

The conjunctiva is infected by mechanically deposited rather than by airborne microorganisms. Flies, fingers and towels play an important role in diseases such as trachoma, and it is significant that the types of *Chlamydia trachomatis* that cause urethritis (see p. 44) also often infect the eye, presumably being borne from one to the other by contaminated fingers. Certain enteroviruses (enterovirus 70, coxsackievirus A24) cause conjunctivitis, and conjunctivitis due to adenovirus 8 is one of the many diseases that can be caused by the physician (iatrogenic diseases). It is transmitted from one patient to the next by the instruments used in extracting foreign bodies from the eye. Foreign bodies in the eye are common in the shipbuilding industry, and the condition has been called "shipyard eye". Microorganisms present in swimming baths have a good opportunity to infect the conjunctiva, water flowing over the conjunctiva depositing microorganisms and at the same time causing slight mechanical and chemical damage. Both the chlamydia and adenovirus 8 have been transmitted in this way. During the birth of an infant gonococci or chlamydia from an infected cervix can be deposited in the eye to cause severe neonatal conjunctivitis.

The Normal Microbial Flora

The commensal microorganisms that live in association with the body surfaces of man have repeatedly been referred to in this chapter. It has been calculated that the normal individual houses about 10^{12} bacteria on the skin, 10^{10} in the mouth and nearly 10^{14} in the alimentary canal. Most of these are highly specialized bacteria,* utilizing available foods, often with

---

* The specialized secretion of the genital mucosa of both sexes (smegma), has its own resident bacterium, *Mycobacterium smegma*, which often contaminates urine. Skin residents include certain yeasts, *Pityrosporum ovale* and *Pityrosporum orbiculare*. *Pityrosporon ovale* appears to be responsible for that widespread but humble human condition dandruff. It is a good parasite, present on most male scalps, feeding on dead skin scales with minimal inconvenience to the host. Fascinating mites (*Demodex folliculorum* and *brevis*) reside unobtrusively in hair follicles or sebaceous glands, feeding on epithelial cells and on sebum. These mites are present in all human beings, and their spectacular success as parasites is reflected by a healthy person's astonishment when shown an adult mite attached to the base of his plucked eyelash. Other mites of the same genus parasitize horses, cattle, dogs, squirrels etc.

mechanisms for attachment to body surfaces, and looking very much as if they have an evolutionary adaptation to a specific host.

Is the normal microbial flora of any value?

There is no doubt that intestinal microorganisms play a vital role in the nutrition of many herbivorous animals. The caecum of the rabbit and the rumen of the cow were referred to on p. 23. The most important beneficial effect in man is probably the tendency of the normal microbial flora to exclude other microorganisms. Intestinal bacteria such as *E. coli*, for instance, fail to establish themselves in the normal mouth and throat, and disturbances in the normal flora induced by long courses of broad spectrum antibiotics may permit the overgrowth of *Candida albicans* in the mouth or staphylococci in the intestine. In one unusual experiment none of 14 volunteers given 1000 *Salmonella typhi* by mouth developed disease (see also p. 19), but one of four did so when the antibiotic streptomycin was given at the same time. Streptomycin probably promoted infection by its bacteriostatic action on commensal intestinal microorganisms. It is known that other *Salmonella* infections of the intestine persist for longer when antibiotics are given.

The composition of the intestinal flora in man is complex, but there are only a small number of predominant types of bacteria. The picture is greatly influenced by diet; for instance, *Sarcina ventriculi*, an intestinal bacterium, is virtually confined to vegetarians, in whom it is present in large numbers. Because of their numbers, the intestinal bacteria have considerable metabolic potential (said to be equal to that of the liver) and products of metabolism can be absorbed. For instance, intestinal bacteria are important in the degradation of bile acids, and glycosides such as cascara or senna taken orally are converted by bacteria into active forms (aglycones) with pharmacological activity. Metabolic products occasionally cause trouble. Substances like ammonia are normally absorbed into the portal circulation and dealt with by the liver, but when this organ is badly damaged (severe hepatitis) they are able to enter the general circulation and contribute to hepatic coma. Adult Bantus, Australian aborigines, Chinese etc. differ from Anglo-Saxons in that the small intestinal mucosa fails to produce the enzyme lactase. This is presumably related to the fact that these people don't normally drink milk as adults. If lactose is ingested, it is metabolized by the bacteria of the caecum and colon, with the production of fatty acids, carbon dioxide, hydrogen etc., giving rise to flatulence and diarrhoea.

The resident bacteria are highly adapted to the commensal life, and under normal circumstances cause minimal damage. They are present throughout life, and avoid inducing the inflammatory or immune responses that might expel them. In the normal individual, the only other microorganisms that can establish themselves are by definition "infectious". These sometimes cause disease and are eventually eliminated. In other words, if it is inevitable that the body surfaces are colonized by microorganisms, it can be regarded as an advantage that colonization should be by specialized nonpathogenic commensals. Human infants like other infants are born germ-free, and the microbial colonization of skin, throat, intestine etc. during and after birth forms a fascinating story.

The traditional way to obtain evidence about the function of something is to see what happens when it is removed. There have been many studies on germ-free animals, including mice, rats, cats, dogs and monkeys. The mother is anaesthetized shortly before delivery, and infants are delivered by caesarean section into a germ-free environment or "isolator" and supplied with sterile air, food and water. Germ-free individuals, not unexpectedly, have a less well developed immune system, because of the absence of microorganisms. Antigens are present in food, but immunoglobulin synthesis occurs at about 1/50th of the rate seen in ordinary individuals. Germ-free animals also show a great enlargement of the caecum, which may constitute a quarter of the total body weight. It can cause death when it undergoes torsion. The enlarged caecum is a feature of germ-free coprophagous animals such as rabbits or mice, and does not occur in cats, dogs or monkeys. It rapidly diminishes to normal size when bacteria are fed to the germ-free individual. Otherwise, the germ-free individual seems better off and generally has a longer life span. Even caries is not seen, because this requires bacteria (see Ch. 1). At one time it was a fashionable belief that the normal intestinal microorganisms produced "toxins" that were harmful, and large segments of colon were removed from patients with diseases attributed to the action of these toxins. Toxins, especially endotoxin, are indeed absorbed from the intestine, but under normal circumstances this is not now thought to have harmful effects. On the other hand, there have been suggestions that carcinogenic substances, formed from the cholic acid in bile by intestinal bacteria, are important in cancer of the intestine, especially when the bowel contents move slowly (e.g. on low-fibre diets) and carcinogens have longer encounters with epithelial cells. Also, bacterial overgrowth in the stomach results in increased production of nitrites which can combine with amines to form carcinogenic nitrosamines.

It must be remembered that pathogenic as well as commensal microorganisms are absent from the germ-free animal, and in experimental animals it is possible to eliminate only the specific microbial pathogens, leaving the normal flora intact. This can be done by obtaining animals (mice, pigs etc.) by caesarean section and rearing them without contact with others of the same species, but not in a germ-free environment. Alternatively germ-free animals can be selectively contaminated with commensal microorganisms.

These specific pathogen-free (SPF) animals have increased body weight, longer lifespan and more successful reproductive performance, with more litters, larger litters and reduced infant mortality. Furthermore, it has long been known that chickens, pigs etc. grow larger when they receive broad-spectrum antibiotics in their food, presumably because certain unidentified microorganisms are eliminated. But even if we were to conclude that the normal microbial flora, as opposed to the pathogens, on the whole does more harm than good this conclusion, although of great interest, would have little practical significance. Colonization by commensal microorganisms is the unavoidable fate of all normal individuals, and the germ-free life will remain an impossibly artificial condition; expensive, technically demanding and psychologically crippling for an intelligent animal.*

The elimination of specific pathogenic microorganisms, however, is a less theoretical matter. Specific pathogen-free mice are routinely maintained in laboratories and are much superior to non-SPF animals, as mentioned above. The population of the developed countries of the world (USA, Canada, northern Europe) can be likened to SPF mice, most of the serious microbial pathogens having been eliminated by vaccines, quarantine and other public health measures, or kept in check by good medical care and antibiotics. The peoples of the developing countries of the world, on the other hand, are comparable to the conventionally reared, non-SPF mice, who are exposed to all the usual murine pathogens. The comparison is complicated by the often inadequate diet of those in the developing world. A WHO survey of 23 countries showed that in developing countries the common pathogenic infections such as diphtheria, whooping cough, measles and typhoid have respectively 100, 300, 55 and 160 times the case mortality seen in developed countries. Compared with those in the developed countries those in the developing countries often tend to be smaller, with a shorter lifespan, and poorer reproductive performance (abortions, neonatal and infantile mortality). They are the non-SPF people.

Opportunistic infection

There is one important consequence of the existence of the normal microbial flora. These microorganisms are present as harmless commensals, their need to feed and multiply having been achieved in relation to the resistance

---

* A boy who developed aplastic anaemia when 9 years old was maintained in a 2.5 m × 2.7 m germ-free type isolator, shielded from contact with the microbial hazards of the outside world. Life was not easy, although he felt less abnormal when he was able to wear his protective astronaut-type suit at a science fiction convention. He was spared from infection and died at the age of 17 years, from complications of repeated blood transfusions.

of the host to invasion and damage. They are normally well-behaved. If, in a given individual, this balance is upset and there is a decrease in the normal level of resistance, then the commensal bacteria are generally the first to take advantage of it. Thus damage to the respiratory tract upsets the balance and enables normally harmless resident bacteria to grow and cause sinusitis or pneumonia. Minor wounds in the skin enable skin staphylococci to establish small septic foci, and skin sepsis is particularly common in poorly controlled diabetes. This is probably due to defective chemotaxis and phagocytosis in polymorphs, which show impaired energy metabolism. High concentrations of blood sugar and the presence of ketone bodies may play a part, but a more direct effect of diabetes is suggested by the recent observation that adding insulin to diabetic polymorphs *in vitro* rapidly restores their bactericidal properties. Commensal faecal bacteria infect the urinary tract when introduced by catheters, and commensal streptococci entering the blood from the mouth can cause subacute bacterial endocarditis if there are abnormalities in the heart valves or endocardium. The tendency of commensal bacteria to take opportunities when they arise and invade the host is universal. These infections are therefore called opportunistic infections.

Opportunistic infections are common nowadays. This is partly because many specific microbial pathogens have been eliminated, leaving the opportunistic infections relatively more numerous than they were. Also, modern medical care keeps alive many people who have impaired resistance to microbial infections. This includes those with congenital immunological or other deficiencies, those with lymphoreticular neoplasms, and a great many patients in intensive care units or in the terminal stages of various illnesses. Modern medical treatment also often requires that host immune defences are suppressed, as after organ transplants or in the treatment of neoplastic and other conditions with immunosuppressive drugs. Also, certain virus infections (e.g. cat leukemia, AIDS in man) can cause a catastrophic depression of immune responses (see Ch. 7). In each case opportunistic microorganisms tend to give trouble.

There are other opportunistic pathogens in addition to the regular commensal bacteria. *Candida albicans*, a common commensal, readily causes troublesome oropharyngeal or genital ulceration. *Pseudomonas aeruginosa* is essentially a free-living species of bacteria, sometimes present in the intestinal tract. In hospitals it is now a major source of opportunistic infection. This is because it is resistant to many of the standard antibiotics and disinfectants, because its growth requirements are very simple, and because it is so widely present in the hospital environment. It multiplies in eyedrops, weak disinfectants, corks, in the small reservoirs of water round taps and sinks, and even in vases of flowers. *Pseudomonas aeruginosa* causes infection especially of burns, wounds, ulcers, and the urinary tract after instrumentation.* It is a common cause of respiratory illness in patients with cystic fibrosis.† When resistance is very low it can spread systematically through the body, and nowadays this is a frequent harbinger of immunological collapse. Viruses also act as opportunistic pathogens. Most people are persistently infected with cytomegalovirus, herpes simplex virus, varicella-zoster virus etc. (see Ch. 10), and these commonly cause disease in immunologically depressed individuals. Cytomegalovirus, for instance, is activated within the first six months after most renal transplant operations, as detected by a rise in antibody titre, and may cause hepatitis and pneumonia. The protozoan parasite *Pneumocystis carini* is an extremely common human resident, normally of almost zero pathogenicity, but can contribute to pneumonia in immunosuppressed individuals.

Exit of Microorganisms from the Body

After an account of the entry of microorganisms into the body, it seems appropriate to mention their exit. General principles were discussed in the first chapter. Nearly all microorganisms are shed from the body surfaces (Fig. 2). The transmissibility of a microorganism from one host to another depends to some extent on the degree of shedding, on its stability, and also on its infectiousness, or the dose required to initiate infection (see Table 30, p. 271). For instance, when 10 bacteria are enough to cause oral infection (*Shigella dysenteriae*) the disease will tend to spread from person to person more readily than when 10^6 bacteria are required (salmonellosis, Table 23, p. 197). The properties that give increased transmissibility are not the same as those causing pathogenicity. There are strains of influenza virus that are virulent for mice, but which are transmitted rather ineffectively to other mice, transmissibility behaving as a separate genetic attribute of the virus. For other microorganisms also, such as staphylococci and streptococci, transmissibility may vary independently of pathogenicity. Types of transmission are illustrated in Fig. 7.

---

* *Pseudomonas* recently demonstrated its versatility by causing a profuse rash in users of a hotel Jacuzzi (whirlpool). The bacteria multiplied in the hot, recirculated, inadequately treated water, and probably entered the skin via the orifices of dilated hair follicles.

† Cystic fibrosis, the most common fatal hereditary disease in Caucasians (about 1 in 20 carry the gene), involves defects in mucus-producing cells. The lung with its viscid mucus becomes infected with *Staphylococcus aureus*, and *Haemophilus influenzae*, but the presence of *Pseudomonas aeruginosa* is especially ominous. *Pseudomonas* strains from cystic fibrosis patients often produce a jelly-like alginate rather than the regular "slimy" type of polysaccharide (Table 6, p. 76), and this may physically interfere with the action of phagocytes.

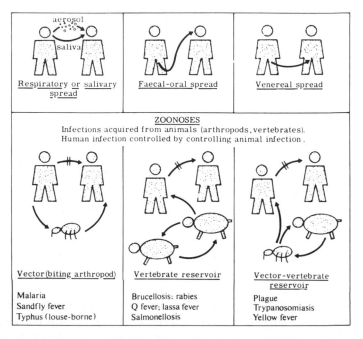

Fig. 7. Types of transmission of infectious agents. Respiratory or salivary spread—not readily controllable. Faecal–oral spread—controllable by public health measures. Venereal spread—control difficult because it concerns social factors. Zoonoses—human infection controlled by controlling vectors, or by controlling animal infection.*

Respiratory tract

In infections transmitted by the respiratory route, shedding depends on the production of airborne particles (aerosols) containing microorganisms. These are produced to some extent in the larynx, mouth and throat during speech and normal breathing. Harmless commensal bacteria are thus shed, and more pathogenic streptococci, meningococci and other microorganisms are also spread in this way, especially when people are crowded together inside buildings or vehicles. There is particularly good aerosol formation during singing and it is always dangerous to sing in a choir with patients suffering from pulmonary tuberculosis. Microorganisms in the mouth, throat, larynx and lungs are expelled to the exterior with much greater

---

* Although man to man transmission does not normally occur in the zoonoses, direct contact with blood or secretions from infected individuals occasionally can lead to infection of nurses, doctors etc. (e.g. Lassa fever).

efficiency during coughing; shedding to the exterior is assured when there are increased mucus secretions and the cough reflex is induced. Tubercle bacilli in the lungs that are carried up to the back of the throat are mostly swallowed and can be detected in stomach washings, but a cough will project bacteria into the air.*

Efficient shedding from the nasal cavity depends on an increase in nasal secretions and on the induction of sneezing. In a sneeze (Fig. 8) up to 20 000 droplets are produced† and during a common cold, for instance, many of them will contain virus particles. The largest droplets (1 mm diameter) fall to the ground after travelling 4 m or so and the smaller ones evaporate rapidly, depending on their velocity, water content and on the relative humidity. Many have disappeared within a few feet and the rest, including those containing microorganisms, then settle according to size. The smallest (1–4 μm diameter), although they fall theoretically at 0.3–1.0 m h^{-1}, in fact stay suspended indefinitely because air is never quite still. Particles of this size are likely to pass the turbinate baffles (see above) and reach the lower respiratory tract. If the microorganisms are hardy, as in the case of the tubercle bacillus and smallpox virus, people coming into the room later on can be infected. Many other microorganisms are soon inactivated by drying of the suspended droplet or by light, and for transmission of measles, influenza, the common cold or the meningococcus, fairly close physical proximity is needed. Conversely, foot and mouth disease virus spreads by air and wind over surprisingly long distances.‡

Shedding from the nasal cavity is much more effective when fluid is produced and, among the viruses that are shed from this site, evolution has

---

Mycobacterium leprae multiplies in nasal mucosa and 10^8 bacilli a day can be shed from the nose of patients with lepromatous leprosy. The bacteria are shed as plentifully as from patients with open pulmonary tuberculosis, and also survive in the dried state.

†Most of the droplets in fact originate from the mouth, but larger masses of material ("streamers") as well as droplets are expelled from the nose when there is excess nasal secretion. A cough, in contrast, produces no more than a few hundred particles. Talking is also a source of airborne particles, especially when the consonants f, p, t and s are used. It is perhaps no accident that the most powerfully abusive words in the English language begin with these letters, so that a spray of droplets (possibly infectious) is delivered with the abuse.

‡Pigs infected with foot and mouth disease virus excrete in their breath 100 million infectious units each day. With relative humidity of more than 65% the airborne virus survives quite well, and can be carried in the wind across the sea from France to the Channel Islands or England where cattle, who inhale 150 m^3 air a day, become infected. Outbreaks of this disease are often explained by studying air trajectories and other meteorological factors.

In humans, legionellosis (see Glossary) can spread by air over shorter distances. An outbreak in Glasgow affected 33 people and had its source in a contaminated industrial cooling tower, cases occurring downwind up to a distance of 1700 m.

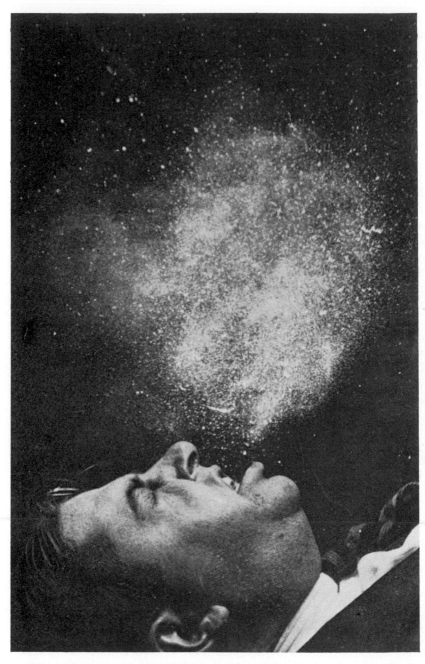

Fig. 8. Droplet dispersal following a violent sneeze. Most of the 20 000 particles seen here are coming from the mouth. The authors used oblique illumination, to give a dark field effect, and high speed (1/30 000 s flash) photography. Particles as small as 5–10 μm could be seen; images are larger than actual particle size, and objects out of focus are magnified. (From Jennison, M. W. (1947). "Aerobiology" p. 102, A.A.A.S. No 17. Washington, DC.)

favoured those that induce a good nasal discharge.* In the crowded conditions of modern life, with unprecedented numbers of susceptible individuals
in close physical proximity and with only temporary nasal immunity (see Ch.
6), there is rapid selection for the virus strains that spread most effectively.
There are more than 100 antigenically different common cold viruses, and
there are signs that these infectious agents are entering their golden age,
with little hope of control by vaccination or chemoprophylaxis.

Saliva

Microorganisms reach the saliva during upper or lower respiratory tract
infections and may be shed during talking and other mouth movements as
discussed above. Certain viruses, such as mumps, EB virus, herpes simplex
and cytomegalovirus in man infect the salivary glands. Virus is present in the
saliva, and shedding to the exterior takes place in infants and young children
by the contamination of fingers and other objects with saliva. Adolescents
and adults who have escaped infection earlier in life exchange a good deal of
saliva in the process of kissing, particularly "deep" kissing. In developing
countries, EB virus infects mainly infants and children, and at this age causes
little or no illness. In developed countries, however, infection is often
avoided during childhood, and primary infection with EB virus occurs at a
time of life when sexual activity is beginning. At this age it gives rise to the
more serious clinical conditions included under the heading of glandular
fever. In animals also, saliva is often an important vehicle of transmission,
depending on social and sexual activities such as licking, nibbling, grooming,
fighting. Rabies, foot and mouth disease virus, and the various types of
cytomegalovirus and other herpes viruses may be present in large amounts
in saliva.

Spitting is an activity practised only by man and a few animals including
camels, chameleons and certain snakes. Chimpanzees soon learn to do it.
Microorganisms resistant to drying, such as the tubercle bacillus, can be
transmitted in this way. The expectorated material contains saliva together
with secretions from the lower respiratory tract. In the days when pulmonary
tuberculosis was commoner, spitting in public places came to be frowned
upon and there were laws against it. It is perhaps better for the chronic
bronchitic to discharge his voluminous secretions discreetly into a receptacle

---

*Nasal secretions are inevitably deposited (directly or via handkerchiefs) onto hands, which
can then be a source of infection. Contamination of other people's fingers, and thus of their nose
and conjunctiva, might be as important as aerosols in the transmission of these infections.

rather than swallow them, but the expectoration of mere saliva in public places, now becoming commoner again, is a regrettable reversion to the unaesthetic days of the spittoon.

Skin

Shedding of commensal skin bacteria takes place very effectively. Skin bacteria are mostly shed attached to desquamated skin scales, and an average of about 5×10^8 scales, 10^7 of them carrying bacteria, are shed per person per day, the rate depending very much on physical activity. The fine white dust that collects on surfaces in hospital wards consists to a large extent of skin scales. The potentially pathogenic *Staphylococcus aureus* colonizes especially the nose (nose-picking area), fingers and perineum. Shedding takes place from the nose and notably from the perineal area. Males tend to be more effective perineal shedders than females, and this is partly hormonal and partly because of friction in this area; shedding can be prevented by wearing occlusive underpants. A good staphylococcal shedder can raise the staphylococcal count in the air from less then 36 m^{-3} to 360 m^{-3}. Although people with eczema or psoriasis shed more bacteria from the skin it is not known why some normal individuals are profuse shedders; the phenomenon is important for cross infection in hospitals.

For microorganisms that cause skin lesions (see Table 9, p. 113), however, shedding to the environment is not necessarily very important. Shedding takes place only if the skin lesion breaks down, as when a vesicle ruptures or a dried scab is shed (smallpox), or if the microorganism penetrates through to the outer layers of the epidermis (wart virus). Even then, spread of infection is often by direct bodily contact, as with herpes simplex, syphilis or yaws, rather than by shedding into the environment. Smallpox is a very stable virus and used to be shed from scabs and vesicles, but shedding from the respiratory tract was a more important mechanism of transmission in epidemics.

Intestinal tract

All microorganisms that infect the intestinal tract are shed in faeces. Those shed into the bile, such as hepatitis A (an enterovirus) and typhoid bacilli in the typhoid carrier, also appear in the faeces. Microorganisms swallowed after growth in the mouth, throat or respiratory tract can also appear in the faeces, but most of them are not resistant to acid, bile and other intestinal substances and are inactivated. Faeces are the body's largest solid contribution to the environment,* and although the microorganisms in faeces are nearly all harmless commensals, it is an important source of less harmful microorganisms. During an intestinal infection, intestinal contents are often hurried along and the faeces become fluid. There is no exact equivalent to the sneeze, but diarrhoea certainly leads to increased faecal contamination of the environment and spread to other individuals. In animal communities and in primitive human communities, there is a large-scale recycling of faecal material back into the mouth. Contamination of food, water and living areas ensure that this is so, and the efficiency of this faecal–oral movement is attested to by the great variety of microbes and parasites that spread from one individual to another by this route. If microorganisms shed into the faeces are resistant to drying and other environmental conditions, they remain infectious for long periods. Protozoa such as *Entamoeba histolytica* produce an especially resistant cyst which is the effective vehicle of transmission, and *Clostridia* form resistant spores that contaminate the environment and remain infectious for many years. The soils of Europe are heavily seeded with tetanus spores from the faeces of domestic animals, and these spores can infect the battlefield wound or the gardening abrasion to give tetanus. Viruses have no special resistant form for the hazardous journey to the next host, but they show variable resistance to thermal inactivation and drying. Poliovirus, for instance, is soon inactivated on drying.

Many microorganisms are effectively transmitted from faeces to mouth after contamination of water used for drinking. The great water-borne epidemics of cholera are classical examples,† and any faecal pathogen can be so transmitted if it survives for at least a few days in water. In densely inhabited regions faecal contamination of water is inevitable unless there is adequate sewage disposal and a supply of purified water. Two hundred years ago in England there were no water closets and no sewage disposal; human excrement was deposited in the streets. There was nowhere else to put it,

---

*Herbivorous animals make a bigger and less well controlled contribution than do human beings. The output of a pig is about three times and a cow 10 times that of a man. We are less fussy about the disposal of animal sewage and this can be important for instance in transfer of salmonellosis (p. 195). The amount from an individual animal seems less important than its quality and site of deposition when we consider the apalling canine contribution to public parks and paths in dog-ridden cities.

†Dr. John Snow, a London physician, charted the cases of cholera on a street map during an outbreak in 1854. After observing that all cases had used water from the same pump in Broad Street, Soho, he removed the handle of this pump. The outbreak terminated dramatically, and the mode of transmission was thus demonstrated nearly 40 years before Koch identified the causative organism.

although one enterprising Londoner in 1359 was fined twelve pence for running his sewage by a pipe into a neighbour's cellar. Water supplies came from rivers and from wells, of which there were more than 1000 in London. Efficient sewage disposal and piped water supplies are a comparatively recent (nineteenth century) development. Nowadays the map of the London sewage system resembles that of the London Underground (subway) system. Water for domestic use is collected into vast reservoirs before being shared out to tens of thousands of individuals. This would give great opportunities for spread once pathogens entered the water supply, but water purification and chlorination ensures that this spread remains at almost zero level. Life in present-day urban society depends on the large-scale supply of pure water and the large scale disposal of sewage. Both are complex and vital public services of which the average citizen or physician is profoundly ignorant. Largely as a result of these developments the steady flow of faecal materials into the mouth that has characterized much of human history has been interrupted.

Urinogenital tract

Urine can contaminate food, drink and living space, and the same things can be said as have been said about faeces. Urine in the bladder is normally sterile, and is only contaminated with skin bacteria as it is discharged to the exterior. The pathogens regularly present in urine include a specialized group that are able to spread through the body and infect the kidney or bladder. The leptospiral infections of rats and other animals are spread in this way, sometimes to man. *Leptospira** survive in water, can penetrate the skin, and people are infected following contact with contaminated canals, rivers, sewage, farmyard puddles and other damp objects. Polyoma virus spreads naturally in colonies of mice after infecting tubular epithelial cells in the kidney and being discharged to the exterior in urine. Mice carrying lymphocytic choriomeningitis virus shed the virus in urine and can thus infect people in mouse-infested dwellings. Humans infected with their own polyoma virus, or with cytomegalovirus, excrete the virus in urine. Urinary carriers of typhoid have a persistent infection in the bladder, especially when the bladder is scarred by *Schistosoma* parasites, and typhoid bacilli are shed in the urine.

---

*There are about 10 different serotypes, carried by mice, rats, swine, dogs, cattle, and leptospirosis is the most widespread zoonosis (see p. 36) in the world. In the UK nowadays, cases of rat-born leptospirosis occur in the bathers, canoeists etc. who use canals and rivers rather than in sewer workers or miners, and leptospirosis from cattle continues to cause a mild disease in farmers and cowmen.

Microorganisms shed from the urethra and genital tract generally depend for transmission on mucosal contacts with susceptible individuals. Herpes simplex type 2 can infect the infant as it passes along an infected birth canal during delivery, and gonococci or chlamydia infect the infant's eye in the same way. Venery, however, gives far greater opportunities for spread, as was discussed in Ch. 1. If there is a discharge, organisms are carried over the epithelial surface and transmission is more likely to take place.

The transmission of microorganisms by mucosal contact is determined by social and sexual activity (see also p. 2). In animals, licking, nuzzling, grooming and biting can be responsible for the transmission of micro-organisms such as rabies and herpes viruses. In recent years there have been major changes in man's social and sexual customs, and this has had an interesting influence on certain infectious diseases. Generally speaking there has been less mucosal contact in the course of regular social life. In modern societies saliva is exchanged less freely between children (as noted on p. 39) or within a family, and children are more likely to escape infections that are spread via saliva such as those due to EB virus. Things are different when we consider sexual activity. For adolescents and adults mucosal contacts are possibly increasing in frequency, but more importantly they are being made with a greater number of different partners. Sexual activity is now considered less sinful, and the fact that it is safer (pregnancy avoidable and disease treatable) means that multiple partners are commoner than they used to be. Furthermore, infectious agents are transmitted with much greater efficiency now that many couples use oral rather than mechanical contraceptives. All these things have led a great flowering of sexually transmitted diseases, which with respiratory infections are now the com-monest communicable diseases in the world. Their incidence is rising. The four most frequent sexually transmitted diseases in England today are nonspecific urethritis (largely due to *Chlamydia*), gonorrhoea, candidiasis, and genital warts.* It seems likely that AIDS (caused by HIV, see p. 162) is going to have an impact on sexual promiscuity. Although it was initially a disease largely restricted to male homosexuals, drug addicts and haemophiliacs, an apparently identical infection is spreading rapidly in Central Africa by means of regular (vaginal) heterosexual intercourse. It now looks as if a phase of heterosexual transmission is beginning in

---

*This is not to say that promiscuity is a new thing. The well charted sexual adventures of Casanova (1725–1798) brought him four attacks of gonorrhoea, five of chancroid, and one of syphilis, while Boswell (1740–1795) experienced 19 episodes of (mainly gonococcal) urethritis. These activities of course were not restricted to those who became famous or wrote books. But the extraordinary increase in man's mobility has transformed social life and, together with the factors mentioned above, has had a major impact on the sexual transmission of infectious diseases.

Table 3. Principal sexually transmitted diseases in man[a]

	Microorganism	Disease	Comments
Viruses	Herpes simplex type 2	Genital herpes	Very common—reactivates
	Human papillomavirus	Genital warts	Very common—involvement in cervical and penile cancer makes them more than ornamental appendages
	Poxvirus	Molluscum contagiosium	Uncommon
	Cytomegalovirus	Ill defined	Virus presence in semen and cervix suggests sexual transmission
	HIV[b] (HTLV$_3$)	AIDS	Common in male homosexuals, transmitted perhaps by anal intercourse. But in Africa, HIV spreads by heterosexual (vaginal) intercourse
	Hepatitis B	Hepatitis	
Chlamydia	*C. trachomatis* (types D–K)	Nonspecific urethritis	Responsible for more than half of cases; causes eye infection in newborn
	C. trachomatis (types L1–L3)	Lymphogranuloma inguinale	Ulcerating papule plus lymph node suppuration Commoner in tropics and subtropics
Mycoplasmas	*Ureoplasma* spp.	Nonspecific urethritis	Importance not clear. Require 10% urea for growth, which would direct them to urogenital tract
Bacteria	*Neisseria gonorrhoeae*	Gonorrhoea	Acute and more severe urethritis in male; chronic pelvic infection in female; eye infection in newborn
	Treponema pallidium	Syphilis	Syphilis was name of infected shepherd in Frascator's poem (1530) describing disease

Table 3. (*Cont.*)

	Microorganism	Disease	Comments
	Haemophilus ducreyi	Chancroid	Genital sore, lymph-node suppuration, commoner in subtropics
	Donovania granulomatis	Granuloma inguinale	Commoner in subtropics Ulcerative lesions
Fungi	*Candida albicans*	Vulvovaginitis (balanoposthitis in male)	Asymptomatic vaginal carriage common
Protozoa	*Trichomonas vaginalis*	Vulvovaginitis (urethritis in male)	Disease worse in female (compare gonorrhoea)

[a] More than half of all infections occur in people under the age of 24 years. In addition, there are special "at risk" groups, such as tourists, long-distance lorry drivers, seamen, homosexuals.
[b] Human Immunodeficiency Virus.

developed countries. In the sadly afflicted homosexual population, promiscuity has already been curtailed, as indicated for instance by falling gonorrhoea infection rates. The threat of such a serious infection, with no vaccine and no treatment, in which 10–20% of those infected develop AIDS, will probably act as a restraining influence on heterosexual promiscuity and encourage the use of barrier contraceptives.*

A list of sexually transmitted diseases is given in Table 3. Even the more serious diseases such as syphilis and gonorrhoea have been difficult to control. A small number of sexually active individuals, if they evade the public health network, can be relied upon to infect many others.

Because almost all mucosal surfaces in the body can be involved in sexual activity, microorganisms encounter a number of interesting opportunities to infect new bodily sites. Thus, *Neisseria meningitidis*, a resident of the nasopharynx, is occasionally recovered from the cervix, the male urethra and the anal canal. *Neisseria gonorrhoea* infects the throat and the anal region. *Chlamydia* can at times be recovered from the rectum and pharynx as well as the urethra. Genito–oro–anal contacts in promiscuous homosexual communities give chances for intestinal microorganisms to spread between

---

*Condoms have been shown to reliably retain herpes simplex virus, HIV, chlamydia, and gonococci in simulated coital tests of the syringe and plunger type.

individuals in spite of good sanitation and sewage disposal (see p. 2).* There have been examples of transmission of *Salmonella, Gardia lamblia*, hepatitis A, pathogenic amoebae and *Shigella*, constituting what has been referred to as the "gay bowel syndrome".†

Blood

Most of the microorganisms that are transmitted by blood-sucking arthropods such as mosquitoes, fleas, ticks, sandflies or mites, have to be present in blood. This is true for arthropod-borne viruses, rickettsiae, malaria, trypanosomes and many other infectious agents. In these diseases transmission is biological (see p. 11). The microorganism is ingested with the blood meal, multiplies in the arthropod and then is discharged from the salivary gland or intestinal tract of the arthropod to infect a fresh host. To infect the arthropod vector, the blood of the vertebrate host must contain adequate amounts of the infectious agent. Microorganisms can be said to have been shed into the blood.

Miscellaneous

Microorganisms rarely occur in semen, which is not designed by nature for shedding to the environment. Perhaps it is because of the superb opportunities for direct mucosal spread during venery that only an occasional microorganism, such as cytomegalovirus in man, has made use of semen as a vehicle for transmission. Milk, in contrast, is a fairly common vehicle for transmission. Mumps virus and cytomegalovirus are shed in human milk, although perhaps not very often transmitted in this way, but the mammary tumour viruses of mice are certainly partly transmitted via milk. Cows' milk containing *Brucella abortus*, tubercle bacilli or Q fever rickettsia is a source of human infection.

No shedding

In a very few instances transmission takes place without any specific shedding of microorganisms to the exterior. Anthrax, for instance, infects

---

* In Western societies intestinal pathogens can also spread by more innocent pathways, as when amoebiasis was transmitted to 15 patients who received colonic irrigation in a clinic in Colorado.

† It should be noted that these conditions, like other sexually transmitted infections, are confined to homosexuals of the male variety. Female homosexuals, in contrast, enjoy more discreet, less promiscuous, relationships which are infection-free because that necessary instrument for transmission, the penis, is absent.

and kills susceptible animals, and the corpse as a whole then contaminates the environment. Spores are formed aerobically, where blood leaks from body orifices, and they remain infectious in the soil for very long periods. It seems that spores are only formed during the terminal stages of the illness or after death, so that death of the host can be said to be necessary for the transmission of this unusual microorganism. Again, kuru (see p. 263) is only transmitted after death when the infectious agent in the brain is introduced into the body via mouth, intestine or fingers during cannibalistic consumption of the carcass.

Finally, certain microorganisms such as leukaemia and mammary tumour viruses spread from parent to offspring directly by infecting the egg or the developing embryo. If sections from mice congenitally infected with LCM virus are examined after fluorescent antibody staining, infected ova can be seen in the ovary (Fig. 17, p. 100). Also ovum transplant experiments show that similar infection occurs with murine leukaemia virus, and the embryos of most strains of mice have leukaemia virus antigens present in their cells. All progeny from the originally infected individuals are infected and there is no need for shedding to the exterior. Some other mode of spread would be necessary if there were to be infection of a fresh lineage of susceptible hosts.

References

Beachey, E. H. (1981). Bacterial adherence: adhesin-receptor interactions mediate the attachment of bacteria to mucosal surfaces. *J. Inf. Dis* **143**, 325–345.

Buckley, R. M. *et al.* (1978). Urine bacterial counts after sexual intercourse. *New Engl. J. Med.* **298**, 321–323.

Cockburn, W. C. and Assaad, F. (1974). Some observations on the communicable diseases as public health problems. *Bull. W.H.O.* **49**, 1–12.

Donaldson, A. I. (1983). Quantitative data on airborne foot and mouth disease virus: its production, carriage and deposition. *Phil. Trans. R. Soc. London, B* **302**, 529–534.

Duguid, J. P. (1946). The size and duration of air carriage of respiratory droplets and droplet nuclei. *J. Hyg., Camb.* **44**, 471.

Gordon, H. A. and Pesti, L. (1972). The gnotobiotic animal as a tool in the study of host–microbial relationships. *Bact. Rev.* **35**, 390–429.

Hentges, D. J. (Ed.) (1983). "Human Intestinal Microflora in Health and in Disease." Academic Press, New York and London.

Hinds, C. J. (1985). Medical hazards from dogs. *Brit. Med. J.* **291**, 760.

Mackowiak, P. A. (1982). The normal microbial flora. *N. Engl. J. Med.* **307**, 83.

Mims, C. A. (1981). Vertical Transmission of Viruses. *Microbiol. Rev.* **45**, 267–286.

Newhouse, M. *et al.* (1976). Lung defense mechanisms. *New Engl. J. Med.* **295**, 990, 1045.

Noble, W. C. (1981). "Microbiology of the Human Skin", 2nd edn. Lloyd-Luke, London.

Owen, R. L. (1977). Sequential uptake of horseradish peroxidase by lymphoid follicle epithelium of Peyer's patches in the normal unobstructed mouse. *Gastroenterology* **72**, 440–451.

Peterson, P. K. and Quie, P. G. (1981). Bacterial surface components and the pathogenesis of infectious diseases. *Ann. Rev. Med.* **32**, 29.

Savage, D. C. (1977). Microbial ecology of the GI tract. *A. Rev. Microbiol.* **31**, 107–133.

Schachter, J. (1978). Chlamydial infection. *New Engl. J. Med.* **298**, 428–435, 490–495, 540–549.

Scully, C. (1981). Dental caries: progress in microbiology and immunology. *J. Infection* **3**, 101–133.

Shuster, S. (1984). The aetiology of dandruff and mode of action of therapeutic agents. *Brit. J. Dermatol.* **111**, 235–242.

Ward, M. E. and Watt, P. J. (1972). Adherence of Neisseria gonorrhoea to urethral mucosal cells: an electron microscopic study of human gonorrhoea. *J. Inf. Dis.* **126**, 601–604.

Wilcox, R. R. (1981). The rectum as viewed by the venereologist. *Br. J. Ven. Dis.* **57**, 1–6.

3

Events Occurring Immediately After the Entry of the Microorganism

Growth in Epithelial Cells

Some of the most successful microorganisms multiply in the epithelial surface at the site of entry into the body, produce a spreading infection in the epithelium, and are shed directly to the exterior (Table 4). This is the simplest, most straightforward type of microbial parasitism. If the infection progresses rapidly and microbial progeny are shed to the exterior within a few days, the whole process may have been completed before the immune response has had a chance to influence the course of events. It takes at least a few days for antibodies or immune cells to be formed in appreciable amounts and delivered to the site of infection. This is what seems to happen with a variety of respiratory virus infections, especially those caused by rhinoviruses, corona viruses, parainfluenza viruses and influenza viruses. Epithelial cells may be destroyed, and inflammatory responses induced, but there is little or no virus invasion of underlying tissues. The infection is terminated partly by nonimmunological resistance factors, and partly because most locally available cells have been infected. Interferons are important nonimmunological resistance factors. They are low molecular weight proteins, coded for by the cell, and formed in response to infection with nearly all viruses (see Ch. 9). The interferon formed by the infected cell is released and can act on neighbouring or distant cells, protecting them from infection. Freshly formed virus particles from the first infected epithelial cell enter the fluids bathing the epithelial surface and are borne away to initiate fresh foci of infection at more distant sites. Interferons too can reach these sites, and as more and more interferon is formed on the epithelial sheet more

Table 4. Microbial infections that are generally confined to epithelial surfaces of the body

Microbe	Respiratory tract and conjunctiva	Urinogenital tract	Skin	Intestinal tract
Viruses	Influenza Parainfluenza 1–4 Rhinoviruses Coronaviruses	Certain papillomas	Papillomas (warts) Molluscum contagiosum	Rotaviruses of man, mouse etc.
Chlamydias	Trachoma Inclusion conjunctivitis	Nonspecfic urethritis	—	—
Mycoplasma	*Mycoplasma pneumoniae* (atypical pneumonia)	T strains (nonspecific urethritis)	—	—
Bacteria	*Bordetella pertussis* Corynebacterium *diphtheriae* *Streptococci*	Gonococcus	Staphylococci *Corynebacterium minutissimum*[a]	Most Salmonellae; Shigellae *Campylobacter* sp.
Rickettsias	—	—	—	—
Fungi	*Candida albicans* (thrush)	*Candida albicans*	*Trichophyton* spp. (athlete's foot, ringworm etc.)	—
Protozoa	—	*Trichomonas vaginalis*	—	*Entamoeba coli* *Giardia lamblia*

[a] This bacterium commonly infects the stratum corneum and causes erythrasma, a scaly condition of the axilla, groin and between toes.

and more cells are protected, so that the infectious process is slowed and finally halted. Other unknown antiviral factors probably play a part, and the immune response itself comes into action in the final stages. Interferons are produced a few hours after infection of the first epithelial cell at a site where they are needed and without the delay characteristic of the immune response. The immune response provides resistance to subsequent re-infection, but it does not appear to be of primary importance in recovery from respiratory infections of this type.

The spread of infection is very rapid on epithelial surfaces that are covered with a layer of liquid, because of the ease with which the microorganism in the fluid film encounters cells and is disseminated over the surface. This is true for the respiratory infections mentioned above, and also for infections of intestinal epithelium, such as those caused by the human diarrhoea viruses. The argument does not apply, however, to local infections of the skin. In this case, where the microorganism is not carried across the epithelial surface in a liquid film to establish fresh foci of infection, the whole process takes a much longer time. Papilloma (wart) viruses, for instance, cause infection in a discrete focus of epidermal cells; indeed a wart consists of a clone of cells produced by the division of a single initially infected cell. The inevitably slow evolution of single virus-rich lesions means that immune responses have the opportunity to play a more important part in the infection. Only small amounts of interferon are produced and these viruses are in any case often relatively resistant to its action. But wart virus escapes the attention of the immune system as follows. In the basal layer of the epidermis, adjacent to the antibodies and immune cells that arrive from dermal blood vessels, the virus infection is incomplete; in this layer of the epidermis, virus antigens are not formed on the cell surface and no virus particles are produced. The infected basal cell is therefore not recognized and not a target for the immune response. As the cells move further away from these immune forces, approaching the epidermal surface and becoming keratinized, more and more virus is produced for liberation to the exterior. Neither antibodies nor immune cells are present on this dry surface to influence virus multiplication and shedding.

The respiratory viruses described above have a hit and run type of infection of epithelial cells, and are very successful parasites. We may ask if there is anything that prevents them invading subepithelial tissues and spreading systemically in the host. A number of other viruses, including measles and smallpox, infect inconspicuously via the respiratory tract, then spread systemically through the body and only emerge again to cause widespread respiratory infection and shedding to the exterior after a prolonged incubation period. The limitation of rhinoviruses and human coronaviruses to the surface of the upper respiratory tract is at least partly determined by their optimum growth temperature. Many of them replicate successfully at 33°C, the temperature of nasal epithelium, but not very well at the general body temperature (37°C). Thus they do not spread systemically nor to the lung. Viruses of the influenza and parainfluenza groups can infect the lung as well as the nasal mucosa, but they are generally limited to the epithelial surfaces. This is certainly to a great extent due to their inability to infect other cells, but the limitation is not absolute. Occasionally in adults and more often in infants, influenza and parainfluenza viruses infect the heart, striated muscle or the central nervous system.

The spread of infection from epithelial surfaces is also controlled by the site of virus maturation from cells. Influenza and parainfluenza viruses are liberated (by budding) only from the free (external) surface of epithelial cells, as is appropriate for infection limited to surface epithelium. A similar restriction in the topography of budding is seen with rabies virus in the infected salivary gland (p. 164). However, vesicular stomatitis virus (p. 301) is released only from the basal surface of the epithelial cell, from whence it can spread to subepithelial tissues and then through the body: topographical restriction in the site of virus release from epithelial cells reflects the polarization of function in these cells and is not seen with fibroblasts.

Many bacterial infections are more or less confined to epithelial surfaces (Table 4). This is a feature, for instance, in diphtheria and streptococcal infections of the throat, gonococcal infections of the conjunctiva or urethra, and most *Salmonella* infections of the intestine. To a large extent this is because host antibacterial forces, to be described at a later stage, do not permit further invasion of tissues. Under most circumstances these bacteria are not able to overcome the host defences, but gonococci and streptococci at least often spread locally through tissues and occasionally systemically through the body. Bacteria such as gonococci and streptococci have some ability to counteract host defences (see Ch. 7), and a certain amount of subepithelial spread is inevitable. Gonococci cause a patchy infection of the columnar epithelium of the male urethra, reaching subepithelial tissues 3–4 days after infection; the yellow discharge consists of desquamated epithelial cells, inflammatory exudate, leucocytes and gonococci. Subepithelial spread probably takes the infection to other parts of the urethra and to local glands.

Most Gram-negative bacteria have only a very limited ability to invade a given host. In man, *E. coli*, *Proteus* spp. and *Pseudomonas aeruginosa* are only capable of invasion when defences are impaired or when bacteria are inadvertently introduced into a suitable site in the body (see Ch. 2). They cause systemic infection in debilitated, malnourished, or immunosuppressed patients; they produce sepsis in the uterus after abortion, and when they are introduced into the body by intravascular devices or catheters. Certain Gram-negative bacteria penetrate the intestinal epithelium but get no further, as in *Shigella* dysentery and salmonellosis (see p. 195). One or two highly specialized Gram-negative bacteria penetrate intestinal epithelium, enter lymphatics and spread systemically through the body to cause enteric or typhoid fever (*Salmonella typhi* and *paratyphi*).

A few bacteria show a temperature restriction similar to that described above for rhinoviruses, which prevents anything more than local spread. For instance, the lesions in leprosy (*Mycobacterium leprae*) are confined to cooler parts of the body (skin, superficial nerves, nasal mucosa, testicles etc.). Other mycobacteria (*Mycobacterium ulcerans* and *marinum*) occur in water and enter human skin through superficial abrasions, especially in warm countries, and cause chronic skin ulcers. These bacteria, which also infect fish, have an optimum growth temperature of 30–33°C and remain restricted to the skin.

Table 5. Examples of infections in which microorganisms enter across epithelial surfaces and subsequently spread through the body

Microbe	Respiratory tract and conjunctiva	Urinogenital tract	Skin	Intestinal tract
Viruses	Measles Rubella Varicella	Herpes simplex 2	Arboviruses	Enteroviruses Certain adeno- viruses
Chlamydias	Psittacosis	Lympho- granuloma venereum	—	—
Mycoplasmas	—	—	—	—
Bacteria	*Mycobacterium tuberculosis Pasteurella pestis*	*Treponema pallidum*	*Bacillus anthracis*	*Salmonella typhi*
Rickettsias	Q fever	—	Typhus	Q fever?
Fungi	Cryptococcosis Histoplasmosis	—	Maduromycosis	Blastomycosis
Protozoa	Toxoplasmosis	—	Malaria Trypanosomiasis	*Entamoeba histolytica*

Fungi of the dermatophyte group (ringworm, athlete's foot*) infect skin, nails and hair, but are restricted to the dead keratinized layers of epithelium. Fungal antigens are absorbed from the site of infection and immune (including allergic) responses are generated, which at least partly account for the failure to invade deeper tissues.

Intracellular Microorganisms and Spread Through the Body

Some of the important microorganisms that regularly establish systemic infections after traversing epithelial surfaces are listed in Table 5.

There is one important distinction between intracellular and extracellular microorganisms. If an obligate intracellular microbe is to spread systemically from the body surface, it must first enter the blood or lymph. This means gaining access to the lumen of a subepithelial lymphatic or blood vessel, either as a free microorganism, or alternatively after entering a mobile cell (leucocyte) that will carry it to other parts of the body. The microorganism cannot replicate until it reaches a susceptible cell, and the absence or shortage of such cells except at the body surface would prevent or seriously hinder its spread through the body. Thus rotaviruses and rhinoviruses

---

* Fungi causing this condition flourish in a moist environment, and athlete's foot is restricted to those who encase their feet in shoes. However, those who do not wear shoes (e.g. tropical Africa) are vulnerable to other fungi that enter skin at sites of injury and cause deeper lesions called mycetomas.

replicate at the epithelial surface but cannot infect leucocytes, and in any case would be unlikely to find susceptible cells elsewhere in the body if they entered blood or lymphatic vessels. Certain viruses (yellow fever, poliovirus) spread through the body to reach susceptible target organs (liver, central nervous system) after free virus particles have entered vessels below the skin or intestinal epithelium. Measles virus, or tubercle bacilli infect leucocytes which carry them through the body to organs such as the liver, spleen, skin and lung.

If, on the other hand, the microbe is able to replicate outside cells and does not have to find a susceptible cell, it can in principle multiply locally, in the blood and lymph, and in whatever part of the body it gets to. Extracellular replication, however, itself conveys a serious disadvantage, because the microorganism is forever naked and exposed to all the antimicrobial forces that the body can summon up. Indeed bacteria and other microorganisms that are capable of extracellular replication generally advertize their presence by releasing a variety of products into surrounding fluids, many of which cause inflammation and thus bring antibacterial agents such as immunoglobulins, complement and leucocytes to the site of the infection. Lymphatics are also dilated, and carry the infecting organisms to lymph nodes for further exposure to antibacterial and immune forces. Intracellular microorganisms in contrast, although exposed to the infected cell's own defence mechanisms, are directly exposed to the general bodily defences only during transit from one infected cell to another. However, if the infected cell is recognized as such by the immune defences, it can be destroyed (see Chs 6 and 9). A number of bacteria and protozoa, such as *Mycobacterium tuberculosis*, *Brucella abortus*, or *Leishmania donovani* carry out much of their multiplication in macrophages that have ingested them. Although they are not obligate intracellular parasites, this shifts the host–microbe battlefield into the cell. The battle is then waged in the infected macrophage, whose antimicrobial powers (Ch 4) and participation in immune defences (see Chs 6 and 9) become of critical importance.

Subepithelial Invasion

After traversing the epithelial cell layer, a microorganism encounters the basement membrane. The basement membrane acts as a filter and can to some extent hold up the infection, but its functional integrity is soon broken by inflammation or epithelial cell damage.

The invading microorganism has now reached the subepithelial tissues (Fig. 9), and here it is exposed to three important host defence systems. These are (i) the tissue fluids, (ii) the lymphatic system leading to the lymph nodes and (iii) phagocytic cells.

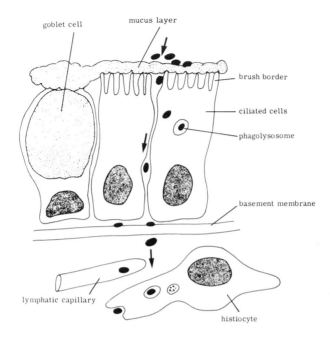

Fig. 9. Microbial invasion across an epithelial surface.

These three host defence mechanisms are of supreme importance and come into play whatever part of the body is infected, whether the nasal mucosa, meninges, urethra, cardiac muscle or liver lobule. Each depends for its action on the inflammatory response, because this response brings the phagocytes and serum factors to the site of infection and promotes drainage from the site by the lymphatic system. Therefore a short account of the inflammatory response will be given, and after this each of the three antimicrobial factors will be considered separately. Table 5 shows some of the important microorganisms that regularly spread through the body in spite of these antimicrobial factors.

The inflammatory response

The capillary blood vessels supplying a tissue bring oxygen and low molecular weight materials to the cells, taking away carbon dioxide and metabolic or secretory products. There is also a constant passage of plasma proteins and leucocytes from capillaries into normal tissues, and these are returned to the blood via the lymphatic system after entering lymphatic capillaries (see below). Indeed, their presence in tissues is inferred from their presence in lymphatics draining these tissues. The cells are nearly all lymphocytes, which leave blood capillaries by actively passing through endothelial cells. After moving about and performing any necessary tasks in the tissues, the lymphocytes penetrate lymphatic capillaries and thus enter the lymph. The lymph, with its content of proteins and cells, then passes through the local lymph nodes and generally at least one more lymph node before entering the thoracic lymph duct and being discharged into the great veins in the thorax or abdomen. Blood lymphocytes also enter lymph nodes directly and in larger numbers through postcapillary venules. The constant movement of lymphocytes from blood to tissues or lymph nodes, and back via lymphatics to the blood again, is called *lymphocyte recirculation*. Circulating lymphocytes are mostly T-cells, and in the course of their continued entries into tissues and lymph nodes they have regular opportunities to encounter any microbial antigens that may be present. There is in fact a regular monitoring of tissues by lymphocytes, and this is referred to as *immune surveillance*.

The various plasma proteins occur in the tissues in much the same proportion as in plasma, the actual concentrations depending on the structure of the capillary bed. As determined by concentrations in local lymphatics, the leaky sinusoids of the liver let through 80–90% of the plasma proteins into liver tissue, the less leaky fenestrated capillaries of the intestine admit 40–60% into intestinal tissues, and capillaries of skeletal muscle with their continuous lining only 10–30% (see Fig. 10). Thus, immunoglobulins, complement components etc. occur regularly in normal tissues, but in lesser concentrations than in blood. There is some discrimination against very large molecules because the largest immunoglobulins (IgM) do not leave the blood vessels and are not detectable in afferent lymph.

There is a prompt and vigorous change in the microcirculation when tissues are damaged or infected. Capillaries and post-capillary vessels are dilated, gaps appear between endothelial cells, and the permeability of these vessels increases, allowing leakage from the blood of a protein-rich fluid. Increased amounts of immunoglobulins, complement components and other proteins are then present in tissues and fibrinogen, for instance, may be converted into fibrin so that a diffuse network of fibrils is laid down. Circulating leucocytes (especially polymorphs and monocytes) adhere to endothelial cells, and this is followed by active passage (diapedesis) of leucocytes between endothelial cells and out into tissues. The affected part now shows the four cardinal signs of inflammation, being RED and WARM (vasodilation), SWOLLEN (vasodilation, cell and fluid exudate) and often PAINFUL (distension of tissues, presence of pain mediators).

Lymphatic capillaries also become dilated, taking up the inflammatory fluids and carrying them to local lymph nodes. There is a greatly increased turnover of plasma components in the inflamed tissue. Initially, the predo-

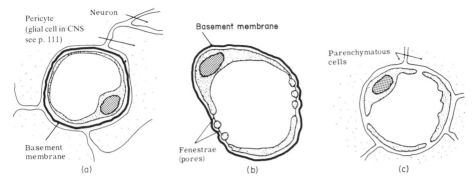

Fig. 10. Diagram to show types of blood–tissue junction in capillary, venule, or sinusoid. (a) Continuous endothelium (transport of tissue nutrients and metabolites): central nervous system, connective tissue, skeletal and cardiac muscle, skin, lung. (b) Fenestrated endothelium (transport of secreted, excreted or digested materials): renal glomerulus, intestinal villi, choroid plexus, pancreas, endocrine glands. (c) Sinusoid (reticuloendothelial system); liver, spleen, bone marrow, adrenal, parathyroid.

minant cell is the polymorph, a reflection of the situation in the blood, but polymorphs only live for a day or two in tissues, and as the acute inflammatory state subsides mononuclear cells become more prominent, especially macrophages, which phagocytose dead polymorphs and tissue debris.

The initial stages of the inflammatory response tend to be much the same, whatever the nature of the tissue insult, and this is partly because the changes are caused by the same mediators of acute inflammation. These include histamine (released from mast cells lying close to blood vessels), kinins (polypeptides derived from precursors in plasma; see Glossary) and complement activation products (C3a and C5a; see pp. 145–7). Some of the kinins are highly active and kallidin, for instance, a decapeptide formed from kallidinogen (an a_2 globulin) is about 15 times more active (on a molar basis) than histamine in causing inflammation. Most bacteria form inflammatory materials during their growth in tissues. Inflammatory responses, like other powerful tissue responses, must be controlled and terminated, and the mediators of inflammation not only have a variety of inhibitors but are also inactivated locally (e.g. kinins inactivated by kininases). At a later stage prostaglandins (a family of 20-carbon fatty acid molecules) and leukotrienes (a group of biologically active lipids) come into play. They are produced from leucocytes, endothelial cells and platelets and they both mediate and control the response.

If inflammation is due to infection with one of the pyogenic bacteria and the infection continues, then the continued supply of inflammatory and chemotactic products from the multiplying bacteria (see below) maintains vasodilation and the flow of polymorphs to the affected area. It is a polymorph exudate.* There is an increase in the number of circulating polymorphs, because of an increase in the rate of release from the bone marrow. The bone marrow holds a vast reserve supply with 20 times as many polymorphs as are present in the blood. If the tissue demand continues, the rate of production in the bone marrow is increased, and circulating polymorphs may remain elevated in persistent bacterial infections such as subacute bacterial endocarditis. Polymorph production in the bone marrow is regulated by certain colony-stimulating factors, and it is a serious matter if something goes wrong and the marrow supplies are exhausted. A fall in circulating polymorphs (neutropenia) during a bacterial infection is of ominous significance.

Viruses produce inflammatory products in tissues in the form of necrotic host cell materials or antigen–antibody complexes, but these are less potent than bacterial products, and the acute inflammatory response is of shorter duration, polymorphs being replaced by mononuclear cells. Mononuclear infiltrates are also favoured in virus infections because the infected tissues themselves are often one of the sites for the immune response, with mononuclear infiltration and cell division.

After extravasation from blood vessels, leucocytes would not automatically move to the exact site of infection. Polymorphs show random movement in tissues, and also a directional movement (chemotaxis) in response to chemical gradients produced by chemotactic substances. Monocytes show little or no random movement, but they too respond to similar chemotactic substances. Chemotactic substances such as leukotrienes, C3a and C5a (see above) are formed during the inflammatory response itself. Also, many bacteria, such as *Staphylococcus aureus* or *Salmonella typhi*, form chemotactic substances and thus automatically betray their presence and attract phagocytic cells. It would obviously be an advantage to an infectious agent if no inflammatory or chemotactic products were formed, but for most large microorganisms (bacteria, fungi, protozoa) these products seem an almost inevitable result of microbial growth and metabolism.

The early stages of the inflammatory response in particular are known to have an important protective effect against microorganisms. In experimental staphylococcal skin infections, for instance, if the early inflammatory response is inhibited by adrenalin, and the early delivery of plasma factors and leucocytes to the site of infection thus reduced, bacteria multiply more rapidly and produce a more severe lesion. Perhaps it is not surprising that *Staphylococcus aureus* can suppress the early inflammatory response, prob-

---

* Human polymorphs can be labelled with the gamma-emitter Indium III and reinfused into a patient. Within 30 s they localize in hidden foci of infection and inflammation, which can then be located with a body scanner.

ably by means of α-haemolysin which causes local vasoconstriction.* Other staphylococcal products inhibit the movement of polymorphs, and lesions are thus enhanced.

If inflammation becomes more severe or widespread it is generally modulated by increased output of corticosteroid hormones (see p. 288), but at the same time it is backed up by a general metabolic response in the body. This is called the *acute phase response*. The liver releases proteins such as haptoglobulins (α_2 glycoproteins), protease-inhibitors, fibrinogen, serum amyloid protein and C-reactive protein (see p. 240). The exact function of these *acute phase proteins* is not clear, but their presence is associated with an increased erythrocyte sedimentation rate (ESR; see p. 240). The patient may develop headache, muscle pains, fever, anaemia, with decreased iron and zinc and increased copper and ceruloplasmin in the serum. Proteins in muscle are broken down, partly to provide energy required during fever and fasting, and partly to provide amino acids needed by proliferating cells and for the synthesis of immunoglobulins and acute phase proteins.

Many of the features of the acute phase response appear to be due to the action of interleukin 1 (see Glossary) released from macrophages. It is a complex response, which on the whole would be expected to serve useful purposes, although some less obviously beneficial "side effects" may be unavoidable.

Tissue fluids

Tissue fluids normally contain variable amounts of plasma proteins, including IgG antibodies discussed above. In the absence of specific antibodies and complement, tissue fluids make a good culture medium for most bacteria, but bacterial multiplication almost inevitably causes some inflammation. As soon as there is inflammation, larger amounts of IgG as well as activated complement components, will be present in tissue fluids. At a later stage secretory products from phagocytes (lysosomal enzymes, oxygen radicals, lactoferrin etc.) will also be present, and finally tissue breakdown products and additional antimicrobial substances liberated from dead platelets, polymorphs and macrophages.

Lymphatics and lymph nodes

A complex network of lymphatics lies below the epithelium at body surfaces. After reaching subepithelial tissues, foreign particles of all kinds, including

---

*By shutting down local blood vessels the α-haemolysin can increase the severity of staphylococcal mastitis in cows and sheep, leading to gangrenous mastitis (black udder).

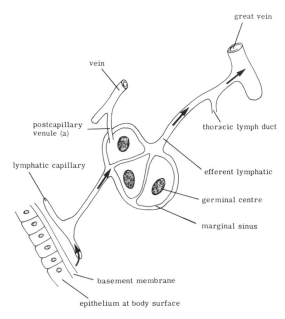

Fig. 11. Diagram of lymphatic system, showing pathways from body surface to venous system. (a) indicates site of lymphocyte circulation from blood to lymph node.

microorganisms, rapidly enter lymphatic capillaries after uptake by or passage between lymphatic endothelial cells. There is a particularly rich superficial plexus of lymphatics in the skin and in the intestinal wall. Microorganisms scratched or injected into the skin inevitably enter lymphatics almost immediately. The intestinal lymphatics not only take up microorganisms that have breached the epithelial surface, but also have an important role in the uptake of fat in the form of chylomicrons.

Microorganisms in peripheral lymphatics are born rapidly (within minutes) to the local lymph nodes strategically placed to deal with the flow of lymph before returning to the blood. The rate of flow of lymph is greatly increased during inflammation, when there is increased exudation of fluid from local blood vessels and the lymphatics are dilated. Microorganisms carried to the node in the lymph are exposed to the macrophages lining the marginal sinus (Fig. 11), and these cells take up particles of all types from the lymph and thus filter it. The efficiency of filtration depends on the nature of the particles, on the physiological state of the macrophages, and also on the particle concentration and flow rate, the efficiency falling off at high particle concentrations or high flow rates (see Ch. 5).

All infecting microorganisms are handled in the same way and delivered via lymphatics to the local lymph node. When there has already been microbial multiplication at the site of initial infection, very large numbers may be delivered to the node. The efficiency of the node as a defence post depends on its ability to contain and destroy microorganisms rather than allow them to replicate further in the node and spread to the rest of the body. The antimicrobial forces are the macrophages of the node, the polymorphs and serum factors accumulating during inflammation, and the immune response which is initiated in the node. Under normal circumstances, as the first trickle of microorganisms reaches the node the most important event is the encounter with macrophages in the marginal sinus. Microorganisms escaping phagocytosis by these cells enter the intermediate sinuses where they run the gauntlet of a further set of macrophages before leaving the node. If there is an inflammatory reaction in the node, a substantial migration of polymorphs into the sinuses greatly increases the phagocytic forces and thus the filtering efficiency. There is usually a further node to be traversed before the lymph is discharged into the venous system.

As well as functioning as filters, the lymph nodes, of course, are sites where the immune response comes into play. The lymphatic system takes invading microorganisms that have penetrated the body surfaces and delivers them directly to phagocytic cells and to the immune system. Soon after infection, as inflammatory products of microbial growth arrive in the node, there is some swelling and inflammation. The microbial antigens, some of which are already associated with antigen-presenting cells encountered at the body surface (see p. 124), generate an immune response, and there is further swelling of the node as cells divide and additional lymphoid cells are recruited into the node from the blood. The ability of viruses and other intracellular microorganisms to bypass the defences of the node and spread to the blood stream is discussed in Ch. 5.

Phagocytic cells

Specialized phagocytic cells are divided into two main types: the macrophages, scattered through all the major compartments of the body (see Ch. 4) and the circulating neutrophil polymorphonuclear granulocytes (polymorphs, or microphages). The phagocytic cells to which microbes are exposed in the subepithelial tissues are the local macrophages (histiocytes) and also the cells arriving from the small blood vessels during inflammation. These comprise the blood monocytes which become macrophages after extravasation, and the polymorphs.

From the time of the Russian zoologist Elie Metchnikoff, who described phagocytosis in 1883, the importance of the phagocyte in defence against disease organisms has been accepted, and children have learnt of the white blood cells that act both as scavengers and policemen, removing debris, foreign particles and microorganisms. Since the 1920s, however, phagocytes had suffered a long period of neglect by research workers, and after the pioneer studies very little had been added to our understanding. In recent years there has been almost a rediscovery of phagocytosis as a central and relevant phenomenon in infectious diseases. This has quickened the interest of investigators and modern biochemical, immunological and ultrastructural techniques are now fruitfully being applied to the subject of phagocytosis. Because of this blossoming of interest and understanding, and because of the central importance of the phagocytic defence mechanisms, the subject will receive a chapter to itself.

References

Dinarello, C. A. (1984). Interleukin-1 in the pathogenesis of the acute phase response. *New Engl. J. Med.* **311**, 1413–1418.

Rodriguez-Boulan, E. and Sabatini, D. D. (1978). Asymmetric budding of viruses in epithelial monolayers. Model systems for epithelial polarity. *Proc. Natn. Acad. Sci. U.S.A.* **75**, 5071–5075.

Ryan, G. B. and Majno, G. (1977). Acute inflammation. *Am. J. Pathol.* **86**, 183–276.

Taussig, M. J. (1984). "Processes in Pathology and Microbiology", 2nd Edn, Blackwell Scientific Publications.

Yoffey, J. M. and Courtice, F. C. (1970). "Lymphatics, Lymph and the Lymphomyeloid Complex". Academic Press, London and New York.

4

The Encounter of the Microbe with the Phagocytic Cell

The phagocyte is the most powerful and most important part of the host defences that can operate without delay against the invading microorganism after the epithelial surface has been breached. There are two types of specialized phagocytic cells, the macrophage and the polymorphonuclear leucocyte. In the subepithelial tissues there are local resident macrophages (histiocytes), and as soon as an inflammatory response is induced, polymorphonuclear leucocytes arrive in large numbers after passing through the walls of small blood vessels. The inflammatory cells include also monocytes and lymphocytes.

Polymorphonuclear leucocytes arise in the bone marrow and are continuously discharged in vast numbers into the blood. The 3×10^{10} polymorphs that are present in normal human blood carry out their functions after leaving the circulation and entering sites of inflammation in tissues. These cells live for a few days only and each day about 10^{11} disappear from the blood, even in the absence of significant inflammation. Indeed, at any given time about half of them are adherent to or moving slowly along the walls of capillaries and postcapillary venules. This daily loss is balanced by entry into the blood from the bone marrow, and to make some provision for sudden demands the bone marrow contains an enormous reserve of about 3×10^{12} polymorphs.

Monocytes are circulating precursors of macrophages. They arise from stem cells in the bone marrow, and as soon as they leave the circulation and begin to carry out their phagocytic duties in tissues they become macrophages. Macrophages are widely distributed throughout the body, but they are not as numerous as polymorphs, and there are no great reserves of macrophages in tissues. Fixed macrophages line the blood sinusoids of the liver (Kupffer cells), spleen, bone marrow, adrenals, and monitor the blood for effete cells, microorganisms or other foreign particles. Macrophages lining lymph sinuses in lymph nodes monitor the lymph, and the alveolar macrophages in the lung monitor the alveolar contents. The peritoneal and pleural cavities also contain large numbers of macrophages. Macrophages, in fact, are strategically placed throughout the body to encounter invading microorganisms. Alveolar macrophages deal with those entering the lung when they are deposited in the alveolus, beyond the mucociliary defences. Those in subepithelial sites in the skin, intestine etc. meet invading micro-organisms once epithelial surfaces are breached, and those lining lymphatics and blood sinusoids come into play if there is spread of the infection via lymph or blood. Macrophages in the peritoneal and pleural cavities form a first line of defence in these vulnerable cavities.

Lymphocytes have an immunological function to be described more fully later. When they encounter microbial antigens to which they are by nature or by previous experience sensitized, they undergo profound changes. B (bursa-derived) cells are stimulated to differentiate into antibody-producing (plasma) cells and T (thymus-derived) cells differentiate into lymphoblasts, divide, and release lymphokines in the course of carrying out the cell-mediated immune response. Lymphokines induce further inflammatory or immunological changes and have profound effects on the function of macrophages, activating them, promoting their accumulation in the tissue and indeed "focusing" them onto the site of infection (see Ch. 6).

Phagocytosis is a basic type of cell function, and is not restricted to macrophages and polymorphs. For instance, epidermal cells in the skin take up injected carbon particles, and intestinal epithelial cells and vascular endothelial cells also ingest certain marker particles, but this is on a very restricted scale compared with the professional phagocytes. Mere phagocytosis is not enough. If the ingestion of a microorganism is to be of service to the infected host, it must be followed by killing and preferably intracellular digestion of the microorganism. The specialized phagocytic cells are therefore equipped with a powerful array of antimicrobial weapons and lysosomal enzymes.

Phagocytosis in Polymorphonuclear Leucocytes

Polymorphs generally carry out their functions after leaving the blood-stream, but they can under certain circumstances adhere to the endothelium of small blood vessels, especially in the lungs, and act as "fixed" phagocytes. This happens, for instance, when Gram-negative bacteria or endotoxin enter the blood stream, and probably depends on the action of complement.

There are three types of polymorphonuclear leucocytes: the neutrophils, the basophils and the eosinophils, each serving separate functions and distinguished by the staining reactions of their prominent cytoplasmic granules. The granules are lysosomes, consisting of membrane-lined sacs containing enzymes and other materials.

The neutrophils are the most numerous, comprising 70% of the total leucocytes in blood, and are the cells generally referred to as "polymorphs". They contain two or three types of granules, whose enzymes include peroxidase, alkaline phosphatase, acid phosphatase, ribonuclease, deoxyribonuclease, nucleotidases, glucuronidase, lysozyme and cathepsins.

The eosinophils (1% of the leucocytes) are less effective than polymorphs in the phagocytosis and killing of microbes but they are especially active in the phagocytosis of immune complexes. For every circulating eosinophil there are 300–500 in the extravascular tissues, and they are especially numerous in the submucosal tissues of the intestinal and respiratory tracts. Their granules probably contain, in addition to various enzymes, blockers of the inflammatory mediators (histamine, kinins and serotonin) and a major basic protein generated by immune complexes (see Ch. 6). A rise in the number of circulating eosinophils is a feature of certain parasitic and allergic diseases, and they are attracted into tissues by eosinophil chemotactic factor released from mast cells. They bear C3b and Fc receptors and attach to and kill certain parasites (e.g. schistosomula) that are coated with specific antibody, probably by discharge of the major basic protein.*

Basophils comprise 0.5% of the total blood leucocytes, and their granules are especially rich in histamine and heparin. They closely resemble the mast cells seen in submucosal tissues and round blood vessels, and bear Fc receptors for IgE antibody. When antigen binds to IgE antibody on their surface the granules are discharged, and this leads to various "allergic" inflammatory changes.

After extravasation from blood vessels, polymorphs would not automatically congregate at the exact site of microbial infection without any guidance. When seen in time-lapse cinephase movies, they display very active cell movement, travelling at up to $40 \ \mu\text{m} \ \text{min}^{-1}$. One type of movement is random, in all planes, and to some extent this would bring the cells to the scene of infection. They also show chemotaxis, which is a directional cell movement in response to chemical gradients formed by the release of certain chemotactic materials in tissues. Many soluble bacterial products attract polymorphs in this way, as do the mediators generated by C3 and C5

---

*The polymorph also is a small cell and large numbers may attach to the surface of the schistosomula, which is too big to be phagocytosed. Killing takes place if enough damage is inflicted in this combined assault. When polymorphs kill opsonized *Trichinella spiralis*, dozens of them may be seen attached to the surface of the parasite.

components after antigen–antibody interactions (see Ch. 6), and various substances derived from host tissue.

Before phagocytosis can take place there must be a preliminary attachment of the object to the phagocytic cell surface. Divalent cations such as Ca^{2+} or Mg^{2+} are required for phagocytosis, and this indicates that electrostatic forces are important in the initial attachment; these cations are universally present in tissues. The firm attachment and certainly the ingestion of particles is facilitated by serum substances called opsonins. Opsonins include acquired or naturally occurring antibodies, and complement. Opsonin comes from a Greek word meaning sauce or seasoning; it makes the microbe more palatable and more easily ingested by the phagocyte. The action of opsonins and the triggering of phagocytosis depends on the Fc portion of the immunoglobulin combining with specific Fc receptors on the surface of the phagocytic cell. In man, all IgG immunoglobulins except the IgG_2 subclass attach to (are cytotrophic for) polymorphs. Phagocytic cells thus have a special affinity for microorganisms coated with antibody.* If complement (C3b fragment) is present on the microbe (following antibody-mediated or alternative pathway activation of complement) it can react with C3b receptors for this on the cell and thus provide further assistance for attachment and ingestion. Ordinary tissue cells differ from professional phagocytes and do not have these specific receptors; they consequently fail to adsorb and ingest opsonized microorganisms. Although phagocytosis is strikingly enhanced by opsonins, and sometimes depends entirely on opsonins, there are a variety of objects including starch grains, yeasts, bacteria and polystyrene particles, that adsorb to the polymorph surface and are phagocytosed without apparent need for serum factors. Some of this may be explained by phagocytes attaching to particles that are more hydrophobic or more negatively charged than themselves. Also, phagocytes can attach to bacteria when sugars present on either of them bind to certain proteins also present on either phagocyte or microbe. These sugar-binding cross-linking proteins are referred to as lectins (e.g. the protein on *E. coli* that attaches to D-mannose on host cells; p. 20).

Phagocytosis is a familiar event in physical terms (Fig. 12). The infolding of the plasma membrane to which particles are attached is due to the contraction of actin and myosin filaments ("muscles") anchored to a skeleton of microtubules in the cytoplasm. The process is triggered off by the attachment of particles to the receptors on the plasma membrane. Phagocytosis is associated with energy consumption involving oxidation of

---

*During chemotactic movement of polymorphs the Fc receptor that will mediate attachment and ingestion of opsonized materials (see below) are appropriately localized at the leading edge of the cell.

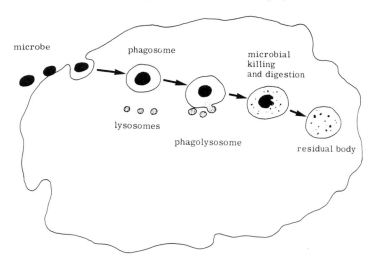

Fig. 12. Diagram to show phagocytosis and intracellular digestion.

glucose via the hexosemonophosphate pathway. There is a 10–20-fold increase in respiratory rate of the cell. There is also an increased turnover of membrane phospholipids. This is hardly surprising, because the multiple infoldings of the cell surface during active phagocytosis, in which up to 35% of the plasma membrane may be internalized, obviously requires synthesis of extra quantities of cell membrane.

As a result of phagocytosis, microorganisms are enclosed in membrane-lined vacuoles in the cytoplasm of the phagocytic cell, and subsequent events depend on the activity of the lysosomal granules (Fig. 12). These move towards the phagocytic vacuole (phagosome), fuse with its wall to form a phagolysosome, and discharge their contents into the vacuole, thus initiating the intracellular killing and digestion of the microorganism. The loss of lysosomal granules is referred to as degranulation. The process of ingestion, killing and digestion of a nonpathogenic bacterium by polymorphs can be followed biochemically by radioactive labelling of various bacterial components, and structurally by electron microscopy. When *E. coli* are added to rabbit polymorphs *in vitro*, phagocytosis begins within a few minutes. Nearly all polymorphs participate, each one ingesting 10–20 bacteria. Polymorph granules then move towards the phagocytic vacuoles and fuse with them, delivering their contents into the vacuoles. The pH of the vacuoles become acid (pH 3.5–4.0), and this alone has some antimicrobial effect. Bacteria are killed (in the sense that they can no longer multiply when freed from the phagocytic cell) a minute or two later, before there is detectable biochemical breakdown of bacteria. Digestion then proceeds, first the bacterial cell wall

OXYGEN-DEPENDENT

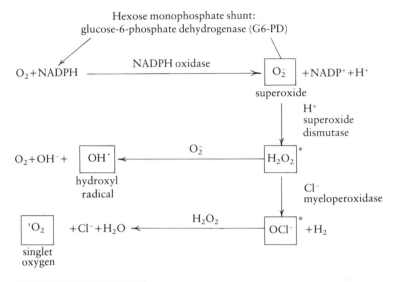

OXYGEN INDEPENDENT

* Acid pH
* Lysozyme—dissolves the cell wall of certain Gram positive bacteria.
  Cationic proteins*—bactericidal activity?
  Lactoferrin
  Vitamin B-12-binding protein } bacteriostatic activity?
  Acid hydrolases—post-mortem digestion of microorganisms?

Fig. 13. Antimicrobial mechanisms in the neutrophil polymorph (* = probably important in killing).

components (detectable by the release from bacteria of radioactively labelled amino acids) and subsequently the contents of the bacterial cell. By electron microscopy the bacterial cell wall appears "fuzzy" rather later, after about 15 minutes. The early killing is presumably associated with impaired functional integrity of the bacterial cell wall, the gross digestion of the corpse being detectable biochemically at a later stage, and changes in ultrastructural appearances later still.

The biochemical basis for the killing of bacteria and other microorganisms is complex and is still poorly understood. The present state of knowledge is outlined in Fig. 13. The brief burst of respiratory activity that accompanies phagocytosis is needed for killing rather than for phagocytosis itself, and membrane-associated NADPH oxidase is activated after phagocytosis has occurred. The following events taking place within the vacuole are important. The oxygen produced gives rise to superoxide by the addition of one electron, and two superoxide molecules may interact (dismutate) and form hydrogen peroxide, either spontaneously or with the help of superoxide dismutase. The hydrogen peroxide in turn can be reduced to give the hydroxyl radical (OH·). It can also undergo myeloperoxidase-mediated halogenation to generate hypophalite (OCl^-) which not only disrupts bacterial cell walls by halogenation, but also reacts with H_2O_2 to form singlet oxygen, which is possibly antimicrobial. Thus, free hydroxyl (OH·) and superoxide (O_2^-) radicals, H_2O_2, OCl^- and singlet oxygen ($'O_2$) are all produced in polymorphs in the wall of the phagosome, mostly by means of an electron transport chain, and involving cytochrome b. But it is not clear whether some or all of these products are responsible for killing or whether it also depends on other activities of the electron transport chain.

But oxygen-dependent killing is not the whole story. Polymorphs often need to operate at low oxygen tension, for instance where relatively anaerobic bacteria are multiplying, and such microorganisms are killed quite effectively in the absence of oxygen. There are a number of possible mechanisms. First, within minutes of phagocytosis the pH within the vacuole falls to about 3.5 and this would itself have an antimicrobial effect. Also the granules delivered to the phagocytic vacuole contain certain antimicrobial substances. There are "specific" granules and "azurophil" granules, as well as the regular lysosomes. These contain not only myeloperoxidase, mentioned above, but also lactoferrin, lysozyme, a vitamin B12-binding protein, a variety of cationic proteins and acid hydrolysases. Lactoferrin, which binds iron very effectively, even at a low pH (see p. 293) would not kill but would deprive the phagocytosed microorganism of iron. The cationic proteins bind to bacteria and under alkaline conditions have a pronounced but unelucidated antibacterial action; they would need to act early, before the pH becomes acid. The acid hydrolases probably function by digesting the organisms after killing. The enzyme lysozyme hydrolyses the cross links of the giant peptidoglycan molecules that form most of the cell wall of Gram-positive cocci (Fig. 14). The cell wall is rapidly dissolved and the bacteria killed. Gram-negative bacteria have an additional lipopolysaccharide component incorporated into the outer surface of the cell wall, and this gives these bacteria relative resistance to the action of lysozyme.*

Although some of the above components kill bacteria when added to them *in vitro*, their significance in the phagocyte is not known. we are still profoundly ignorant of the ways in which polymorphs attempt to kill and then to digest the great variety of microorganisms that are ingested.

---

*Granule proteins generally have to bind to the bacterial surface if killing is to occur, and a longer polysaccharide chain makes binding less effective.

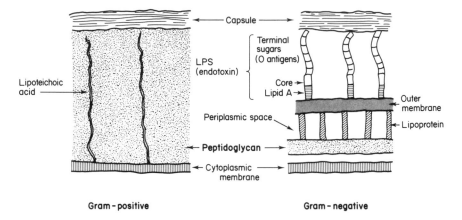

Fig. 14. Comparison of Gram-positive and Gram-negative bacterial cell wall. Pili and flagella (the latter bearing H antigens in Gram-negative bacilli) are not shown. Peptidoglycan (= mucopeptide) has lipoteichioic acid molecules extending through it, ± teichoic acid linked to peptidoglycan. The capsule may be protein or polysaccharide and is the site of the K antigen of Gram-negative bacilli.

Fusion of lysosomal granules with phagosomes is the morphological basis for intracellular digestion in phagocytes, and is closely comparable with the process by which a free-living protozoan such as *Amoeba* digests its prey. In both cases, the phagocytic vacuole becomes the cellular stomach. Under certain circumstances, polymorph granules fuse with the cell surface rather than with the phagocytic vacuole, and the contents of the granule are then discharged to the exterior, producing local concentrations of lysosomal enzymes in tissues and often giving rise to severe histological lesions. Antigen–antibody complexes induce this type of response in polymorphs, and the resultant tissue damage is exemplified in the blood vessel wall lesions in a classical Arthus response. On other occasions lysosomes fuse with the phagocytic vacuole before phagocytosis is completed and the vacuole internalized. Lysosomal enzymes then pass to the exterior of the cell to give what is referred to as "regurgitation after feeding". This occurs after exposure to certain inert particles or to antigen–antibody complexes. Since polymorphs live for no more than a day or two, their death and autolysis inevitably leads to the liberation of lysosomal enzymes into tissues. When this occurs on a small scale, macrophages ingest the cells and little damage is done, but on a larger scale the accumulation of necrotic polymorphs and other host cells, together with dead and living bacteria, and autolytic and inflammatory products, forms a localized fluid product called pus. This product, resulting from the age-old battle between microorganism and phagocyte, can be thin and watery (streptococci), thick (staphylococci), cheesy (*Mycobacterium tuberculosis*), green (*Pseudomonas aeruginosa* pigments), or foul-smelling (anaerobic bacteria). Before the advent of modern antimicrobial agents, a staphylococcal abscess could contain more than half a litre of pus.

Phagocytosis in Macrophages

The processes of adsorption, ingestion and digestion of microorganisms in macrophages are in general similar to those in polymorphs, but there are important differences.

Macrophages exhibit great changes in surface shape and outline, but do not have the polymorph's striking ability to move through tissues. They show chemotaxis, but the chemotactic mediators are different from those attracting polymorphs. This contributes to the observed local differences in macrophage and polymorph distribution in tissues. Macrophages also have a different content of lysosomal enzymes, which varies with the species of origin, the site of origin in the body and the state of activation (see Ch. 6). They do not contain the cationic proteins found in polymorph granules, nor the same oxygen-dependent antimicrobial system. This gives rise to differences in their ability to handle ingested microorganisms. Thus, although the fungus *Cryptococcus neoformans* is phagocytosed by human polymorphs and then killed by chymotrypsin-like cationic proteins and the oxygen-dependent system, the same fungus survives and grows readily after phagocytosis by human macrophages. The antimicrobial armoury of human polymorphs also gives them a major role in the killing of the fungus *Candida albicans*, whereas macrophages are much less effective. Indeed, for many bacteria polymorphs show a bactericidal activity that is superior to that of monocytes and macrophages. This is because opsonized phagocytosis is often more rapid in polymorphs, and there is a greater generation of the antibacterial species of oxygen mentioned on pp. 68–9. On the other hand, macrophages live for long periods (months, in man) compared with polymorphs (days, in man). Polymorphs are very much "end cells", delivered to tissues with a brief life span and limited adaptability, whereas macrophages are capable of profound changes in behaviour and biochemical make up in response to stimuli (see Ch. 6). When polymorphs have discharged their lysosomal granules into phagosomes the cells rather than the granules, are renewed. Macrophages, on the other hand, retain considerable synthetic ability, so that they can be stimulated to form large amounts of lysosomal and other enzymes. Also, because of their longer life in tissues, it is common to see macrophages loaded with phagocytic vacuoles whose contents are in all stages of digestion and degradation. Certain materials, particularly the cell walls of some bacteria, are only degraded very slowly or incompletely by macrophages.

Macrophages bear on their plasma membrane trypsin-resistant receptors for the Fc portion of IgG and IgM immunoglobulins, and trypsin-digestible receptors for complement, so that immune complexes or particles coated with immunoglobulins and complement are readily adsorbed. Macrophages also have the ability to recognize and adsorb to their surface various altered and denatured particles, such as effete or aldehyde-treated erythrocytes. This could be important in the phagocytosis of microorganisms, and opsonins are not always necessary. But opsonins make a big difference. When microbes that have reacted with antibody or complement are bound to Fc or C3b receptors this triggers off a distinct set of lysosomal antimicrobial events following uptake. Mere adsorption of microorganisms to the cell surface does not necessarily lead to phagocytosis. Certain mycoplasma, for instance, attach to macrophages and grow to form a "lawn" covering most of the cell surface, but are not phagocytosed unless antibody is present.

Macrophages are also secretory cells, and liberate about 60 different products ranging from lysosyme to collagenase. These may be important in antimicrobial defence as well as in immunopathology (see Ch. 6).

Microbial Strategy in Relation to Phagocytes

As has been discussed earlier, microorganisms invading host tissues are first and foremost exposed to phagocytes, and the encounter between microbe and phagocyte has played a vital role in the evolution of multicellular animals, all of which, from the time of their origin in the distant past, have been exposed to invasive microorganisms. The central importance of this ancient and perpetual warfare between the microbe and the phagocytic cell was clearly recognized by Metchnikoff a hundred years ago.

Microorganisms that readily attract phagocytes, and are then ingested and killed by them, are by definition unsuccessful. They fail to cause a successful infection. Phagocytes, when functioning in this way, have an overwhelming advantage over such microorganisms. Most successful microorganisms, in contrast, have to some extent at least succeeded in interfering with the antimicrobial activities of phagocytes, or in some other way avoiding their attention. The contest between the two has been proceeding for so many hundreds of millions of years that it can be assumed that if there is a possible way to interfere with or otherwise prevent the activities of phagocytes, then some microorganisms will almost certainly have discovered how to do this.

Therefore the types of interaction between microorganisms and phagocytes will be considered from this point of view.

The larger microorganisms, including bacteria, fungi and protozoa, display metabolic activity in the extracellular environment and produce many soluble substances. Some of these substances are irrelevant products of metabolism and growth with no effect on the host except in so far as they may induce an immune response. Others have been found to have a "toxic" activity, usually demonstrable in some artificial test sytem. In three classical instances (diphtheria, tetanus and botulism) bacterial toxins were shown in the nineteenth century to be not only important, but actually responsible for the disease (see Ch. 8). Since then, a great variety of soluble products have been described, some of them toxic, and some not toxic. Unfortunately very few have been shown to have a well-defined role in pathogenesis. Although biochemical and pathophysiological studies are now characterizing such toxins and defining their activity, we still have little understanding of their significance in the infected host. A toxin may have what appears to be a useful antiphagocytic action but that does not mean that it is produced in large enough quantities in infected tissues, or that the antiphagocytic activity is important in pathogenicity. Thus, while on the one hand the biochemical basis of bacterial pathogenicity in the disease cholera has now been unravelled, the role of endotoxin in Gram-negative bacterial infections remains to a large extent an enigma (see Ch. 8).*

In spite of these uncertainties, the microbial factors that would appear on the face of it to favour pathogenicity will most of the time be referred to as if they in fact do so. It will be many years before these matters are clarified so that we know exactly which toxins matter and which do not matter. Many of them will be mentioned merely to illustrate the important principle that the disease depends on the interplay between the invasive pathogenic powers of the microbe and the defence reactions of the host. Microbial factors that damage the host or actively promote the spread of infection are often called *agressins*. Such factors have a "toxic" activity that is demonstrable in a suitable test system. In many instances, however, microbial factors inhibit the operation of host defence mechanisms without actually doing any damage. There is no "toxic" activity, and Professor Alan Glynn has called such factors *impedins*.

Microbes that are noninfectious for man are dealt with and destroyed by the phagocytic defence system just as in the case of the nonpathogenic bacteria in polymorphs as described above. Nearly all microorganisms,

---

* Genetic engineering will unravel some of these problems. For instance, the genes controlling the K1 capsular polysaccharides of *E. coli* which confer resistance to phagocytosis (see p. 81) have now been cloned. The role of K1 in virulence and invasiveness can be determined by transferring the genes to other strains of *E. coli*.

indeed, are noninfectious, and it is only a very small number that can infect the vertebrate host, and an even smaller number that are significant causes of infection in man. The ways in which microorganisms meet the challenge of the phagocyte will be classified, for simplicity (Fig. 15, Table 6).

Killing the phagocyte

The most straightforward antiphagocytic approach is to kill the phagocyte, and many successful infectious bacteria do this. Some, as they multiply in tissues, release soluble materials that are lethal for phagocytes. Part of the success of pathogenic streptococci and staphylococci is attributable to their ability to kill the phagocytes that pour into foci of infection. Pathogenic streptococci release haemolysins (streptolysins) which lyse red blood cells and are much more active weight for weight than haemolysins such as bile salts or saponin, but which also have a more important toxic action on polymorphs and macrophages. The mechanism of toxicity is of some interest. Streptolysin O probably binds to cholesterol in cell membranes, and within 1–2 min of its addition to polymorphs, the polymorph granules explode and their contents are discharged into the cell cytoplasm. The lysosomal enzymes, when confined to a phagocytic vacuole, help the cell by performing valuable digestive functions, but when enough are released into the cell cytoplasm in this way, they act on cell components and within a minute or two the cytoplasm liquefies and the cell dies. The streptolysin, by damaging the lysosomes, makes them function as "suicide bags". Streptolysin S has an even more potent action on membranes. Various haemolysins are released also by pathogenic staphylococci, and these too can kill phagocytes. They are of uncertain significance in staphylococcal infections. In addition, there is a nonhaemolytic leucocidin whose production is related to staphylococcal virulence. It consists of two antigenically distinct proteins, acting synergistically on the leucocyte membrane and causing discharge of lysosomal granules just as with streptolysin O. *Listeria monocytogenes* releases rather similar cytolytic toxins. In general, polymorphs are more readily killed by toxins than are macrophages, possibly because their lysosomes are more easily discharged. Invaders with good lysosomal weaponry of their own, such as virulent strains of the protozoan parasite *Entamoeba histolytica*, can kill polymorphs by mere contact. Others exert their toxic action on the phagocyte after phagocytosis has taken place, releasing cytotoxic substances which pass directly through the vacuole wall and into the cell. The phagocyte can be said to have died of food poisoning. For instance, virulent shigellas kill mouse macrophages after phagocytosis whereas avirulent shigella fail to do so and are themselves killed and

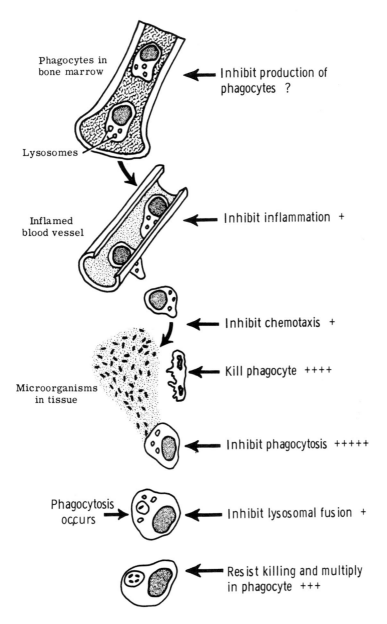

Fig. 15. Antiphagocytic strategies available to microorganisms. Extent to which strategies are actually used by microorganisms are indicated by plusses.

Table 6. Showing types of interference with phagocytic activities

Microorganism[a]	Type of interference[b]	Mechanism (or responsible factor)
Streptococcus pyogenes	Kill phagocyte	Streptolysin induces lysosomal discharge into cell cytoplasm
	Inhibit polymorph chemotaxis	Streptolysin
	Resist phagocytosis	M substance on fimbriae;
	Resist digestion	hyaluronic acid capsule
Staphylococci	Kill phagocyte	Leucocidin induces lysosomal discharge into cell cytoplasm
	Inhibit opsonized phago- cytosis	Protein A blocks Fc portion of Ab; polysaccharide capsule in some strains
	Resist killing	Cell wall mucopeptide; production of catalase?
Bacillus anthracis	Kill phagocyte	Toxic complex
	Resist killing	Capsular polyglutamic acid
Haemophilus influenzae *Strepococcus pneumoniae* *Klebsiella pneumoniae*	Resist phagocytosis (unless Ab present) Resist digestion	Polysaccharide capsule
Pseudomonas aeruginosa	Kill phagocyte	Exotoxin A kills macrophages; also cell-bound leucocidin, mol. wt. 27,500
	Resist phagocytosis (unless Ab present) Resist digestion	"Surface slime" (polysaccharide)
Escherichia coli	Resist phagocytosis (unless Ab present)	O antigen (smooth strains) K antigen (acid polysaccharide)
	Resist killing	K antigen
Salmonella typhi	Resist phagocytosis (unless Ab present) Resist killing	Vi antigen
Clostridium perfringens	Inhibit chemotoxis	θ toxin
	Resist phagocytosis	Capsule
Cryptococcus neoformans	Resist phagocytosis	Polysaccharide capsule (polymer containing uronic acid)
Treponema pallidum	Resist phagocytosis	Polysaccharide capsular material

Table 6. (*Cont.*)

Microorganism[a]	Type of interference[b]	Mechanism (or responsible factor)
Yersinia pestis	Resist killing	Protein–carbohydrate cell wall
Mycobacteria	Resist killing and digestion	Cell wall component
	Inhibit lysosomal fusion	Unknown
Brucella abortus	Resist killing	Cell wall substance
Toxoplasma gondii	Inhibit attachment to polymorph	Unknown
	Inhibit lysosomal fusion	Unknown
Plasmodium berghei	Resist phagocytosis	Capsular material

[a] Often it is only the virulent strains that show the type of interference listed.
[b] Sometimes the type of interference listed has been described only in a particular type of phagocyte (polymorph or macrophage) from a particular host, but it generally bears a relationship to pathogenicity in that host.

digested. Certain chlamydia multiply in macrophages after phagocytosis and destroy the cell by inducing the discharge of lysosomal contents into the cytoplasm. Virulent intracellular bacteria of the *Mycobacterium*, *Brucella* and *Listeria* groups owe much of their virulence to their ability to multiply in macrophages. The macrophage is often destroyed in the end, but the mechanism is not known.

Inhibition of chemotaxis or the mobilization of phagocytic cells

Various substances released from bacteria attract phagocytes, but their activity is generally weak. Other bacterial substances react with complement to generate chemotactic factors such as C5a. Microorganisms can avoid the attentions of phagocytic cells by inhibiting chemotaxis, and as a result of this the host is less able to focus polymorphs and macrophages into the exact site of infection. Substances produced by *Staphylococcus aureus*, for instance, inhibit the locomotion of polymorphs and macrophages. The streptococcal streptolysins which kill phagocytes can suppress polymorph chemotaxis in even lower concentrations, apparently without adverse effects on the polymorph. Random mobility is not affected. *Clostridium perfringens* β toxin has a similar action on polymorphs. There are good methods available for the quantification of chemotaxis, and it is possible that other pathogenic bacteria will be shown to produce inhibitors.

Both polymorphs and macrophages arise from stem cells in the bone marrow, and their rate of formation is greatly increased during infection, so that blood leuocyte counts reach 2–4 times normal levels. This is associated with increased blood levels of certain factors that stimulate colony formation by leucocyte precursors. Four of these *colony stimulating factors*, which are glycoproteins active at very low concentrations (10^{-11}–10^{-13} molar), have been identified. They are produced in many tissues, and their concerted action is needed for the production and final differentiation of polymorphs (also eosinophils) and macrophages. They also help control the activity of differentiated cells. Little is known of the factors regulating their production, or of the influence of microbial products. Clearly if it were possible for microorganisms to release substances that inhibited the formation or action of colony stimulating factors, and thus seriously impair the phagocytic response to infection, some of them might be expected to do so. There is a decrease rather than an increase in blood polymorphs during certain infections such as typhoid and brucellosis, but there is so far no evidence that this is due to effects on colony stimulating factors. *Listeria monocytogenes* is so-called because it causes an *increase* in circulating monocytes by means of a cell-wall component of molecular weight 22 000, but the significance of this is not known.

Inhibition of adsorption of microorganism to surface of phagocytic cell

Many microorganisms tend to avoid phagocytosis without being obviously toxic for phagocytes. As a rule, it is not possible to distinguish between a failure to adsorb and a failure to ingest the microorganism. Since our understanding of adsorption is so slight (see above), our understanding of failure to adsorb is equally inadequate. Yet the distinction can sometimes be made, as when pilated (virulent) gonococci attach to polymorphs but are not ingested or killed. *Mycoplasma hominis* remains extracellular when added to human polymorphs *in vitro*, and it appears that there is no firm adsorption of the mycoplasmas to the polymorph surface, although in the presence of antibody to the mycoplasmas there is adsorption, ingestion and digestion. The reason for the failure in adsorption is not clear, but it may be because the mycoplasmas damage the polymorph, which shows increased oxidation of glucose and defective killing of phagocytosed *E. coli*. If polymorphs are added to the protozoan parasite *Toxoplasma gondii* (see Glossary) *in vitro*, the mobile polymorphs are seen to turn aside from the toxoplasmas, indicating perhaps a failure of attachment. Antibody-coated or dead toxoplasmas, on the other hand, are successfully phagocytosed and digested by polymorphs. Macrophages, it may be noted, ingest the live parasite and support its growth (see below).

It must be remembered that intracellular microorganisms, far from avoiding adsorption, *must* be adsorbed to the susceptible cell if they are to enter it and multiply. In the case of bacteria and fungi the susceptible cell tends to be a phagocyte, perhaps because that is the type of cell that invading microorganisms have always had the opportunity to infect after being phagocytosed. Intracellular bacteria such as *Mycobacterium tuberculosis*, *Brucella abortus* and *Listeria monocytogenes* grow in the macrophages that phagocytose them, and their success as infectious agents depends on this. It is not known whether there are special receptors on the macrophage for such intracellular bacteria. Many viruses will not adsorb to, and therefore cannot infect, a cell unless a specific receptor is present on the cell surface (see Ch. 2). When the virus cannot grow in the phagocyte it would be an advantage to avoid being taken up and destroyed, but so far it has not been possible to associate avoidance of phagocytosis with virus pathogenicity. When, however, a virus infects and grows in the phagocytic cell this may be an important part of the infectious process (see Ch. 5), especially if the phagocyte is so little affected that it carries the infecting virus from one part of the body to another.

Inhibition of phagocytosis — opsonins

Microbial products that kill phagocytes (see above) may at lower concentrations interfere with their locomotion or their phagocytic activity, for instance by inhibiting protein synthesis. A more direct challenge to the phagocyte is provided by the various microorganisms whose surface properties prevent their phagocytosis. As mentioned above, it is not usually possible to distinguish between inhibition of adsorption to the phagocytic cell and inhibition of phagocytosis which follows adsorption.

Many important pathogenic bacteria bear on their surface substances that inhibit phagocytosis (see Table 6). Clearly it is the bacterial surface that matters. The phagocyte physically encounters the surface of the microorganism, just as the person knocked down by a car encounters the hard metal exterior of the vehicle, and the phagocyte has no more immediate interest in the internal features or antigens of the microorganism than the person knocked down has of the upholstery or luggage inside the car. Resistance to phagocytosis is sometimes due to a component of the bacterial cell wall, and sometimes it is due to a capsule enclosing the bacterial wall, secreted by the bacterium. Classical examples of antiphagocytic substances on the bacterial surface include the M proteins of streptococci and the polysaccharide capsules of pneumococci. These bacteria owe their success to their ability to survive and grow extracellularly, avoiding uptake by phagocytic cells. Certain M proteins on the surface and the pili of streptococci are undoubtedly associated with resistance to phagocytosis and with virulence, but it is not clear how these act (see also p. 170). Streptococci appear to slither off the surface of polymorphs that are attempting to engulf them, suggesting the absence of specific adsorption factors. When the M protein is covered with antibody (opsonized), the Fc portion of the antibody molecule attaches to receptors on the polymorph surface and phagocytosis takes place (see later). It must be remembered that although attachment to the phagocyte is to be avoided, it is advantageous to attach to cells at the body surface (see pp. 21-2). The pili, accordingly, contain not only M protein but also lipoteichoic acid which mediates attachments to epithelial cells.

The polysaccharide capsule of the pneumococcus is likewise associated with resistance to phagocytosis and with virulence. It takes less than 10 encapsulated virulent bacteria to kill a mouse after injection into the peritoneal cavity, but 10 000 bacteria are needed if the capsule is removed by hyaluronidase. As with pathogenic streptococci, phagocytosis takes place more readily via Fc and C3b receptors, when the bacterial surface has been coated with specific antibody and C3b deposited. Unencapsulated strains of bacteria are coated with C3b without the need for antibody, after activation of the alternative pathway (see p. 147), but this is inhibited by sialic acid components of the capsule. If a mouse is rendered incapable of forming antibodies to the capsule, infection with a single bacterium is then enough to cause death. It is not clear why the capsule confers resistance to phagocytosis; perhaps its slimy polysaccharide nature makes the phagocytic act difficult for purely mechanical reasons. Although antibody is needed for phagocytosis in a fluid medium, it is known that phagocytosis takes place without antibody on the solid surface lining of an alveolus or lymphatic vessel (or on a piece of filter paper!), where the physical act of phagocytosis is favoured, and the phagocyte can "corner" and get round the bacterium. Pathogenic bacteria with similar polysaccharide capsules include *Haemophilus influenzae* and *Klebsiella pneumoniae*. Patients with agammaglobulinaemia have repeated infections particularly with streptococci and these encapsulated bacteria. Their polymorphs fail to take up and destroy bacteria because opsonizing antibodies cannot be produced. Polysaccharide capsules are not necessarily associated with virulence, since they occur in free-living nonparasitic bacteria. Presumably they have functions other than the antiphagocytic one, perhaps giving protection against phages and colicins (see Glossary).

Anthrax and plague bacteria also have capsules that are associated with virulence. Bacteria of the *Bacteroides* group are normally commensal, but can form abscesses, often together with other microorganisms, and they have polysaccharide capsules. Pathogenic strains of *E. coli* and *Salmonella typhi* have thin capsules consisting of acidic polysaccharide (K antigen), which in some way make phagocytosis difficult. Perhaps this is because (in the absence of antibody) the encapsulated strains do not activate complement via the alternate pathway, and are therefore poorly opsonized. Gram-negative bacteria also have cell walls containing a lipopolysaccharide complex (endotoxin), and the somatic (O) antigens occur in the polysaccharide side chains (Fig. 14). Bacteria with certain types of O antigen have a colonial form designated as smooth, and they show an associated virulence, with resistance to phagocytosis except in the presence of antibody. Rough colonial forms lack these particular antigens, which are determined by immunodominant sugars in the polysaccharide side chains, and are not virulent, showing no resistance to phagocytosis.

The parasitic trypanosomes causing African sleeping sickness circulate in the blood, from which they are transmitted to fresh hosts by biting tsetse flies. The bloodstream forms have a pronounced surface coat with an outer carbohydrate layer, which perhaps inhibits phagocytosis of the parasites by reticuloendothelial cells (see Ch. 5) and enables the parasitaemia to continue.

There is one other everyday example of a possible mechanism for inhibition of phagocytosis. Virulent strains of staphylococci produce a coagulase that forms fibrin strands when added to plasma in the presence of certain accessory plasma factors. The fibrin network may help form a wall round the staphylococcal infection site, but the advantage to the bacteria is not clear. Infiltration by polymorphs still occurs on a large scale, and at least for streptococci, virulence is associated with breakdown rather than formation of tissue barriers. A slightly more convincing, though unproven, role for staphylococcal coagulase is that it precipitates fibrin in the immediate vicinity of the bacteria, thus impeding the final access of phagocytic cells, as well as depositing host fibrin on the bacterial cell wall, which therefore presents a less foreign surface to phagocytic cells.

Some microorganisms pose purely mechanical problems for the phagocytic cell without specifically preventing phagocytosis. There are difficulties with motile microorganisms, whether motility is due to flagella (Gram-negative bacteria, *Trichomonas vaginalis*) or to amoeboid movement (*Entamoeba histolytica*). Imobilizing antibodies may be necessary. The sheer size of a microorganism can be a problem. A single macrophage will be unable to phagocytose a large microorganism, and macrophages attempting to phagocytose the advancing tip of fungal hyphae are just carried along by the hyphal growth. In such situations several macrophages must cooperate and if necessary form syncytial giant cells, as in the response to fibres and other large foreign objects (see also p. 65).

As mentioned above, both polymorphs and macrophages have specific surface receptors for the Fc fragment of IgG and IgM antibodies and also for the C3b product of complement activation (see Ch. 6). This ensures that microorganisms coated with antibody or complement are opsonized, i.e. effectively attached to the surface of the phagocytic cell and phagocytosed. Cells other than polymorphs and macrophages lack these receptors and here attachment and phagocytosis of particles coated with antibody is not promoted but even inhibited. Opsonized microbes are not only taken up but also killed more rapidly in the phagocyte. For instance, in the early stages of typhus, the rickettsiae multiply in macrophages after phagocytosis, but later, when antibodies have formed, the antibody-coated rickettsiae are rapidly phagocytosed and killed, and eventually digested.

Opsonization without specific antibody takes place following deposition of C3b on the bacterial surface after activation of the alternative complement pathway (see p. 147) and attachment to the C3b receptor on the phagocyte. It is an important host defence early in infection, before antibodies are formed, and the following can be considered as microbial "strategies" to prevent this type of opsonization. Encapsulated strains of *Staphylococcus aureus* appear to activate and bind complement without the need for antibody, but are not opsonized and phagocytosed. It is thought that C3b is somehow hidden by the bacterial capsule and cannot attach to C3b receptors on phagocytes. In the case of Group A streptococci the outer covering of M protein prevents complement activation by the alternative pathway. Strains of *E. coli* with K1 capsular polysaccharide are pathogenic for newborn infants and show an associated resistance to opsonization by the alternative complement pathway. Finally, gonococci become resistant to killing by normal serum (presumably involving alternative pathway activation) if they have a receptor for an IgG antibody present in normal serum that blocks the killing action.

There are a number of ingenious ways in which bacteria and other microorganisms avoid inactivation by host antibodies, or even avoid eliciting antibodies (see Ch. 7). One example will be given here, since it involves phagocytosis. A substance called protein A is present in the cell wall of *Staphylococcus aureus*. Each molecule of protein A binds strongly to two molecules of IgG via the Fc portion, and there are about 80 000 binding sites on each bacterium. It is tempting to suppose that such a molecule is not there by accident, and that it interferes with the opsonization and phagocytosis of staphylococci. Similar IgG binding molecules are present on many streptococci. The gene coding for protein A has been cloned and sequenced and its role will be clearer when it has been introduced into a nonpathogenic staphylococcus to see whether this results in an increase in pathogenicity.

Inhibition of fusion of lysosome with phagocytic vacuole

Clearly if the phagocytosed microorganism is not exposed to intracellular killing and digestive processes, it has the opportunity to survive and multiply.Those parts of the oxygen-dependent killing mechanisms that do not require myeloperoxidase (see pp. 68–9) will operate without fusion of lysosomes with the phagocytic vacuole, but if there were a way in which fusion could be prevented, some microorganisms might be expected to have accomplished this. One instance where this seems to occur is when virulent *Mycobacterium tuberculosis* is ingested by mouse macrophages. There is a failure of lysosomal fusion. Many phagocytic vacuoles remain free from lysosomal enzymes, the lysosomes keeping their distance in the cytoplasm, and the bacteria remain intact and grow. Certain sulphatides on the bacteria, and also ammonium ions, have the same effect. This is in contrast to the events after uptake of nonvirulent *M. tuberculosis*, when lysosomal fusion is general, phagocytic vacuoles receive lysosomal contents, and bacilli are killed. The forces that move lysosomes towards vacuoles and then cause fusion are not known, so that little can be said about mechanisms except that a soluble inhibitor is presumably released from vacuoles by the virulent bacteria. This is not a general inhibition of fusion in the phagocyte, but a failure to fuse with the particular vacuoles containing the microorganism.

The intracellular protozoan parasite *Toxoplasma gondii* (see Glossary) is phagocytosed by macrophages, inducing its own engulfment by actively inserting a specialized 35 mm diameter cylinder into the macrophage.* But in a large proportion of the vacuoles there is no lysosomal fusion, and the toxoplasmas multiply, eventually killing the cell. Mitochondria and lengths of endoplasmic reticulum surround these vacuoles, presumably in response to chemical stimuli arising from the toxoplasmas, and perhaps playing a part in nourishment of the parasite. Other instances of nonfusion of lysosomes are known, such as when the fungus *Aspergillus flavus* enters the alveolar macrophages of susceptible (cortisone-treated) mice, when *Chlamydia psittaci* enter macrophages in culture, or when *Staphylococcus aureus* is phagocytosed by Kupffer cells in the perfused liver *in vitro*. Inhibition of fusion is an active process, and does not generally occur when microorganisms are killed or coated with antibody beforehand.

Escape from the phagosome

After capture in a phagosome, a microorganism can still evade antimicrobial forces by escaping at an early stage from the phagosome and entering the

---

* *Toxoplasma gondii* can also invade a large variety of nonphagocytic cells. Little is known about attachment mechanisms or receptors, but the parasite secretes substances that help penetration, and the process is an active one, help being given by the host cell!

cytoplasm. Although this is a logical strategy, it has not been thoroughly studied. For viruses it involves fusion of the virus envelope with the phagosome wall so that the nucleocapsid core is set free in the cytoplasm, and this is discussed on p. 88. There is evidence that the phenomenon also occurs with *Mycobacterium leprae*, *Rickettsia mooseri*, and the trypomastigote form of *Trypanosoma cruzi*. These can be seen free, often multiplying, in the cytoplasm of macrophages. Escape from the phagosome has not been followed in detail and little is known of mechanisms, but it is generally prevented when the microorganism is coated with antibody.

Resistance to killing and digestion in the phagolysosome

Many successfully infectious microorganisms resist killing and digestion in the phagocytic vacuole. For those whose multiplication is for the most part extracellular this ability to survive rather than suffer death and dissolution in the phagocyte may possibly add to their success in the infected host. Other microorganisms, however, are specialists in intracellular growth and some of them grow in phagocytes. Certain viruses depend for their success on infecting the phagocyte after avoiding killing and digestion in the phagolysosome; macrophages rather than polymorphs are important (see below). In the case of reoviruses, exposure to lysosomal enzymes actually initiates the "uncoating" of the virus particle in the cell and thus helps virus multiplication. The cells susceptible to reoviruses, however, are not necessarily specialized phagocytes. Many other viruses have specialized mechanisms for entering susceptible nonphagocytic cells (see receptors, below); their fate in phagocytic cells is not necessarily important. Polio- and rhinoviruses, for instance, are taken up, killed and digested in phagocytic cells, but they nevertheless successfully infect target cells in the upper respiratory tract and alimentary canal and are shed profusely from these sites.

Bacteria, as a result of phagocytosis, enter phagocytic cells more commonly than any other type of host cell, and intracellular bacteria cannot establish a successful infection unless they resist killing and then grow in the phagocyte. Thus, macrophages are important sites of bacterial growth in infections with *Mycobacteria*, *Brucella*, *Listeria*, *Trypanosoma*, *Nocardia* and *Yersinia pestis*.* In some instances the microorganism escapes from the

---

* *Yersinia pestis* is the causative agent of the plague (L plaga, a blow), an often lethal infection transmitted to man by fleas from infected rats or other rodents, which can also spread from man to man by the respiratory route. In the fourteenth century epidemics of the Black Death it is estimated to have killed a third of the people of Europe. The bacteria are able to grow in the phagolysosome of macrophages when Ca^{2+} concentrations reach low levels ($<100 \mu M$), and produce several potent toxins.

phagosome or inhibits lysosomal fusion (see above), but *Mycobacterium lepraemurium*, *Listeria monocytogenes*, *Y. pestis* and virulent strains of *Salmonella typhimurium* can grow in the phagosome in spite of lysosomal fusion. Polymorphs are less important sites of microbial growth, partly because of their short life span, but their powerful lysosomal enzymes take a heavy toll of ingested bacteria that show no particular resistance to killing and digestion.

Once a microorganism has been phagocytosed the most important thing is whether or not it is killed in the phagocyte. It should be remembered that by definition microorganisms are dead when they are incapable of multiplying. When nonvirulent *E. coli* is phagocytosed by polymorphs it is soon killed, but bacterial macromolecular machinery proceeds for a while after death of the bacterium. Most microorganisms are killed after phagocytosis, but the bacteria or protozoa that infect phagocytes must allow themselves to be taken up by these cells, and their success hinges in the first place on their resistance to killing (Table 6). We know almost nothing about resistance to killing, except that it is likely to depend on the outer surfaces of the microorganism, or on the secretion of substances that interfere with the action of lysosomal enzymes.

After the microorganism has been killed, the subsequent disposal of the corpse is only of concern to the host. Most microorganisms are readily digested and degraded by lysosomal enzymes. But the microbial properties that give resistance to killing, sometimes also give resistance to digestion and degradation, because the cell walls or capsules of certain pathogenic bacteria are digested with difficulty. Group A streptococci, for instance, are rapidly killed once they have been phagocytosed, but the mucopeptide–polysaccharide complex in the cell wall resists digestion, and streptococcal cell walls are sometimes still visible in phagocytes a month or so after the infection has terminated.* The waxes on the outer surface of certain mycobacteria are not readily digested by lysosomal enzymes and it is possible that this is why such bacteria are difficult to kill. *Mycobacterium lepraemurium* is particularly resistant to lysosomal enzymes, and grows in phagocytic vacuoles even after extensive fusion with lysosomes. It has a hydrophobic mycoside as a capsule, and although saprophytic mycobacteria have a similar type of covering, it may have particular properties in *Mycobacterium lepraemurium*.

Many pathogenic bacteria show a degree of resistance to killing and sometimes also to digestion in the phagolysosome, as indicated in Table 6.

---

*Because the capsules or cell walls of streptococci, pneumococci, mycobacteria, *Listeria* and other bacteria pose problems for lysosomal enzymes and are not readily digested in phagocytes, bacterial fragments are sometimes retained in the host, for long periods. This can lead to interesting pathological or immunological results (see Ch. 8).

Catalase, by destroying H_2O_2 might protect bacteria from killing, and catalase-rich strains of staphylococci and *Listeria monocytogenes* show better survival inside polymorphs. Superoxide dismutase, on the other hand, generates H_2O_2, but there is no correlation between production of this enzyme by bacteria and their survival in polymorphs. Studies of these matters have only just begun, and because so very little is known about killing and digestion we are equally ignorant about resistance to killing and digestion.

Growth in the Phagocytic Cell

The ways in which microorganisms avoid being phagocytosed and killed have been discussed above. An equally satisfactory victory over the phagocyte is achieved when the microorganism uses it as a site of growth. The microorganism must now allow itself to be phagocytosed, but resist killing and digestion, and then multiply, deriving nourishment from the phagocytic cell. As was pointed out in the preceding section, polymorphs have such a brief life span that they are rarely important sites for microbial growth. Virulent bacteria tend to remain viable if they are phagocytosed by polymorphs, but intracellular growth is generally slight compared with the growth of bacteria in extracellular fluids. Macrophages, by comparison, live for long periods. Many microorganisms have as it were come to accept eventual phagocytosis by macrophages as inevitable, and are able to multiply inside the cell (Table 7). They have learnt how to induce the macrophage to protect and feed them, rather than destroy and digest them. This ability to grow in macrophages is often a key property of successful invasive microorganisms (see Ch. 5).

Certain viruses grow in macrophages, and in a few instances, such as the highly successful lactic dehydrogenase virus of mice (see Glossary), the macrophage is the only cell in the body that is infected. The mechanisms of virus growth are probably basically similar to the mechanisms of growth in other types of cell, although differing in details. The infecting virus generates specific RNA messengers and the metabolic machinery of the host cell is utilized to synthesize progeny virus particles. When larger and more complex microorganisms such as rickettsias, bacteria, fungi or protozoa parasitize macrophages, they usually multiply inside phagocytic vacuoles. Nourishment of the parasite takes place across the wall of the vacuole and host materials must be made available to the parasite. Certain coccidias, for instance, induce the host cell to extrude material into the vacuole and then take it up by endocytosis (see Glossary). In a few instances (*Trypanosoma cruzi, Mycobacterium leprae*) the microorganism appears to escape from the

Table 7. Examples of microorganisms that regularly multiply in macrophages

Viruses	Herpes-type viruses
	Hepatitis viruses of mice
	Measles, distemper
	Poxviruses
	LCM
	Lactic dehydrogenase virus of mice
	Aleutian disease of mink (see Glossary)
Rickettsias	*Rickettsia rickettsi*
	Rickettsia prowazeki
Bacteria	*Mycobacterium tuberculosis*
	Mycobacterium leprae
	Listeria monocytogenes
	Brucella spp.
	Legionella pneumophila
Fungi	*Cryptococcus neoformans*
Protozoa	Leishmanias
	Trypanosomes
	Toxoplasmas

vacuole and multiplies free in the cytoplasm. For most of the microorganisms that parasitize macrophages, including leprosy bacilli, tubercle bacilli, *Leishmania* and *Toxoplasma*, little or nothing is known about microbial nutrition inside the cell. Macrophages parasitized by *Toxoplasma gondii* appear to be giving biochemical support to the invader in a most hospitable fashion. Microvilli from the host cell extend into the vacuole which is surrounded by strips of endoplasmic reticulum and mitochondria.

Entry into the Host Cell other than by Phagocytosis

Although the usual way in which a particle enters a cell is by phagocytosis, so that the particle is enclosed in a phagocytic vacuole, there are other methods of entry. Electron microscope studies indicate that some bacteria, for instance, adsorb to the cell surface and enter the cytoplasm directly after inducing a local breakdown in the plasma membrane. The plasma membrane is reformed immediately. Shigellas and pathogenic salmonellas appear to enter intestinal epithelial cells in this way, and other bacteria show the same behaviour in tissue culture cells. It may be a less frequent occurrence in specialized phagocytic cells. Protozoa have a complex structure and can utilize their own lysosomal enzymes to penetrate host cells. Trypanosomes,

*Eimeria,** *Toxoplasma gondii* and *Entamoeba histolytica* enter susceptible cells by active penetration, and the active end of the parasite has vesicles containing lysosomal enzymes that aid the penetration process. When a malaria parasite penetrates a red blood cell, a specialized projection (conoid end) on the malarial merozoite makes contact with the red cell surface. The parasite then injects a lipid-rich material from special glands (rhopteries), and it seems that this material is inserted into the red cell membrane, whose area is thus increased. As the merozoite actively enters the red cell, the membrane stays intact, but there is now enough of it to form an invagination and accommodate the advancing parasite.

There has long been a controversy as to whether viruses enter the susceptible cell via the phagocytic vacuole or directly through the surface membrane of the cell. Certain enveloped viruses such as Sendai (parainfluenza I) are adsorbed to the cell surface, and a special "fusion protein" in the viral envelope then mediates fusion with the plasma membrane so that viral contents are set free in the cytoplasm. The risks of entering a phagocytic vacuole and being exposed to lysosomal enzymes are thus eliminated, and this might be of some advantage in the infection of most types of cell. The risks of such exposure, however, are necessarily higher in a specialized phagocytic cell, where there is rapid uptake of virus particles into phagocytic vacuoles. Virus particles have a simple structure compared to bacteria, with no capsule and no extracellular metabolic activity or products. The possibilities of chemical inhibition of lysosomal fusion or resistance to digestion in the phagosome are therefore limited. If, therefore, most viruses are inevitably killed in the phagolysosome, the only way of avoiding this is by initiating intracellular infection almost immediately after ingestion, before lysosomal fusion.† Lysosomal fusion can take place within minutes, but it is known that ingested virus particles can enter the cytoplasm through the phagosome wall as early as this.

Most of the discussion had dealt with the ways in which microorganisms can avoid intracellular digestion. There are one or two instances where exposure to lysosomal enzymes is actually necessary for the multiplication of microorganisms. Reoviruses require a preliminary breakdown of the outer viral coat by lysosomal hydrolases before the viral core can enter the cytoplasm and initiate infection, and spores of *Clostridium botulinum* are

---

* Various species of *Eimeria* (a protozoan parasite) cause contagious enteritis, or coccidiosis, in all domestic animals. Ingested oocysts invade intestinal epithelial cells and the entire life cycle with schizonts, merozoites and gametocytes takes place in these cells.

† Sometimes (as with influenza virus) a viral envelope protein acts as a "fusion protein" only when exposed to the low pH that is established within a minute or two in the phagolysosome.

said to germinate in cells only after the stimulus of exposure to lysosomal contents.

Consequences of Defects in the Phagocytic Cell

The importance of the phagocytic cell in defence against microorganisms is illustrated from observations on diseases where there are shortages or defects of phagocytic cells. A serious shortage of polymorphs, with less than $1000 \, mm^{-3}$ in the blood (normal 2000–$5000 \, mm^{-3}$), is seen in acute leukaemia or after X-irradiation, and predisposes to infection with Gram-negative and pyogenic Gram-positive bacteria. There are also one or two inherited shortages. Blood polymorph counts are about one-tenth of normal in Yemenite jews, although surprisingly they seem little the worse for it except for a susceptibility to periodontal disease. But certain naturally occurring defects in the function of phagocytes have more serious consequences, and recent studies of these defects have thrown much light on normal phagocyte function. Unfortunately the defects are often multiple so that interpretation is not easy.

Children with chronic granulomatous disease, usually an X-linked recessive trait, have polymorphs that look normal and show normal chemotaxis and phagocytosis, but there is defective intracellular killing of bacteria. The gene that is abnormal has recently been cloned, and it appears to code for an essential component in the phagocyte's NADPH-oxidase system. The superoxide radical and H_2O_2 are therefore not generated (see Fig. 13, p. 68), and associated with this there is increased susceptibility especially to staphylococcal and Gram-negative bacterial infections. In spite of undiminished immune responses to infection, patients suffer recurrent suppurative infections with bacteria of low-grade virulence such as *E. coli*, *Klebsiella* sp. staphylococci and micrococci, and usually die during childhood. Polymorphs are present in foci of infection but cannot kill the microorganisms, and are eventually taken up by macrophages, leading to the formation of a chronic inflammatory lesion called a granuloma (see Ch. 8). Interestingly, the patients have normal resistance to streptococcal infections because streptococci are catalase-negative and can themselves generate the H_2O_2 required for their destruction after phagocytosis. As might be expected, patients with severe G6-PD (glucose 6-phosphate dehydrogenase) deficiency also suffer from infection with catalase-positive organisms, because they too fail to generate superoxide and hydrogen peroxide. Patients with myeloperoxidase deficiency show delayed killing of bacteria in polymorphs but normal resistance to bacterial infections and surprisingly an increased susceptibility to *Candida albicans*.

Another example of a polymorph defect is seen in Chediak-Higashi disease, which occurs in mice, mink, cattle, killer whales and man, and here too there is increased susceptibility to certain infections. Polymorphs contain anomalous giant granules (lysosomes) and the basic defect is probably in microfilaments. Phagocytosis and even lysosomal enzyme content appear normal, but there is defective chemotaxis, defective lysosomal fusion and delayed bacterial killing.

As well as shortages or defects in the quality of phagocytic cells, there may also be defects in the delivery system by which phagocytes are focused and assembled in the infectious foci where they are needed. Polymorphs show defective chemotaxis (as well as phagocytosis) in a variety of rare conditions such as the lazy leucocyte syndrome, due to a disorder of the cell membrane, and the actin dysfunction syndrome where actin is not polymerized as normally to form microfilaments so that the "muscle" system of the cell is defective. Impaired digestion and disposal of microbial antigens is likely to be associated with immunopathology, but little is known of this aspect of phagocyte function.

Abnormalities in phagocyte function are not uncommon in certain acute infections such as Gram-negative bacteraemia and also in otherwise normal patients with recurrent staphylococcal infections. Presumably the abnormality could cause the infections, but at times it reflects the antimicrobial activities of the infectious agent.

Some of the clinical conditions are complex and of varied origin, often with multiple defects. In chronic mucocutaneous candidiasis, for instance, some patients have impaired cell-mediated immunity and others defective macrophage function. They suffer from persistent and at times severe infection of mucous membranes, nails and skin with the normally harmless yeast-like fungus *Candida albicans*.

Summary

In summary, the encounter between the microorganism and the phagocytic cell is a central feature of infection and pathogenicity. Phagocytes are designed to ingest, kill and digest invaders, and the course of the infection depends on the success with which this is carried out.

Virulent microorganisms have developed a great variety of devices for countering or avoiding the antimicrobial action of phagocytes. Although substances produced by or present on microbes may at first sight appear to have a useful function, not all will prove to be of practical importance in the infected host. Studies on microbial killing and digestion in phagocytes are still poorly understood, but it is important to conceive logically of the ways in which microorganisms can avoid being ingested, killed and digested.

References

Armstrong, J. A. and Hart, P. D. (1971). Response of cultured macrophages to Mycobacterium tuberculosis, with observations on fusion of lysosomes with phagosomes. *J. Exp. Med.* **134**, 713–740.

Bannister, L. H. (1979). The interaction of intracellular protista and their host cells, with special reference to heterotrophic organisms. *Proc. R. Soc. B* **204**, 141–163.

Bannister, L. H., Mitchell, G. H., Butcher, G. A. and Dennis, E. D. (1986). Lamellar membranes associated with rhopteries in erythrocyte merozoites of *Plasmodum knowlesi*: a clue to the mechanism of invasion. *Parasitology* **92**, 291–303.

Beaman, L. and Beaman, B. L. (1984). The role of oxygen and its derivatives in microbial pathogenesis and host defence. *Ann. Rev. Microbiol.* **38**, 27–48.

Eissenberg, L. G. and Wyrick, P. B. (1981). Inhibition of phagolysosome fusion is localized to Chlamydia psittaci-laden vacuoles. *Infect. Immunity* **32**, 889–898.

Elsbach, P. (1980). Degradation of microorganisms by phagocytic cells. *Rev. Inf. Dis.* **2**, 106–128.

Hirsch, J. G. *et al.* (1963). Motion picture study of the toxic action of streptolysins on leucocytes. *J. Exp. Med.* **118**, 223–228.

Segal, A. W. (1985). Variations on the theme of chronic granulomatous disease. *Lancet* (June 15), 1378.

Silver, R. P. *et al.* (1981). Molecular cloning of the K1 capsular polysaccharide genes of *E. coli. Nature, Lond.* **289**, 696–698.

Van Epps, D. E. and Anderson, B. R. (1974). Streptolysin O inhibition of neutrophil chemotaxis and mobility: non-immune phenomenon with species specificity. *Inf. Immunity* **9**, 27–33.

Wilkinson, P. C. (1980). Leucocyte locomotion and chemotaxis; effects of bacteria and viruses. *Rev. Inf. Dis.* **2**, 293–319.

5

The Spread of Microbes through the Body

When invading microorganisms have traversed one of the epithelial surfaces and arrive in subepithelial tissues, it is almost inevitable that they enter local lymphatics, as discussed in Ch. 3. They are then delivered to the filtration system and immune forces in the local lymph node. Sometimes this serves to disseminate rather than confine the infection and spread from local to regional lymph nodes, and eventually to the blood, takes place. It is also possible, though not common, for the invading microorganism in subepithelial tissues to enter small blood vessels directly. This occurs when the microorganism damages the vessel wall, when viruses grow through the vessel wall, or when the initial act of infection, whether by injury or insect bite (see Ch. 2), introduces microorganisms directly into blood vessels.

Spread via lymphatics and the blood is rapid, enabling microorganisms to reach distant target organs or tissues within a few days. Thus poliovirus and *Salmonella typhi* infect the intestine and enter the blood stream within a few days, silently reaching the central nervous system (polio) or causing disease by multiplication in reticuloendothelial cells and liberation into the blood (typhoid).

Direct Spread

Microorganisms that fail to spread via the circulating body fluids in this way are confined to the site of initial entry into the body, except in so far as there is local extension of the infection into neighbouring tissues. The extent of the local spread depends on the outcome of the encounter between microbe and host defences mentioned in Chs 3 and 4, but some spread is common. When

92

vaccinia virus is introduced into the dermis during vaccination against smallpox it establishes infection in epidermal and dermal cells and spreads radially by infecting and being released from successive groups of cells. The rate of progress is slow, and within a week an epidermal area about a centimetre in diameter has been infected. Spread in the subepithelial tissues of the dermis is slightly more rapid, with infection of histocytes and fibroblasts, but the extracellular connective tissue matrix is a hydrated gel and does not give free movement to virus particles. Bacteria that spread effectively in this tissue tend to produce spreading factors (see below) and conditions become more fluid (oedematous) once an inflammatory response has been induced.

If microbes infect epithelial surfaces that are covered with fluid, their progeny are liberated onto these surfaces and can establish fresh sites of infection elsewhere on the epithelium (see Ch. 2). This form of local spread takes place with respiratory infection, when ciliary action moves micro-organisms from the initial site of infection in the direction of the throat, giving fresh opportunities to establish infection *en route*. If cilia are not functioning properly or if there is too much fluid for them to transport, there is a flow by gravity to other parts of the respiratory tract. During upper respiratory tract infections excess nasal secretions tend to drain or are sniffed backwards and downwards, and during lower respiratory infections gravity inevitably plays some part in the movement of excess secretion, especially during sleep (see p. 294). Coughing and sneezing redistribute the infectious agent over uninfected epithelial areas. Sometimes larger amounts of fluid and mucus are coughed up and reinhaled before reaching the back of the throat. Anaesthesia or alcoholic stupor favour the drainage or aspiration of secretions from the throat to the lower respiratory tract.

The same type of local spread takes place easily in the intestine because of the continuous flow of intestinal contents; salmonellas and shigellas that have established initial foci of infection are thereby carried into more distal parts of the intestine. Local spread in the urethra, conjunctiva or vagina is likewise facilitated by movement of microorganisms in the fluid covering the epithelial surface.

The skin, on the other hand, with its dry surface, is less suitable for this type of local spread. It is not an easily infected surface (see Ch. 2) and most mammals are in any case covered with a generous layer of fur which itself impedes the local spread of microorganisms. There are only a few animals that are more or less naked, and these include the pig, elephant, man and rhinoceros. It is in man that there are best opportunities for spread from one part of the skin to another, because microorganisms are readily transferred by the scratching and rubbing activities of the fingers. The constant attention of fingers to the face promotes the local spread of various bacteria, and can help to distribute over the face the staphylococci or streptococci responsible for impetigo. Warts are spread in the skin by scratching or by the rubbing together of naturally opposing areas of skin ("kissing" warts), and vaccinia virus used to be readily transferred by fingers from the inoculation site to other skin areas. The skin has a moister covering of sweat and secretions in backwaters such as the armpits or umbilicus, or in the crevices between toes or body folds. Fungi, for instance, spread locally in these areas.

Direct spread also occurs in organs and tissues below the body surfaces, extending the focus of infection and sometimes accounting for striking complications. When infection in the lung spreads towards the surface of this organ it causes inflammation or actual infection of the pleura (pleurisy). Similarly, infection in the appendix or elsewhere in the intestines causes inflammation or infection of the peritoneum (peritonitis) if it spreads towards the serosal surfaces. The direct spread of infection from the middle ear to neighbouring structures gives rise to meningitis, cerebral abscess etc.

Microbial Factors Promoting Spread

Direct spread of microorganisms through normal subepithelial tissues is not easy, being limited physically by the gel-like nature of the connective tissue matrix. Certain bacteria produce soluble substances with an effect on the physical properties of this connective tissue matrix, and at first sight these substances would appear to promote the spread of infection. Invasive streptococci liberate hyaluronidase, an enzyme that liquefies the hyaluronic acid component of the connective tissue matrix. Streptococcal skin infections, accordingly, often spread rapidly through the dermis causing the condition erysipelas. Hyaluronidase was originally referred to as the "spreading factor", but it is certainly not a necessary factor, because bacteria such as *Brucella* are highly invasive in the absence of hyaluronidase. Moreover *Staphylococcus aureus* produces plenty of hyaluronidase without being particularly invasive. Indeed, there is evidence suggesting that unless a microorganism is highly virulent it gains advantages if after entry into the body it first multiplies locally before spreading. A bacterial inoculum that causes a local lesion after intradermal injection often fails to produce a lesion if hyaluronidase is injected with the bacteria. Early local spread perhaps favours the host by diluting out infecting microorganisms and exposing them more effectively to host defences (see p. 58). As if to warn us against naive conclusions staphylococci produce a coagulase that lays down a fibrin network in tissues (see Ch. 4), but at the same time form a fibrinolysin. Streptococci also produce a fibrinolysin (streptokinase) in addition to hyaluronidase. Doubtless these enzymes have functions other than those connected with local spread in the purely mechanical sense. Bacteria in general produce a great variety of enzymes, including proteinases, collagenases, lipases and nucleases, but only very few of them have been clearly shown to be of any pathogenic significance. Many of these enzymes presumably have functions related to bacterial nutrition or metabolism rather than a relation to some theoretically important role in the infectious process.

Spread via Lymphatics

Proteins and particles in tissue fluids enter lymphatic capillaries rather than blood capillaries, and are transported to the nearest lymph node. Virus particles or bacteria injected into the skin, for instance, reach local lymph nodes within a few minutes. A rich lymphatic network lies below the epithelium in the nasopharynx, mouth and lung; microorganisms traversing these epithelia enter cervical and pulmonary lymph nodes. The mesenteric nodes receive microorganisms invading from the intestine, and strategically placed nodes occur along the lymphatics draining the urinogenital tract. Lymph nodes receive and monitor the lymph draining most parts of the body. If microorganisms reach the peritoneal cavity, for instance, they are exposed to phagocytosis by large numbers of resident peritoneal macrophages, and also enter subdiaphragmatic lymphatics to reach the retrosternal lymph nodes. A few microorganisms, such as the leprosy bacillus and certain viruses, grow in the endothelium of lymphatic vessels and thus increase their numbers by the time they reach the node in the lymph. The total flow of lymph in the body is considerable, and in the normal man 1–3 litres of lymph enter the blood each day from the thoracic duct. Under certain circumstances the flow rate from an organ is very greatly increased, such as from the pregnant uterus, the lactating mammary gland, or the intestine after a large fatty meal.

Lymph nodes have an important filtering action on account of the phagocytic cells that line the lymph node sinuses, and microorganisms are filtered off rather than allowed to spread to other lymph nodes, the thoracic duct, and the blood (see Fig. 11, p. 60). Inflammatory substances reach the lymph node at an early stage in most bacterial and fungal infections, or when tissues have been damaged in virus infections. As with inflammation elsewhere, blood and lymphatic vessels are dilated and leucocytes are extravasated, so that the node becomes swollen and tender (see Ch. 3). In the normal node the phagocytes are the resident macrophages lining the sinusoids, but in the inflamed node blood-borne polymorphs are also present. The filtering function of lymph nodes is impaired under the following circumstances:

(a) When the lymph flow rate is high, as during inflammation of tissues or exercise of muscles. It has long been a practice to manage infected wounds by immobilization of the affected part of the body, thus reducing lymph flow and increasing filtration efficiency in the draining lymph nodes.

(b) When the concentration of particles is high. Early in infection filtration is efficient, but it may be less so at a later stage when increasing numbers of microorganisms arrive at the node following local multiplication at the site of infection. On the other hand, antibodies to the microorganisms reach inflamed infected tissues and lymphatics at a later stage, promoting uptake of microorganisms by phagocytic cells in the node.

(c) When phagocytic cells in the node fail to ingest microorganisms. There is discussion in Ch. 4 of the microbial and host factors that impair phagocytosis of microorganisms and thus depress the filtering function of the lymph nodes.

If the lymph node filters out the invading microorganisms but rather than inactivating them supports their multiplication, then the multiplying microorganisms are discharged in the efferent lymph. This occurs with certain bacteria such as *Pasteurella pestis* and *Brucella* and with a variety of nonbacterial infections, including smallpox and typhus. Tubercle bacilli always enter lymphatics at the site of primary infection, and are usually arrested in the local lymph node. Occasionally, especially in children, there is further spread to regional lymph nodes, thoracic lymph duct and blood to give disseminated (miliary) tuberculosis with foci of infection in many organs. Sometimes the infectious agent multiplies in cells in the node without seriously damaging them, and the infected cells can then migrate through the body and disseminate the infection (see below).

After arrival of the first microorganisms in the lymph node the local immune response is set in motion. Microorganisms are phagocytosed by macrophages lining the lymph sinuses and antigenic products are subsequently presented to adjacent lymphoid cells. Antibody and CMI responses are thus built up. Lymphocytes continually circulate through the nodes (see Fig. 26, p. 138) and these are recruited, cell division takes place, and the node enlarges. Within a day or two immunologically stimulated cells emerge in the efferent lymph to spread the response to distant parts of the body. If the efferent lymph from the stimulated node is cannulated and the emerging cells collected, the immune response can be confined to this node.

Changes in the lymph node reflect the inflammatory and immunological phenomena. At one extreme is the picture seen following infection with an invasive bacterium such as a β-haemolytic streptococcus. Bacteria and inflammatory products of bacterial growth arrive in the local node, which rapidly becomes swollen and tender as blood vessels dilate and it is distended with inflammatory cells and exudate. The node becomes the site of a battle between host and parasite, and the determinants of microbial virulence apply in the node as in any other tissue. Virulent bacteria tend to kill phagocytes, resist uptake and inactivation by phagocytes, or multiply in phagocytes (see Ch. 4). While the lymph continues to flow, the invasive streptococci (or the typhus rickettsiae, plague bacilli) have the opportunity to exit via the efferent lymphatics to reach the next node and eventually the blood stream. If the microorganisms are arriving in large numbers from a peripheral site of multiplication, the filtering efficiency of the node falls off and some of these can pass straight through the node. As inflammation and tissue damage in the node become more severe, the flow of lymph ceases, fibrin is formed and the infection is thus localized. Sometimes the swollen node becomes a mere pocket of pus (invasive staphylococci, bubonic plague), a battlefield containing dead and living microorganisms, host cells and inflammatory exudate.

In less severe infections, the changes in the node are less marked, and when entirely avirulent or nonmultiplying microorganisms reach the node, the nodal swelling is barely detectable and is attributable to an uncomplicated immune response. These are many viruses (measles virus, adenoviruses, polioviruses) that have the ability to replicate rather than be destroyed after being filtered out in the lymph node. The infected cells are generally macrophages or lymphocytes, and progeny virus is liberated into the lymph. If the infected cells are not seriously or acutely damaged they can carry virus to distant parts of the body in the course of their normal migratory movements. This last method of spread is of supreme importance for viruses. As a rule, bacteria or protozoa must be rather virulent and pathogenic if they are to spread easily through the body from a peripheral site of growth, but many relatively avirulent viruses such as chickenpox, rubella and mumps accomplish this with consummate ease by way of the lymphatic system. The lymphatic system, faced with a staphylococcus in the dermis, removes it and delivers it to the antibacterial forces assembled in the local lymph node. If, however, the infecting microorganism grows silently in the lymphoid cells or macrophages of the node without setting off the usual alarm system (inflammation), and if immune responses have not yet been initiated the lymph node fails in its function and merely hands on the microorganisms to the efferent lymph, the blood stream, and thus to other susceptible tissues in the body.

In summary, most bacteria, fungi, protozoa, viruses etc. are filtered out and inactivated in lymph nodes. Those that are not dealt with in this way are able to spread through the lymphatic system and into the blood. Certain viruses and rickettsia grow in cells in lymph nodes, the nodes serving as sources for the dissemination of infected cells through the body.

Spread via the Blood

Blood–tissue junctions

The blood is the most effective vehicle of all for the spread of microbes through the body. After entering the blood they can be transported within a minute or two to a vascular bed in any part of the body. In small vessels such as capillaries and sinusoids where blood flows slowly there is an opportunity for the microorganism to be arrested and to establish infection in neighbouring tissues.

In a systemic virus infection* the epithelial surface of the body is traversed and virus reaches the blood at an early stage, either via the lymphatics and lymph nodes as discussed above, or after entering a subepithelial blood vessel. It is then spread through the body via the blood stream, usually without any signs or symptoms. The amount of virus in the blood at any given time may be negligible. This is called a primary viraemia and is a common, silent event often only known to have taken place because of invasion of a distant target organ such as the brain, liver or muscle. After growth of virus in the primary target organs there is sometimes a reseeding of virus into the blood again, to give a secondary viraemia and infection of a fresh set of tissues. The secondary viraemia is of larger magnitude and often easily detectable in blood samples. Thus in measles the infecting virus undergoes minimal growth near the site of infection in the respiratory tract, and then enters the blood via lymphatics and lymph nodes (see Fig. 18). The viraemia is not detectable, but as a result of it certain organs such as the spleen or liver are infected. After further viral growth in these visceral organs there is a secondary viraemia which seeds virus to the epithelial surfaces of the body, where the growth of virus causes a rash and an enanthem. A similar sequence of events takes place in other infections such as yaws, rubella, mumps, with microbial shedding from skin or in respiratory secretions, saliva, urine etc. (Fig. 18). The difference between primary and secondary viraemia or bacteraemia is often not clear, but it is a useful distinction. Clearly, the stepwise spread of infection through the different compartments of the body takes time. Hence the incubation period before disease occurs is longer in these systemic infections than when multiplication and shedding is all accomplished locally at a body surface (see also pp. 50, 133).

Circulating microorganisms generally localize in organs such as the liver and spleen. This is because they are phagocytosed by the macrophages of the reticuloendothelial system lining the sinusoidal blood vessels (see below). Infected leucocytes also tend to be arrested here if they show signs of

---

* Cells infected with viruses can be located and identified with great precision by the fluorescent antibody technique, as described in Fig. 16. Examples of its use in virus infections are shown in Fig. 17.

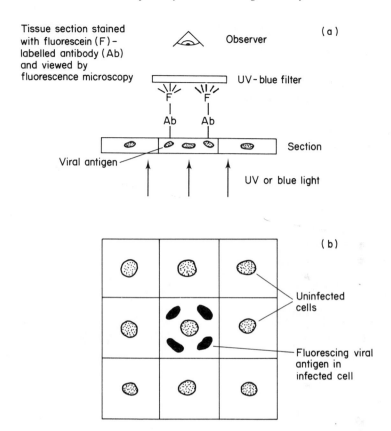

Fig. 16. Antiserum is prepared against the antigens of a given virus. The globulin (antibody) fraction is extracted, and chemically conjugated with fluorescein isothiocyanate. The conjugated antibodies are used to stain unfixed frozen sections of the tissue to be studied. Unattached antibody is removed by washing, the section is examined by fluorescence microscopy, and infected cells are identified. (a) Fluorescent antibody staining. (b) Stained section as seen under fluorescence microscope with infected (antigen-containing) cell. Antigen can also be identified by using antibody coupled to an enzyme (e.g. peroxidase). The enzyme is then made visible by adding substrate to give a coloured product.

damage, or surface changes. However, certain viruses (arthropod-borne viruses for instance) and rickettsias localize in capillary endothelial cells elsewhere in the body (see below).

Bacteria that do not generally cause a systemic infection can enter the blood in very small quantities as an accidental phenomenon, and this is important when it enables them to establish infection elsewhere in the body. Transient bacteraemias are probably not uncommon and under normal circumstances they are of no consequence, circulating bacteria being rapidly removed and inactivated by reticuloendothelial cells. But when host resistance is seriously impaired or when vulnerable tissues are exposed to the

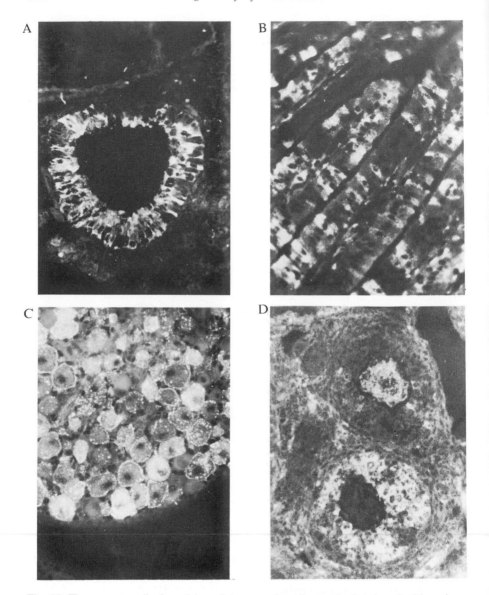

Fig. 17. Fluorescent antibody staining of tissue sections from animals infected with various viruses. (a) Small bronchiole from adult mouse lung 24 h after intranasal infection with Sendai (parainfluenza I) virus, showing infection of nearly all epithelial cells. (b) Intestinal epithelium of LCM virus carrier mouse (congenitally infected), showing several villi with many infected epithelial cells. (c) Dorsal root ganglion of a hamster infected with Lagos bat (rabies-like) virus, showing large numbers of infected neurones. (d) Ovary from LCM virus carrier (congenitally infected) mouse (see p. 154). There are two follicles, one with the ovum infected (above), the other with heavy infection of granulosa cells and an uninfected ovum. ((c) is illustrated here by kind permission of Dr F. A. Murphy.)

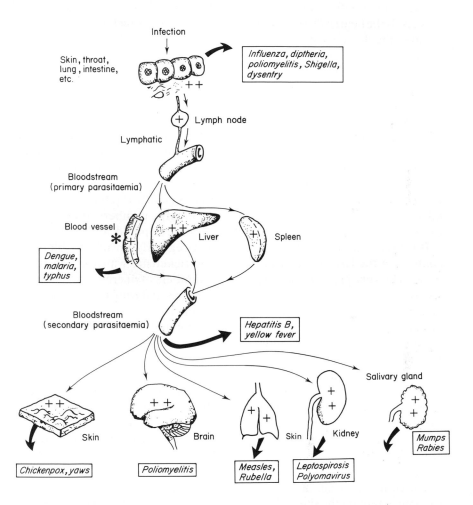

Fig. 18. The spread of infection through the body. + = sites of possible multiplication. Large arrows = sites of possible shedding to the exterior. * Indicates multiplication in blood stream or vascular endothelium rather than in viscera.

circulating bacteria, transient bacteraemias are a more serious matter. Certain bacteria, for instance, particularly those associated with the teeth (e.g. the *Streptococcus viridans* group) readily enter the blood, especially during dental extractions and even during tooth brushing or biting onto hard objects. If the heart valves are abnormal the circulating bacteria settle on them to cause the disease subacute bacterial endocarditis. Trauma to the growing ends of bones promotes the localization of bacteria during transient bacteraemias and thus predisposes to osteomyelitis. Staphylococcal osteomyelitis therefore commonly affects the metaphyses of the long bones of the leg in children. Larger numbers of bacteria sometimes enter the blood during severe infections with bacteria such as pneumococci, meningococci or *Streptococcus pyogenes*, giving rise to the condition called septicaemia. The lung is a common source of bacteria, as in pneumococcal pneumonia, and in the old days of *post partum* sepsis, streptococcal infection of the uterus often led to septicaemia. Finally there are a number of specialized bacteria such as *Bacillus anthracis* and *Salmonella typhi* that regularly establish generalized infections. After entering the blood, often in large numbers, they establish focal infection in organs and cause serious disease (typhoid, anthrax).

But there are few bacteria or fungi that regularly invade the blood, in contrast to the large number of viruses and rickettsias which nearly always do so. The very presence of considerable numbers of microorganisms in the blood causes disease if toxic materials are released during their metabolism and growth. Bacteria and fungi tend to release toxins when multiplying extracellularly, whereas viruses are more commonly being carried passively in the blood, and even when they multiply in cells, toxins are not released. Fungal or bacterial invasion of the blood is thus commonly associated with severe disease, whereas viraemia (e.g. hepatitis B or HIV (HTLV 3) carriers) is often silent. Cell-associated bacteraemia is sometimes silent, even when it continues for long periods. In lepromatous leprosy (see Ch. 9) there is a continuous bacteraemia, nearly all the circulating leprosy bacilli being inside blood monocytes. The bacteraemia persists for some months, but the bacilli remain inside cells, multiplying only very slowly (see Table 20, p. 185) and there are no general or toxic signs.

The course of events after entry of microorganisms into the blood depends to some extent on the site in the body at which entry occurs. After entry into subepithelial blood vessels in the intestine the first slowing down of blood flow is in the sinusoids of the liver, and here microorganisms are exposed to macrophages (Kupffer cells) lining the sinusoids. Many bacterial products and at times intact bacteria enter the portal circulation and are removed by Kupffer cells in the liver, which can thus detoxify or disinfect portal blood before delivering it to the rest of the body. Microorganisms entering small blood vessels in the lung are carried straight to capillary beds in the systemic circulation, and those entering vessels in the systemic circulation are carried first to the pulmonary capillary bed and thence anywhere in the body. Clearly the lung is an important possible site for the localization of circulating microorganisms, as well as an important possible source of microorganisms. Opportunities for localization in other organs will depend to some extent on the blood flow, the kidney for instance, which receives about one-third of the cardiac output, having very good opportunities. Much more than this, localization depends on the form in which the microorganism is carried in the blood, the activity of the reticuloendothelial system, and on the nature of the vascular bed in an organ. These will now be discussed in some detail.

Form in which microorganism is carried in the blood

Microorganisms may be carried free in the plasma, in the formed elements of the blood, or in both compartments (see Table 8).

Free in the plasma

Those carried free in the plasma include viruses such as poliomyelitis and yellow fever, bacteria such as anthrax and the pneumococcus and protozoa such as the trypanosomes. Their localization in organs depends on their ability to adhere to or grow in vascular endothelial cells, and on phagocytosis by reticuloendothelial cells. They must also be resistant to any antimicrobial factors present in the plasma.

Table 8. Carriage of microorganisms in different compartments of blood[a]

| | Free in plasma | Leucocyte associated | | Erythrocyte associated | Platelet associated |
		Mononuclear cells	Polymorphs		
Viruses	Poliovirus Yellow fever Hepatitis B	Measles EB virus Herpes simplex Cytomegalovirus		Colorado tick fever virus	Murine leukaemia virus LCM virus
Rickettsias	All types				
Bacteria	Pneumococci *Leptospira* Anthrax *Borrelia recurrentis*	*Mycobacterium leprae* Listeria *Brucella*	Pyogenic bacteria	*Bartonella baccilliformis*	
Protozoa	Trypanosomes	*Leishmania* *Toxoplasma gondii*		Malaria *Babesia*	

[a] Carriage in more than one compartment is possible, e.g. LCM virus is present in platelets, leucocytes and plasma of infected mice.

White cell associated

Certain microorganisms are carried either in or on white cells. The most important cells are lymphocytes and monocytes. These can be infected with viruses such as herpes simplex, cytomegalovirus, EB virus and measles, and monocytes are also infected with intracellular bacteria such as *Listeria*, tubercle bacilli and *Brucella*. Circulating monocytes are regularly infected by the protozoan parasite *Leishmania donovani* in the condition kala-azar, transmitted by blood-sucking sandflies. If the infected circulating cells remain healthy they protect the microorganism from phagocytosis by reticuloendothelial cells and from antimicrobial factors in the plasma. They can also carry microorganisms with them on their migrations through tissues as they move in and out of the vascular system (see Fig. 26, p. 138). Thus a mononuclear cell infected with measles virus in the subepithelial tissues of the respiratory tract can travel into the blood and then localize in the spleen and initiate infection in a splenic follicle.

Red cell associated

Some microorganisms travel in or on red blood cells. This gives them no opportunity to leave the vascular system, but those that are inside red blood cells are protected from phagocytosis by the reticuloendothelial system as long as the host cell remains normal. Viruses do not infect circulating erythrocytes, which are enucleated, metabolically impoverished cells, unsuitable for virus replication. Colorado tick fever virus (Table 8) is present inside circulating erythrocytes, but probably as a result of having infected precursor cells in the bone marrow. Some viruses adsorb to the red cell surface, a phenomenon demonstrable *in vitro* and forming the basis for haemagglutination tests. Rubella virus haemagglutinates but is not significantly adsorbed to host erythrocytes in the infected individual. The most striking haemagglutinating viruses are those such as parainfluenza and influenza, infecting the respiratory tract. The haemagglutinating factor (haemagglutinin) is a protein subunit on the surface of the virus particle and is the mechanism by which virus adsorbs to specific receptors on susceptible respiratory epithelial cells. Red blood cells happen to have the same receptors, and therefore the viruses cause haemagglutination. Transient viraemias rarely occur in parainfluenza and influenza infections, and would presumably be partly red cell associated. Carriage on red blood cells is a feature of certain arthropod-borne virus infections. Rickettsia are often carried on red blood cells as well in the plasma.

The only bacterium ever found associated with human red cells is *Bartonella bacilliformis*. This occurs in Peru and causes oroya fever, a disease with acute haemolytic anaemia, transmitted by sandflies. Red blood cells are of particular importance in malaria. The malaria parasite lives in the red blood cell, breaking down and utilizing the haemoglobin as it grows and divides, and up to 30 progeny parasites called merozoites are liberated from each red cell into the blood. Within a very short time the liberated merozoites have entered and infected another set of red blood cells by a process which seems similar to phagocytosis although it is not completely understood (see p. 88). During their brief extracellular period in the blood, merozoites are exposed to host antimicrobial forces, but the parasites in red blood cells are protected from the phagocytic reticuloendothelial cells, circulating antibodies and sensitized lymphocytes (see Ch. 6) that might otherwise inactivate or eliminate them. The red cells maintain the parasite in the blood and produce the sexual forms that must be ingested by the transmitting species of mosquitoes. The parasitized red cells undergo various changes before they are lysed. During passage through capillaries they are not deformed as easily as normal red cells and they also adhere more readily to vascular endothelium. As a result of this, and particularly in one type of malaria (*Plasmodium falciparum*), there is a piling up ("sludging") of red cells in the small vessels of various organs, leading to local anoxia and tissue damage. In the brain this gives rise to the serious complication of cerebral malaria. Immunological events are of great importance in malaria (see Ch. 8) and the host–parasite relationship is complex. Each parasitic form is highly differentiated with many antigenic constituents. Parasitized red cells are lysed immunologically, and at times there is large-scale destruction of red cells, including normal ones, the suddenly released haemoglobin spilling over into the urine to give "blackwater fever".

Platelet associated

Platelets are phagocytic and, given the chance, are capable of ingesting microorganisms, but this is not important in infectious diseases. Viruses such as leukaemia viruses and LCM virus in carrier mice infect megakaryocytes, and therefore the circulating platelets derived from these cells are infected. The infected platelets, however, do not appear to be damaged. Microbial transport by platelets is likewise unimportant. Infected platelets could accumulate at a site of blood vessel injury, but they normally remain intravascular.

Reticuloendothelial system (RES)

Macrophages are present in all major compartments of the body, and those lining the sinusoids in the liver, spleen, bone marrow and adrenals monitor the blood, removing foreign particles, microorganisms or effete host cells.

These macrophages consitute the reticuloendothelial system, and the liver macrophages (Kupffer cells) are quantitatively the most important component of the system.* Many studies have been made of the function of reticuloendothelial macrophages, as determined by the removal from the blood of intravenously injected dyes, marker particles such as carbon, viruses and bacteria. Microorganisms entering the circulation, as long as they are free in the plasma, are exposed to phagocytosis by these macrophages. Phagocytosis is influenced by a variety of factors. Larger particles are phagocytosed ("cleared" from the blood) more rapidly than small particles, and many larger viruses and bacteria are cleared completely after a single passage through the liver, so that more than 90% of intravenously injected particles disappear from the blood within a few minutes.† Serum factors can be important, specific antibodies to a microorganism and complement (p. 147) promoting clearance by opsonization (see Fig. 19). Clearance also depends on the nature of the microbial surface (see Ch. 4) and on the physiological state of the macrophages (see "macrophage activation", p. 144). If microorganisms are cleared from the blood, the behaviour of the microorganism in the macrophages becomes of considerable importance. Killing of the microorganism could mean termination of the infection, whereas microbial persistence and growth in the macrophage could lead to infection in the organ harbouring the macrophages, with reseeding of progeny microorganisms into the blood.

Because of their phagocytic activity reticuloendothelial macrophages are inevitably involved in many systemic infections. Foci of infection in liver, spleen and sometimes the bone marrow are features of brucellosis, leptospirosis and typhoid in man. The role of the reticuloendothelial system can be illustrated by examples of the encounter of viruses with liver macrophages. Viruses infecting the liver usually do so by way of the blood, and since the macrophages (Kupffer cells) lining the liver sinusoids form a functionally complete barrier between blood and hepatic cells, no virus has

---

*Macrophages lining the sinusoids in the spleen account for about one-tenth of the total clearance capacity of the RES. After a circulating microorganism or antigen has been phagocytosed by a splenic macrophage, antigenic materials are presented to neighbouring lymphocytes by antigen-presenting cells and an immune response is initiated. Phagocytosis by a liver macrophage, on the other hand, does not have this immunological consequence, except when they are lymphocyte infiltrates (usually periportal) in the liver.

†(See Fig. 19.) Even large numbers of circulating bacteria can be dealt with very effectively by reticuloendothelial macrophages in the normal host. The antibacterial capacity of the peritoneal cavity, by comparison, is poor. If virulent encapsulated pneumococci are injected intravenously into mice about 100 000 bacteria are needed to cause death, but a single bacterium is lethal by the intraperitoneal route. Presumably this is partly because serum factors are important, and partly because there is less efficient phagocytosis in the peritoneal cavity than in a small blood vessel, and the bacteria therefore have more opportunity to multiply.

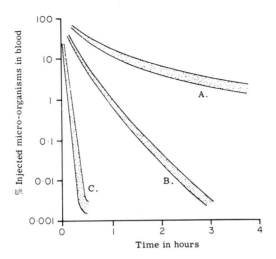

Fig. 19. Clearance of microorganisms from the blood. A, encapsulated pneumococcus or small virus (e.g. T$_7$ bacteriophage, 30 nm diameter). B, encapsulated pneumococcus coated with antibody in complement-depleted animal. C, encapsulated pneumococcus coated with antibody or nonencapsulated bacterium (e.g. *Salmonella*) or large virus (e.g. *Vaccinia*, 250 nm diameter) in normal animals.

access to hepatic cells except through macrophages. There are also distinct endothelial cells lining sinusoids, but the Kupffer cells, being professional phagocytes, are particularly important. Uptake by these cells is a necessary first step in infection of the liver. The *types of virus–macrophage interaction in the liver* can be classified as follows (see Fig. 20):

(a) No uptake by macrophages. This has been described for a few viruses, such as LCM virus from congenitally infected mice, and favours persistence of the viraemia.

(b) Uptake and destruction in macrophages. This is the fate of most viruses circulating in the plasma. If viraemia is to be maintained as much virus must enter the blood as is removed. Thus, in many arthropod-borne virus infections, there must be extensive seeding of virus into the blood to make up for clearance by macrophages and to maintain blood virus levels for ingestion by mosquitoes. Uptake of viruses by reticuloendothelial macrophages is rapid compared with the time taken for localization in capillary vessels in other parts of the body. Hence, if neurotropic viruses such as polio are to reach the central nervous system from the blood, viraemia must be maintained for a period long enough to allow viral localization in cerebral capillaries (see below). As long as virus is being cleared from the blood, a high rate of viral entry into the

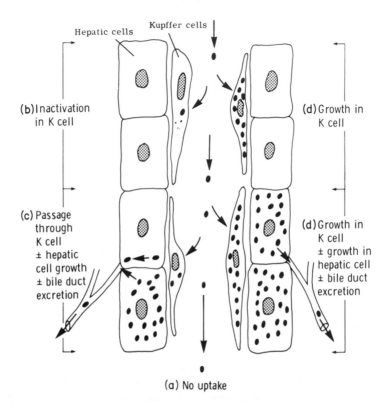

Fig. 20. Diagram to show types of virus behaviour in liver. Endothelial cells have been omitted, as their role is less clear.

blood must be maintained. Experimentally, viraemias can be prolonged and intensified by reducing the rate of virus clearance by reticuloendothelial cells. This is called reticuloendothelial "blockade", and it can be done, for instance, by injecting silica or colloidal thorum dioxide (thorotrast) intravenously. These substances are taken up by reticuloendothelial cells and interfere with their phagocytic activity.

(c) Uptake and passive transfer from macrophages to hepatic cells. Circulating virus particles are taken up by Kupffer cells but fail to establish infection and are passively carried across Kupffer and endothelial cells and presented to adjacent hepatic cells. If the virus cannot then grow in hepatic cells things go no further, although sometimes the hepatic cells excrete virus into the bile. Viruses that infect hepatic cells, however, have an opportunity to cause hepatitis, in spite of their inability to infect macrophages. This is so for certain arthropod-borne viruses such as Rift

Valley Fever virus (see p. 188), and probably for hepatitis A and hepatitis B.

(d) Uptake and growth in macrophages and/or endothelial cells. When this occurs, the progeny virus particles are released in proximity to hepatic cells (Fig. 20d) and hepatitis again becomes a possibility. Liver infection in smallpox and yellow fever is probably caused in this way.

This scheme gives a logical pathogenic background for the development of viral hepatitis, and the possibilities apply also to liver infection by the other microorganisms that grow inside cells. The infection may be restricted to macrophages (*Leishmania donovani*), or involve hepatic cells as with the exoerythrocytic stages of malaria, but microbial behaviour in the liver macrophage will exercise a determining influence on the infection, just as with virus infections. Microorganisms that can grow extracellularly, on the other hand, merely need to lodge in a liver sinusoid and grow. If taken up by a macrophage or a polymorph, their virulence is increased if they destroy the ingesting cell. This will result in an infectious focus containing necrotic cells, with a surrounding zone of inflammatory polymorphs, lymphocytes and macrophages. Such a pattern of liver involvement is seen with the hepatitis produced by *Entamoeba histolytica* or *Leptospira icterohaemorrhagica*.

Haematogenous spread and the nature of the vascular bed

If a circulating microorganism is to invade a tissue without sinusoids, it must first adhere to the endothelium of blood vessels in this tissue, preferably capillaries or venules, where the circulation is slowest and the vessel wall thinnest. The microorganism can then reach tissues by leaking through the vessel wall, being passively ferried across the vessel wall, or by growing through the vessel wall. These alternatives have been studied carefully only in the case of virus infections, especially in relation to the blood–brain junction (see Fig. 10, p. 57). The anatomical nature of the obstacles separating blood from tissue is obviously important. It constitutes the blood–tissue barrier, but because it is not necessarily a barrier it will be referred to as the blood–tissue junction. Protection of tissues from invasion by circulating microorganisms depends to some extent on the anatomical nature of the blood–tissue junction. One of the most important barriers to the spread of virus into an organ is a layer of insusceptible cells that cannot be infected, either the capillary endothelium itself or other cells in extravascular tissues. Even if vascular endothelium is infected, subsequent events may be determined by the topography of budding (see pp. 51–2). Viruses released exclusively from the lumenal surface of the cell would contribute to a viraemia, but unless the cell was destroyed, tissue invasion would depend on liberation of virus from the tissue side of the endothelial cell.

The walls of the sinusoids are lined by macrophages, giving direct access to endothelial or neighbouring tissue cells, as in the case of the liver referred to above. Similar cells line the sinusoids of the spleen and bone marrow, and even when the lining is not complete as seen by electron microscopy, the highly phagocytic cells ensure that it is functionally complete under most circumstances.

Capillaries in the central nervous system, connective tissue, skeletal and cardiac muscles are lined by a continuous layer of endothelium whereas those in the renal glomerulus, pancreas, choroid plexus, ileum and colon have fenestrated gaps in the endothelium (Fig. 10, p. 57). Once micro-organisms have localized in the vessel wall, passage across the endothelium might be expected to be easier when there are fenestrated gaps. In all cases, however, there is a well-defined basement membrane which must also be negotiated if microorganisms are to reach extravascular tissues. The complexity of the basement membrane differs in different organs, but it is less well developed when capillaries are growing ("sprouting") during foetal development or during repair after injury. Since the endothelial cells are not highly phagocytic, localization in capillaries is slow compared with that in the reticuloendothelial cells lining sinusoids. Circulating microorganisms localize readily on the "sticky" capillary endothelium in inflamed areas, but for localization in normal capillaries they must circulate in the blood for long enough and in high enough concentration. Therefore the faster the clearance of viruses from the blood by reticuloendothelial cells the less chance there is for localization in capillaries. Removal of circulating viruses by reticuloendothelial cells, or their inactivation by serum antibody and complement, constitutes the most important barrier to invasion of those organs that have a capillary bed. In a capillary which is not "sprouting" (see above) or inflamed, initial localization of virus presumably depends on attachment to receptors on endothelial cells. Are there differences between capillaries from different organs? Now that endothelial cells from capillaries as well as from large vessels can be cultured *in vitro*, these matters are being investigated.

Removal of circulating bacteria, protozoa etc. by reticuloendothelial cells tends to ensure their localization in the liver, spleen and bone marrow. As with viruses, however, almost nothing is known about the factors governing localization in particular capillary beds. The fact that circulating meningococci tend to localize in meninges, *Salmonella typhi* in the gall bladder and African trypanosomes in the cerebrospinal fluid (sleeping sickness) is of supreme importance, but the reasons for this localization remain wrapped in mystery. Perhaps there are subtle differences in the nature of the capillary beds, or perhaps there is localization in all parts of the body but only some sites provide suitable conditions for microbial growth. Positive activity on the part of a microorganism that is motile may determine localization in a given capillary bed. For instance, the South American trypanosome causing Chagas' disease leaves the blood stream by actively penetrating the capillary wall, nonflagellated end first. The heart, skeletal and smooth muscle, are particularly affected, but the reasons for localization here are not understood. Circulating microorganisms tend to localize more readily in abnormal, inflamed or growing tissues, presumably because of the state of the capillary bed. For instance, circulating gonococci, staphylococci etc. localize more frequently and cause septic arthritis in joints affected by rheumatoid arthritis or other pathological conditions, and circulating staphylococci localize in the growing ends of long bones in young people. The larger bacteria, fungi or protozoa may be large enough to be trapped mechanically in normal capillaries. Tissue invasion is made easier if there is preliminary multiplication or toxin production in the capillary lumen with damage to the vessel wall.

Central nervous system

Circulating viruses often localize more readily in the brains of immature than of adult animals. This is associated with sustained viraemia in the immature host, partly due to increased entry of virus into the blood from peripheral growth sites, and partly to less active reticuloendothelial clearance. Also it may be easier for viruses to traverse the blood–brain junction in the immature host because the basement membrane tends to be much thinner. Certain viruses grow through the walls of cerebral capillaries (herpes simplex, yellow fever, measles) and others leak through or are ferried across (polio). Many capillaries are enveloped by "feet" from glial cells (Fig. 10, p. 57) and the glial feet must be traversed before there can be infection of neurons. A few viruses infect only neurons (rabies) or glial cells (JC virus)* but most viruses that grow in the brain infect both types of cell. Viral encephalitis in man is rare, however, even though the potential viraemic invaders are numerous.

*There is a rare neurological condition in man called progressive multifocal leuco-encephalopathy. A papovavirus (JC virus) has been isolated from the brains of patients, and oligodendroglial cells in the brain are seen by electron microscopy to contain large numbers of virus particles. A related virus (BK virus) has been isolated from the urinary tract of pregnant women and immunosuppressed patients. Most adults have at some time been infected with these viruses because they have antibodies, but little is known about the primary infection and whether or not there is an associated illness.

Bacterial meningitis due to meningococci, pneumococci, *Haemophilus influenza* or *Mycobacterium tuberculosis*, is a tragic and often lethal disease, expecially in developing countries. Almost nothing is known of the factors promoting bacterial localization and invasion across meningeal blood vessels.*

Skeletal and cardiac muscle

Certain viruses infect skeletal or cardiac muscle after passage across the vessel walls, particularly coxsackieviruses, cardioviruses and certain arthropod-borne viruses. This occurs readily in the immature experimental host, and in man coxsackievirus infections can cause severe striated muscle or cardiac involvement. The trypanosomes causing Chaga's disease leave the blood and selectively parasitize the heart, skeletal and smooth muscle (see above), but it is not known how this is done. Circulating bacteria (e.g. the *Streptococcus viridans* group) may localize on abnormal heart valves and cause endocarditis.

The skin

The skin is involved in many systemic infections (Table 9). Rashes are produced after microorganisms or antigens have localized in skin blood vessels, sometimes spreading extravascularly. We do not know why the rash has such a characteristic distribution in many infectious diseases. Inflammation can certainly localize skin lesions, whether produced by sunburn, a tight garter, or pre-existing eczema, but the factors accounting for the characteristic distribution of the rash in chickenpox, smallpox, or hand, foot and mouth disease (caused by certain coxsackie A viruses) remain unknown. The blood–skin junction consists of the endothelial cells forming a continuous lining to dermal capillaries, together with a basement membrane. There may be a fibroblastic cell applied to the basement membrane, and between the capillary and the epidermis lies the connective tissue matrix containing scattered fibroblasts and histiocytes. The skin has its own immune cells, particularly Langerhan's cells (see p. 123), many mast cells (see p. 131), and recirculatory T cells are always present in the dermis.

The skin of man is mostly naked, and is an important thermoregulatory organ, under finely balanced nervous control. It is a turbulent, highly

*The meningococcus, for instance, is present in the oropharynx of 5–30% of normal people, but very occasionally it invades the blood stream, perhaps because of a genetically determined weakness in the capacity to form circulating bactericidal antibodies, and then it has the opportunity to localize, by unknown mechanisms, in meningeal blood vessels and infect the cerebrospinal fluid (see "Vaccines" chapter).

Table 9. Principal rashes in infectious disease in man

Microorganism	Disease	Features
Measles virus	Measles	Very characteristic maculo-papular rash
Rubella virus	German measles	
Echoviruses 4, 6, 9, 16	} Not distinguishable	} Maculopapular rashes not distinguishable clinically
Coxsackie viruses A9, 16, 23		
Varicella-zoster virus	Chickenpox, zoster	
Variola virus	Smallpox	} Vesicular rashes
Coxsackie virus A 16	Hand, foot and mouth disease	
Rickettsia prowazeki and others	Typhus	} Macular or haemorrhagic rash
Rickettsia rickettsiae and others	Spotted fever group of diseases	
Streptococcus pyogenes	Scarlet fever	Erythematous rash caused by toxin
Streptococcus pyogenes	} Impetigo	Vesicles, forming crusts, especially in children
Staphylococcus pyogenes		
Treponema pallidum	Syphilis	} Disseminated infectious rash seen in secondary stage, 2–3 months after infection
Treponema pertenue	Yaws	
Salmonella typhi	} Enteric fever	Sparse rose spots containing bacteria
Salmonella paratyphi B		
Neisseria meningitidis	Spotted fever	Petechial or maculopapular lesions containing bacteria
Dermatophytes (skin fungi)	Dermatophytid or allergic rash	Rash represents hyper-sensitivity to fungal antigens
Blastomyces dermatitidis	Blastomycosis	Papule or pustule develops into granuloma; lesions contain organisms
Leishmania tropica	Cutaneous leishmaniasis	Papules, usually ulcerating to form crusted sores; infectious

reactive tissue, and local inflammatory events are commonplace. At sites of inflammation circulating microorganisms readily localize in small blood vessels and pass across the endothelium. The skin of most animals, in contrast, is largely covered with fur. Skin lesions are a feature of many infectious diseases of animals, but these lesions tend to be on exposed hairless areas where the skin has the human properties of thickness, sensitivity and vascular reactivity. Hence, although virus rashes very occasionally involve the general body surface of animals, it is udders, scrotums, ears, prepuces, teats, noses and paws that are more regular sites of lesions.

For instance, the closely related diseases of measles, distemper and rinder-pest can be compared. Cattle with rinderpest may show areas of red moist skin with occasional vesiculation on the udder, scrotum and inside the thighs. In dogs with distemper the exanthem often occurs on the abdomen and inner aspects of the thighs. Yet in human measles there is one of the most florid and characteristic rashes known, involving the general body surface. Even in susceptible monkeys, the same virus produces skin lesions sparingly and irregularly.

Macules and papules are formed when there is inflammation in the dermis, with or without a significant cellular infiltration, the infection generally being confined to the vascular bed or its immediate vicinity. Immunological factors (see Ch. 8) are often important in the production of inflammation. Measles virus, for instance, localizes in skin blood vessels, but the maculopapular rash does not appear unless there is an adequate immune response. Virus by itself does little damage to the blood vessels or the skin, and the interaction of sensitized lymphocytes or antibodies with viral antigen is needed to generate the inflammatory response that causes the skin lesion. Rickettsia characteristically localize and grow in the endothelium of small blood vessels, and the striking rashes seen in typhus and Rocky Mountain Spotted Fever are a result of endothelial swelling, thrombosis, small infarcts and haemorrhages. The immune response adds to the pathological result. Vascular endothelium is an important site of replication and shedding of viruses and rickettsias that are transmitted by blood-sucking arthropods and which must therefore be shed into the blood. After replication in vascular endothelium, they may be shed not only back into the vessel lumen, but also from the external surface of the endothelial cell into extravascular tissues (see also pp. 109–110). Certain arthropod-borne viruses replicate in muscle or other extravascular tissues, and can then reach the blood after passage through the lymphatic system.

Circulating immune complexes consisting of antibody plus microbial antigen also localize in dermal blood vessels, accounting for the trichophytid rashes of fungal infections and the prodromal rashes seen at the end of the incubation period in many exanthematous virus diseases. Antibodies to soluble viral antigens appear towards the end of the incubation period in people infected with hepatitis B virus and form soluble immune complexes. These localize in the skin causing fleeting rashes and pruritis, and rarely the more severe vascular lesions of periarteritis nodosa (see Ch. 8).

Certain microbial toxins enter the circulation, localize in skin blood vessels, and cause damage and inflammation without the need for an immune response. An erythrogenic toxin is liberated from strains of *Strep-tococcus pyogenes* carrying the bacteriophage β, and the toxin enters the blood, localizes in dermal vessels, and gives rise to the striking rash of scarlet fever.

Vesicles and pustules are formed when the microorganism leaves dermal blood vessels and is able to spread to the superficial layers of the skin. Inflammatory fluids accumulate to give vesicles, which are focal blisters of the superficial skin layers. Virus infections with vesicles include smallpox, varicella, herpes simplex and certain coxsackievirus infections. The circulating virus localizes in dermal blood vessels, grows through the endothelium (herpes, varicella) and spreads across dermal tissues to infect the epidermis and cause focal necrosis. Only viruses capable of extravascular spread and epidermal infection can cause vesicles. Inevitably there is an immunopathological contribution to the lesion, although a primary destructive action on epidermal cells give a lesion without the need for the immune response, as with the oral lesions seen in animals as early as two days after infection with foot and mouth disease virus. A secondary infiltration of leucocytes into the virus-rich vesicle turns it into a pustule which later bursts, dries, scabs and heals. Such viruses are shed to the exterior from the skin lesion. Certain other microorganisms are shed to the exterior after extravasation from dermal blood vessels. They multiply in extravascular tissues and form inflammatory swellings in the skin, which then break down so that infectious material is discharged to the exterior. This occurs and gives rise to striking skin lesions in the secondary stages of syphilis and yaws (caused by the closely related bacteria *Treponema pallidum* and *pertenue*) and is also seen in a systemic fungus infection (blastomycosis) and a protozoal infection (cutaneous leishmaniasis). In patients with leprosy, *Mycobacterium leprae* circulating in the blood localizes and multiplies in the skin, and for unknown reasons superficial peripheral nerves are often involved. The skin lesions do not break down, although large numbers of bacteria are shed from sites of growth on the nasal mucosa. Bacterial growth is favoured by the slightly lower temperature of the skin and nasal mucosa.

Almost all the factors that have been discussed in relation to skin localization and skin lesions apply also to the mucosae of the mouth, throat, bladder, vagina etc. In these sites the wet surface means that the vesicles will break down and form ulcers earlier than on the dry skin. Hence in measles the foci in the mouth break down and form small visible ulcers (Koplik's spots) a day or so before the skin lesions have appeared. Similar considerations apply to the localization of microorganisms and their antigens on the other surfaces of the body (see Fig. 2, p. 9). In smallpox and measles circulating virus localizes in subepithelial vessels in the respiratory tract and after extravasation there is only a single layer of cells to grow through in the nearby epithelium before the discharge of virus to the exterior. Hence in these infections the secretions from the respiratory tract are infectious a few days before the skin rash appears and the disease becomes recognizable. Much less is known about the localization of circulating microorganisms in the intestinal tract. Probably localization here is not often of great importance, but this is a difficult surface of the body to study. In typhoid, secondary intestinal localization of bacteria takes place following excretion of bacteria in bile, rather than from blood. Virus localization in the intestinal tract is a feature in rinderpest in cattle but occurs only to a minor extent in measles. When the patient with measles suffers from protein deficiency, however, it is more important and helps cause the diarrhoea that make measles a life-threatening infection in malnourished children (see p. 285).

The foetus

The blood–foetal junction in the placenta is an important pathway for infection of the foetus. The number of cells separating maternal from foetal blood depends not only on the species of animal, there being four cell sheets for instance in the horse and only one or two in man, but also on the stage of pregnancy. The junction usually becomes thinner, often with fewer cell layers, in later pregnancy. There are regular mechanical leaks in the placenta late in most human pregnancies, and up to 4.0 ml of blood is transferred across the placenta, but this appears to be principally in one direction, from foetus to mother. There is little evidence for the passive carriage of microorganisms across the placenta, and foetal infection takes place by either of two mechanisms. If a circulating microorganism, free or cell associated, localizes in the maternal vessels it can multiply, produce toxins, locally interrupt the integrity of the junction and thus infect the foetus. *Treponema pallidum* and *Toxoplasma gondii* presumably infect the human foetus in this way. Alternatively, a circulating microorganism can localize and grow across the placental junction. This occurs with rubella and cytomegalovirus infections of the human foetus. In both instances, a placental lesion or focus of infection occurs before foetal invasion. The microorganisms causing foetal damage are listed in Table 10 (see also p. 250). These, however, are special cases, and special microorganisms. Nearly always the foetus is protected from microbial as well as from biochemical and physical insults. The factors that localize microorganisms in the placenta are not understood, but blood flow is slow in placental vessels, as in sinusoids, giving maximal opportunities for localization. Once microorganisms are arrested in placental vessels, their growth may be favoured by particular substances that are present in the placenta. Erythritol promotes the growth of *Brucella abortus*, and its presence in the bovine placenta makes this a target organ in infected cows. Susceptibility of infected cattle to abortion thus has a biochemical basis. Microorganisms can damage the foetus without invading foetal tissues. If they localize extensively in placental vessels and cause primarily vascular damage this of course can lead to foetal anoxia, death and abortion. Also the toxic products of microbial growth in

Table 10. Principal microorganisms infecting the foetus

Microorganisms	Species	Effect
Viruses		
Rubella virus	Man	Abortion
		Still birth
		Malformations
Cytomegalovirus	Man	Malformations
Hog cholera virus (vaccine strain)	Pigs	Malformations
Bluetongue virus (vaccine strain)	Sheep	Stillbirths, CNS disease
Equine rhinopneumonitis	Horse	Abortion
Bovine diarrhoea—mucosal disease virus	Cow	Cerebellar hypoplasia
Malignment catarrh virus	Wildebeest	Foetus unharmed
Bacteria		
Treponema pallidum	Man	Stillbirth, malformations
Listeria monocytogenes	Man	Meningoencephalitis
Vibrio fetus	Sheep, cattle	Abortion
Protozoa		
Toxoplasma gondii	Man	Stillbirth, CNS disease

the placenta or elsewhere can reach the foetus and cause damage, and high fever and biochemical disturbances in a pregnant female can adversely affect the foetus.

Miscellaneous sites

There are certain other sites where circulating microorganisms selectively localize. In rats and other animals infected with *Leptospira*, circulating bacteria localize particularly in capillaries in the kidney, and give rise to a chronic local lesion. Infectious bacteria are discharged in large numbers into the urine, which is therefore a source of human infection. Microorganisms that are discharged in the saliva (most herpes-type virus infections in man, rabies in dogs) must localize and grow in salivary glands. Those that are discharged in milk must localize and grow in mammary glands (the mammary tumour virus in mice and *Brucella*, tubercle bacilli, and Q fever rickettsia in cows). A few examples, such as *Haemophilus suis* in pigs and occasionally rubella virus in man, localize in joints. Almost any site in the body, from the feather follicles (Marek's disease) to testicles or epididymis (mumps in man, the relevant *Brucella* species in rams, boars, bulls) can at times be infected. Nothing is known of the mechanism of localization in these organs.

Spread via other Pathways

Cerebrospinal fluid (CSF)

Microorganisms in the blood can reach the CSF by traversing the blood–CSF junction in the meninges or choroid plexus. Capillaries in the choroid plexus have fenestrated endothelium and are surrounded by a loose connective tissue stroma (Fig. 10, p. 57). Inert virus-sized particles and bacteriophages leak into the CSF when very large amounts are injected into the blood. It is assumed that the viruses causing aseptic meningitis in man (polio-, echo-, coxsackie, lymphocytic choriomeningitis and mumps viruses) enter the CSF by leakage or growth across this junction (Fig. 21). Once in the CSF microorganisms are passively carried with the flow of fluid from ventricles to subarachnoid spaces and throughout the neuraxis within a short time. Invasion of the brain itself and spinal cord can now take place across the ependymal lining of the ventricles and spinal canal, or across the pia mater in the subarachnoid spaces. Nonviral microorganisms entering the CSF across the blood–CSF junction include the meningococcus, the tubercle bacillus, *Listeria monocytogenes*, *Haemophilus influenzae*, *Streptococcus pneumoniae*, and the fungus *Cryptococcus neoformans*.

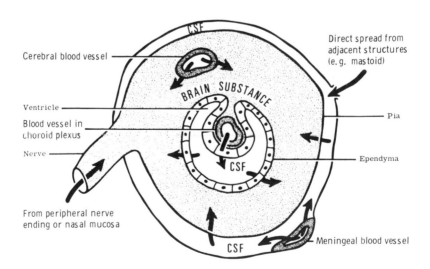

Fig. 21. Routes of microbial invasion of the central nervous system. CSF = cerebrospinal fluid.

Pleural and peritoneal cavities

Rapid spread of microorganisms from one visceral organ to another can take place via the peritoneal or pleural cavity. Entry into the peritoneal cavity takes place from an injury or focus of infection in an abdominal organ. The peritoneal cavity, as if in expectation of such events, is lined by macrophages and contains an antimicrobial armoury, the omentum. The omentum, originating from fused folds of mesentery, contains mast cells and lymphocytes, macrophages and their precursors in a fatty connective tissue matrix. It is movable in the peritoneal cavity and becomes attached at sites of inflammation.* Microorganisms spread rapidly in the peritoneal cavity unless they are taken up and destroyed in macrophages or inflammatory polymorphs. Peritoneal contents drain into lymphatics opening onto the abdominal surface of the diaphragm, so that microorganisms or their toxins are delivered to retrosternal lymph nodes in the thorax, sometimes with slight leakage into the pleural cavity. Inflammatory responses in the peritoneum eventually result in fibrinous exudates and the adherence of neighbouring surfaces, which tends to prevent microbial spread.

Microbes entering the pleural cavity from chest wounds or from foci of infection in the underlying lung have a similar opportunity to spread rapidly. During pneumonia the overlying pleural surface first becomes inflamed, causing pleurisy, and later often infected. Pleurisy occurs in about 25% cases of pneumococcal pneumonia. The pleural cavity, like the peritoneal cavity, is lined by macrophages.

Nerves

For many years peripheral nerves have been recognized as important pathways for the spread of certain viruses and toxins from peripheral parts of the body to the central nervous system (Fig. 21). Rabies, herpes simplex and related viruses travel along nerves at up to 10 mm h^{-1}, but the exact pathway in the nerve was for many years a matter of doubt and debate. Herpes simplex virus, following primary infection in the skin or the mouth, enters the sensory nerves and reaches the trigeminal ganglion (see Ch. 10). Here it remains in latent form until it is reactivated in later life by fever, exposure to sunlight, emotional or other factors. The infection then travels down the nerve to reach the region of the mouth where the skin is once again infected giving rise to a virus-rich cold sore. A similar sequence of events

---

* Because of its ability to attach to sites of inflammation and infection or to foreign bodies the omentum has been referred to as the "abdominal policeman".

explains the occurrence of zoster long after infection with varicella virus. In cattle or pigs infected with pseudorabies, another herpes virus, the infection also travels up peripheral nerves to reach dorsal root ganglia, causing a spontaneous discharge of nerve impulses from affected sensory neurons, and giving rise to the signs of "mad itch". Another herpes virus (B virus) is often present in the saliva of apparently healthy rhesus monkeys, and people bitten by infected monkeys develop a frequently fatal encephalitis, the virus reaching the brain by ascending peripheral nerves from the inoculation site. Rabies virus slowly reaches the central nervous system along peripheral nerves following a bite delivered by an infected fox, jackal, skunk or vampire bat. Poliovirus was long thought to reach the central nervous system via peripheral nerves, but this was a conclusion from studies with artificially neuroadapted strains of virus. In natural infections poliovirus traverses the blood–brain junction (Fig. 10, p. 57). Peripheral nerves are affected in leprosy, the bacteria growing in perineural and epineural cells. This causes a very slow and insidious degeneration of the nerve, but it is certainly not a pathway for the spread of infection. Peripheral nerves are known to transport tetanus toxin to the central nervous system (see Ch. 8).

Possible pathways along nerves include sequential infection of Schwann cells, transit along the tissue spaces between nerve fibres, and carriage up the axon (Fig. 22). The last route is probably an important one, although at first sight it might seem less likely. There is a small but significant movement of marker proteins up normal axons from the periphery to the central nervous system, and in experimental herpes simplex and rabies infections virus particles have been seen in axons by electron microscopy. In experimental infections herpes viruses can also travel in nerves by sequential infection of the Schwann cells associated with myelin sheaths, but this is not a natural route.

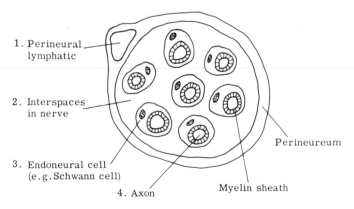

1. Perineural lymphatic

2. Interspaces in nerve

Perineureum

3. Endoneural cell (e.g. Schwann cell)

4. Axon

Myelin sheath

Fig. 22. Possible pathways of virus spread in peripheral nerves.

An alternative neural route of spread to the central nervous system is by the olfactory nerves. Axons of olfactory neurons terminate on the olfactory mucosa, the dendrites projecting beyond the mucosal surface giving a direct anatomical connection between the exterior and the olfactory bulbs in the brain. This route of infection, although at one time a popular postulate, is not often important. Aerosol infection with rabies virus (from the excreta of bats in caves in North America) presumably involves this route, but the anatomical pathway is not clear. *Naegleria fowleri*, a free-living amoeba that can lurk in the sludge at the bottom of freshwater pools, causes a rare but often fatal meningitis in swimmers after infecting by the olfactory route. The meningococci that live commensally in the nasopharynx of 5–10% of normal people, and occasionally cause meningitis, were once thought to spread directly upwards from the nasal mucosa, along the perineural sheaths of the olfactory nerve, and through the cribriform plate to the CSF. More probably, the bacteria invade the blood, sometimes causing petechial rashes ("spotted fever"), and reach the meninges across the blood–CSF junction.

In summary, peripheral nerves are important pathways for the spread of tetanus toxin and a few viruses to the CNS, and for the passage of certain herpes viruses between the central nervous system and the surfaces of the body. The neural route is not generally used by bacteria or other microorganisms.

References

de Voe, I. W. (1982). The meningococcus and mechanisms of pathogenicity. *Microbiol. Rev.* **46**, 162–190.

Drutz, D. J. *et al.* (1972). The continuous bacteraemia of lepromatous leprosy. *New Engl. J. Med.* **287**, 159–163.

Friedman, H. M., Macarek, E. J., MacGregor, R. A. *et al.* (1981). Virus infection of endothelial cells. *J. Infect. Dis.* **143**, 266.

Johnson, R. T. (1982). "Viral Infections of the Nervous System". Raven Press, New York.

Mims, C. A. (1964). Aspects of the pathogenesis of virus diseases. *Bact. Rev.* **28**, 30.

Mims, C. A. (1966). The pathogenesis of rashes in virus diseases. *Bact. Rev.* **30**, 739.

Mims, C. A. (1968). The pathogenesis of virus infections of the foetus. *Prog. Med. Virol.* **10**, 194.

Pearce, J. H. *et al.* (1962). The chemical basis of the virulence of *Brucella abortus* II. Erythritol, a constituent of bovine foetal fluids which stimulates the growth of *Br. abortus* in bovine phagocytes. *B. J. exp. Path.* **43**, 31–37.

6

The Immune Response to Infection

The immune response is conveniently divided into the antibody and the cell-mediated component, the latter being transferable from one individual to another by immune lymphoid cells but not by serum. Antibodies, since they can be tested and assayed without great difficulty, were the first to receive attention with the discovery of antibodies to cholera and diphtheria toxins in the 1890s. Cell-mediated immunity (CMI) in the form of delayed hypersensitivity was described more than 50 years ago, and has received intensive study in the past 20 years. Specific antibodies and CMI are induced in all infections, but the magnitude and quality of these responses varies greatly in different infections. It is not often that the microbial antigens concerned have been individually defined or identified. Generally speaking, the basic knowledge gained in the recent spectacular advances in immunology is only just beginning to be applied to infectious and parasitic diseases.

Most antigens are proteins or proteins combined with other substances, but polysaccharides and other complex molecules also function as antigens. Substances called haptens, often small molecules such as sugars, cannot by themselves stimulate antibody production but do so when coupled to a protein. An antigen stimulates the production of antibodies that react specifically with that antigen. The reaction can be thought of as similar to that between lock and key, and it is specific in the sense that antibody produced against diphtheria toxin does not react with tetanus toxin. An antibody may, however, have weaker reactivity against antigens closely related to the one that stimulated its production. For instance, antibodies produced when human serum is injected into a rabbit will not react with the serum of cows, mice or chickens, but may give a weak reaction with the serum of the gorilla and chimpanzee. The antibodies formed against a given antigen will include representatives from the three main immunoglobulin classes, IgG, IgA and IgM. A single antigen molecule may have several antigenic sites or epitopes, each of which stimulates the formation of a different antibody. Also, different immunoglobulin molecules vary in the firmness (avidity) with which they combine with the antigen, but little is known about antibody avidity in relation to infectious diseases.

The two arms of the immune response are expressed by different types of immunologically reactive lymphoid cells, divided according to their origin into B (bursa or its mammalian equivalent) and T (thymus) dependent cells. These two types of cells are both small to medium sized lymphocytes, only distinguishable by special immunological techniques. B cells are concerned with the antibody response and T cells largely with the cell-mediated immune (CMI) response. B cells bear on their surface immunoglobulin molecules that act as antigen receptors. Different B cells have different antigen-specific receptors. There are about 10^5 receptors per cell; they are spontaneously generated and when almost any antigen enters the body for the first time there will be a few B cells that react with it specifically. When this specific reaction takes place, the B cell differentiates to form a protein-synthesizing plasma cell, and also divides to form a population of cells with the same specific reactivity. B cells are present in spleen, lymph nodes and to a lesser extent in blood. T cells also have specific receptors on their surfaces (10^2–10^3 per cell) and a given T cell responds to an immunologically specific encounter with antigen by dividing, differentiating and often liberating active substances as described below, thus generating a cell mediated immune response.

The above is a simplified picture. Things are more complicated because, nearly always, appropriate responses are produced by cooperation between different types of cell. Macrophages play a central role. Those in lymphoid tissues are strategically placed to encounter microbes or their antigens, and at the same time are in close proximity to lymphoid cells. Microbes and microbial antigens from sites of infection such as the body surfaces are "focused" by afferent lymphatics into macrophages in lymph nodes (see pp. 60–61), and when these materials enter the blood they are taken up by macrophages in lymphoid areas of the spleen. Macrophages in these sites, together with certain non-phagocytic cells called dendritic cells, have a vital immunological function. They "process" microbial and other antigens and present them to immune lymphocytes.* This is separate from the antimicrobial function of macrophages described in Ch. 4 in which infectious agents

---

*Langerhan's cells in the epidermis which send dendritic processes far into the surrounding epithelium have a similar antigen-presenting function. They total 10^9 in man's skin, constituting 2–4% of all epidermal cells, and can migrate into local lymph nodes.

are phagocytosed and killed. The all-embracing word macrophage can be misleading, because not all of them act as antigen-presenting cells and it is clear that separate subpopulations of macrophages carry out the separate functions. For instance, most Kupffer cells are not antigen-presenting cells and therefore the uptake of microorganisms by these cells is generally nonproductive from an immunological point of view (see pp. 106–109).

Antigen-presenting cells (macrophages, dendritic cells, Langerhan's cells) perform their immune function by holding and displaying foreign antigens on their surface in intimate association with Class 2 MHC molecules (see Glossary) which they also carry on their surface. The recognition of a foreign antigen by a T cell, referred to above, is in fact a recognition of antigen plus Class 2 molecule on the surface of an antigen-presenting cell. After this specific recognition event certain T cells cooperate with nearby B cells which have also recognized the foreign antigen and give them the signal for differentiation, proliferation and antibody production.* These T cells, called T helper (Th) or inducer cells, also cooperate with cytotoxic (Tc) and delayed hypersensitivity (Tdth) T cells resulting in proliferation of these specifically reactive cells and generation of cytotoxic and dth cell-mediated responses. Once the response has been generated, the Tc specifically recognize and kill any cells that display the specific foreign antigen in association with Class 1 MHC molecules; specifically reactive Tdth cells, after recognizing the foreign antigen plus Class 1 or Class 2 molecules, release powerful mediators called lymphokines (see below). This simplified summary of immune responses is illustrated in Fig. 23.

When an immune response is initiated, powerful forces are set in motion, which can be advantageous or at times disastrous for the individual (see Ch. 8). So that each response can unfold in a more or less orderly fashion, it is controlled by a combination of stimulatory and inhibitory influences. The latter include antigen control, idiotype controls and suppressor systems. I shall mention these, although their relative significance is unknown. Antigen itself acts as an important regulatory agent. Following its combination with antibody and immunologically nonproductive phagocytosis (see above) it is catabolized and begins to disappear from the body. Since it is the driving force for an immune response this response dies away as antigen disappears. Immune responses can therefore be controlled by controlling the concentration and location of antigen. Both types of lymphocyte bear antigen-binding "receptors" on their surface (see above) and this "receptor" can itself act as an antigen, and is called the idiotype. Each B or T cell has an antigenically

---

*Effective antibody responses to most antigens depend on T cell cooperation, or in other words, most antigens are T-dependent. The so-called T-independent antigens include pneumococcal polysaccharides and endotoxin; IgM rather than IgG antibody is generated.

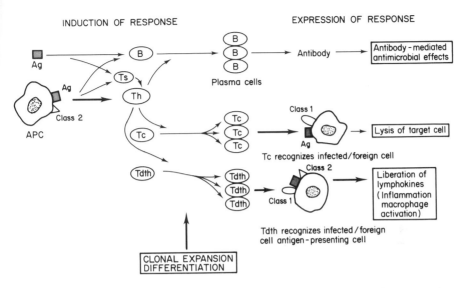

Fig. 23. Events in induction and expression of immune responses. APC = antigen-presenting cell; Ag = foreign antigen.

specific idiotype on its surface which can itself be recognized by appropriately reactive T or B cells in the same individual. This means that lymphocytes, by recognizing the idiotype that is appearing on the surface of increasing numbers of other lymphocytes during the unfolding of an immune response have the opportunity to inactivate these cells and thus control the response. The final inhibitory regulation of immune responses is provided by a distinct subclass of T cells.* These are called suppressor T cells (Ts) and operate by recognizing the antigen and interacting with the helper cells (see Fig. 23). This can lead to an antigen-specific or to a more general suppression of antibody and cell-mediated responses.

In a naturally occurring infection, the infectious dose generally consists of only a small number of microorganisms, whose content of antigen is extremely small compared with that used by immunologists, and quite insufficient on its own to provoke a detectable immune response. But the microorganism then multiplies, and this leads to a progressive and extensive increase in antigenic mass. The classical primary and secondary immune

---

*The importance of immunoregulation is illustrated by noting that many T cells, rather than poised to react with foreign antigens, are responding to signals from within the immune system.

responses merge into one (see Fig. 39, p. 309). Antibodies of various types and reactivities are produced in all microbial infections, and are directed not only against antigens present in the microorganism itself but also against the soluble products of microbial growth, and in the case of viruses against the virus-coded enzymes and other proteins formed in the infected cell during replication. Of the antigens present in the microorganism itself, the most important ones in the encounter between microorganism and host are those on the surface, directly exposed to the immune responses of the host. Responses to internal antigenic components are generally less important, although they are often of great help in detecting past infection, and may play a part in immune complex disease (see Ch. 8).

There are two other important adjuncts to the immune response. These are complement, and phagocytic cells (macrophages and polymorphs), which are described under separate headings below. Each is involved in various types of immune reactions. Antigen-presenting macrophages cooperate with specifically reactive T or B cells in the initiation of the response, as described above. Both macrophages and polymorphs, together with complement, amplify and give expression to the response in tissues.

Antibody Response

Types of immunoglobulin

By the time they reach adult life all animals, including man, have been exposed to a wide variety of infectious agents and have produced antibodies (immunoglobulins) to most of them. Serum immunoglobulin levels reflect this extensive and universal natural process of immunization. The different classes of immunoglobulin, with some of their properties, are shown in Table 11. All are glycoproteins. The major circulating type of antibody is immunoglobulin G (IgG). It has the basic four-chain immunoglobulin structure in the shape of a Y, as illustrated in Fig. 24, and a molecular weight of 150 000. The molecule is composed of two heavy and two light polypeptide chains held together by disulphide bonds. For a given IgG molecule the two light chains are either kappa ($\varkappa$) or lambda (λ), and both heavy chains are gamma (γ). The antigen-reactive ends of the light and heavy chains have a unique amino acid sequence for a given antibody molecule and are responsible for its specificity, while the rest of the chains are identical throughout a given class of antibody. The molecule can be split into three parts by papain digestion. Two of these (Fab) represent the arms of the Y and contain the

Table 11. Properties of immunoglobulin classes in man

Property	IgG	IgM	IgAᵃ	IgE	IgD
Mol. wt	150 000	900 000	385 000 (170 000)	190 000	180 000
Heavy chain	γ	μ	α	ε	δ
Half-life (days)[b]	25	5	(6)[c]	2	2.8
Percentage of total immunoglobulin	80	6	(13)	0.002	0–1
Complement fixation	+	++	±	–	–
Transfer to offspring	Via placenta	No transfer	Via milk	No transfer	No transfer
Proportion in:					
blood	50–60%	90+%	0	V. low	90+%
extracellular fluids	40–50%	<10%	0	–	–
secretions	0[d]	0[d]	100%	High	0[d]
Functional significance	Major systemic immunoglobulin	Appears early in immune response Appears early in development	Present on mucosal surfaces	Allergenic responses e.g. epithelial surfaces	Unknown; most of it present on surface of B cells

[a] Data for secretory IgA; serum IgA in parentheses. In human serum this antibody is mainly a monomer.
[b] Half-life generally shorter for smaller animals.
[c] Strictly speaking, the half-life of secretory IgA on mucosal surfaces is measured in minutes rather than days, because it is soon carried away in secretions of mucus.
[d] Can be increased in inflammation, IgA deficiency.

127

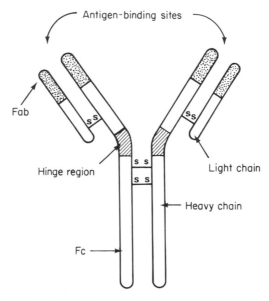

region with variable amino acid sequence in heavy and light chains, conferring antigen specificity.

region with costant amino acid sequence.

Hinge region enables arms to swing out to 180° and bridge antigenic sites. Papain digestion of molecule yields two Fab (fragment antigen-binding) portions, and one Fc (fragment crystalizable) portion which confers biological activity on the molecule (placental passage, binding to phagocytes, etc.).

Fig. 24. Basic Y-shaped (4 chain) structure of immunoglobulin G molecule.

antigen-reactive sites; the third part (Fc) has no antigen-reactive sites but carries the chemical groupings that activate complement and combine with receptors on the surface of polymorphs and macrophages (see below). This last activity of the Fc fragment mediates attachment of antibody coated microorganisms to the phagocyte, giving the antibody opsonic activity. The Fc fragment also contains the groupings responsible for the transport of IgG across the placenta of some mammals. IgG can pass the placenta in primates, including man, but not in rodents, cows, sheep, or pigs. Most IgG antibody is in the blood, but it is also present in smaller concentrations in extravascular tissues including lymph, peritoneal, synovial and cerebrospinal fluids. Its concentration in tissue fluids is always increased as soon as there is inflammation, or when it is being synthesized locally. There are four subclasses of IgG in man, which differ in heavy chains and in biological properties such as placental passage, complement fixation and binding to phagocytes. The amounts present in serum are also different but almost nothing is known of their relative importance in infectious diseases.

IgM is a polymer of five subunits, each with the basic four-chain structure but with a different heavy chain (μ), and has a molecular weight of 900 000. Because it is such a large molecule it is confined to the vascular system. Its biological importance is first that molecule for molecule, it has five times the number of antigen-reactive sites as IgG. It therefore has high avidity and is particularly good at agglutinating microorganisms and their antigens. It also has five times the number of Fc sites and therefore at least five times the complement-activating capacity (see below). A mere 30 molecules of IgM attached to *E. coli* ensure its destruction by complement, whereas 20 times as many IgG molecules are required. Also, IgM is formed early in the immune response of the individual. An infectious disease can be regarded as a race between the replication and spread of the microorganisms on the one hand, and the generation of an antimicrobial immune response on the other. A particularly powerful type of antibody that is produced a day or two earlier than other antibodies may often have a determining effect on the course of the infection, favouring earlier recovery and less severe pathological changes. As each immune response unfolds, the initially formed IgM antibodies are replaced by IgG antibodies, and IgM are thus only detectable during infection and for a short while after recovery. The presence of IgM antibodies to a microbial antigen therefore indicates either recent infection or persistent infection. A pregnant woman with a recent rubella-like illness would have rubella IgM antibodies if that illness was indeed rubella. Measles virus occasionally persists in the brain of children instead of being eliminated from the body after infection, and the progressive growth of virus in the brain causes a fatal disease called subacute sclerosing panencephalitis. The onset of disease may be 5–10 years after the original measles infection, but IgM antibodies to measles are still present because of the continued infection.

IgM antibodies are not only the first to be formed in a given immune response, but are also the first to be formed in evolution. They are the only antibodies found in a primitive vertebrate such as the lamprey. IgM antibodies are also the first to be found during the development of the individual. After the fifth to sixth month of development the human foetus responds to infection by forming almost entirely IgM antibodies, and the presence of raised IgM antibodies in cord blood suggests intrauterine infection.* The only maternal antibodies that can pass the placenta to reach the foetus are IgG in type, and thus the presence of IgM antibodies to rubella virus in a newborn baby's blood shows that the foetus was infected.

---

* A congenital (intrauterine) infection is identified in only about 25% of infants with raised IgM levels. But 50% of the remainder have abnormalities in the central nervous system, liver and elsewhere, and perhaps all have suffered an unidentified infection. Alternatively, it is possible that there are noninfectious causes of raised IgM levels in the neonate.

Secretory IgA is the principal immunoglobulin on mucosal surfaces and in milk (especially colostrum). It is a dimer, consisting of two subunits of the basic four-chain structure with α heavy chains, and as the molecule passes across the mucosal epithelium it acquires an additional "secretory piece". Secretory IgA has a molecular weight of 385 000. It probably has little ability and certainly little opportunity to activate complement (see Ch. 9); complement activation leads to inflammation and chemotaxis in tissues (see below), but there is hardly any complement on mucosal surfaces. It has to function in the alimentary canal, and the secretory piece gives it a greater resistance to proteolytic enzymes than other types of antibody. In the submucosal tissues the IgA molecule lacks a secretory piece, and enters the blood via lymphatics to give increased serum IgA levels in mucosal infections.

In the intestine, that seething cauldron of microbial activity, immune responses are of immense importance but poorly understood. On the one hand commensal inhabitants are to be tolerated, but on the other hand protection against pathogens is vital. Powerful immunological forces are present. The submucosa contains nearly 10^{11} antibody-producing cells, equivalent to half of the entire lymphoid system and in man there are 20–30 IgA cells per IgG cell. Immune responses are probably generated against most intestinal antigens (see p. 22), and the sheer weight of these antigens is formidable. It is a daunting prospect to unravel immune events and understand control mechanisms in this dark, mysterious part of the body. Quite recently it has become clear that in some species most of the intestinal secretory IgA comes from bile. Although some of the IgA produced by submucosal plasma cells attaches to the secretory piece present on local epithelial cells and is then extruded into the gut lumen, most of it reaches the blood. In the liver it attaches to the secretory piece which is present on the surface of hepatic cells, and is transported across these cells (see p. 108) to appear in bile. This is important in the rat, but perhaps less so in man. One consequence of the IgA circulation is that when intestinal antigens reach subepithelial tissues they can combine with specific IgA antibody, enter the blood as immune complexes and then be filtered out and excreted in bile as a result of IgA attachment to liver cells.

There is a separate circulatory system that involves the IgA producing cells themselves. After responding to intestinal antigens some of these cells (B immunoblasts) enter lymphatics and the blood stream, from whence they localize in salivary glands, lung, mammary glands and elsewhere in the intestine. They behave differently from spleen or lymph node immunoblasts and presumably recognize and bind to receptors on vascular endothelium in these areas. In this way, specific immune responses are seeded out to other mucosal areas, where IgA antibody is produced and further responses to antigen can be made.

IgA antibodies are important in resistance to infections of the mucosal surfaces of the body, particularly the respiratory, intestinal and urino-genital tracts. Infections of these surfaces are likely to be prevented by vaccines that induce secretory IgA antibodies (see Addendum) rather than IgG or IgM antibodies. However, most patients with selective IgA deficiencies do not show undue susceptibility to infections of mucosal surfaces, probably because there are compensatory increases in the concentration of IgG and IgM antibodies on these surfaces.* Those that are more susceptible generally have associated deficiencies in certain IgG subclasses.

IgE is a minor immunoglobulin only accounting for 0.002% of the total serum immunoglobulins, and it is produced especially by plasma cells below the respiratory and intestinal epithelia. It has a well marked ability to attach to mast cells, and includes the reagenic antibodies that are involved in anaphylactic reactions (see Ch. 8). When an antigen reacts with antibody attached to a mast cell, mediators of inflammation (serotonin, histamine etc.) are released. Thus, if a microorganism, in spite of secretory IgA antibodies, infects an epithelial surface, plasma components and leucocytes will be focused onto the area as soon as microbial antigens interact with specific IgE on mast cells.

IgD antibodies are for the most part present on the surface of B lymphocytes. The same cells also carry IgM antibody, and it might be expected that IgD had an immunoregulatory function, but this is not clear.

General features

The antibody response takes place mostly in lymphoid tissues (spleen, lymph nodes etc.) and also in the submucosa of the respiratory and intestinal tracts. Submucosal lymphoid tissues receive microorganisms and their antigens directly from overlying epithelial cells, and lymphoid tissues in spleen and lymph nodes receive them via blood or lymphatics (see Ch. 5). Initial uptake and handling is by macrophages, following which macrophages and other antigen-presenting cells deliver antigens to immunocompetent lymphoid cells (see above).

On first introduction of an antigen into the body, the antibody response takes several days to develop. Pre-existing antigen-sensitive (immunoglobu-

---

*Also they may show less deficiency in secretory IgA than in the serum IgA which is usually measured. In any case, the details differ in different species, and in sheep, for instance, IgG figures as prominently as IgA in the secretory immunoglobulins. Finally, it must be remembered that in the lower respiratory tract, at least, local CMI responses can be induced, and may contribute to resistance.

In humans, intestinal antibody is measured in duodenal or jejeunal aspirates, or in faeces ("coproantibody"). Antibody from the entire gut can be sampled by "intestinal lavage", when an isotonic salt solution is drunk until there is a watery diarrhoea, one litre of which is collected, heat inactivated, filtered and concentrated.

lin-bearing) B lymphocytes encounter and recognize the antigen displayed (in association with Class 2 molecules) on antigen-presenting cells. Neighbouring T helper cells also recognize the antigen, and as a result, are stimulated to give additional signals to the B cells. The B cells then:

(1) Divide repeatedly, forming a clone of cells with similar reactivity (clonal expansion), some of which remain after the response is over, as memory cells.
(2) Differentiate, developing an endoplasmic reticulum studded with ribosomes, in preparation for protein synthesis and export. The cytoplasm of the cell therefore becomes larger and basophilic.
(3) Synthesize specific antibody. The fully differentiated antibody-producing cell is a mature plasma cell. Each clone of cells forms immunoglobulin molecules of the same class and the same antigenic specificity.

In a natural infection the initial microbial inoculum is small,* and the immune stimulus increases in magnitude following microbial replication. Small amounts of specific antibody are formed locally within a few days, but free antibody is not usually detectable in the serum until about a week after infection. As the response continues and especially when only small amounts of antigen are available, B cells producing high-affinity antibodies are more likely to be triggered, so that the average binding affinity of the antibody increases as much as 100-fold. The role of antibody in recovery from infection is discussed in Ch. 9, the relative importance of antibody and cell-mediated immunity depending on the microorganism. On re-exposure to microbial antigens later in life there is an accelerated response in which larger amounts of mainly IgG antibodies are formed after only one or two days. The capacity to respond in this accelerated manner often persists for life, and depends on the presence of "memory cells".

Antibodies to a given microbial antigen remain in the serum, often for many years. Since the half-life of IgG antibody in man is about 25 days, antibody forming cells are continually active. In some instances (herpes viruses, tuberculosis) microorganisms remain in the body after the original infection, and can continuously stimulate the immune system. In other instances it seems clear that antibody levels are kept elevated partly by repeated re-exposure to the microbe, which gives subclinical re-infections and boosts the immune response. This is known to occur with whooping cough, measles and other infections. Sometimes, however, antibodies remain present in the serum for very long periods in the absence of persistent infection or re-exposure. For instance, five of six individuals who suffered an attack of yellow fever in an epidemic in Virginia, USA in 1855 were found to

---

*Remember that every infection is a race between the ability of the invading microbe to multiply and cause disease and the ability of the host to mobilise specific and non specific defences—a delay of a day or so on the part of the host can be critical.

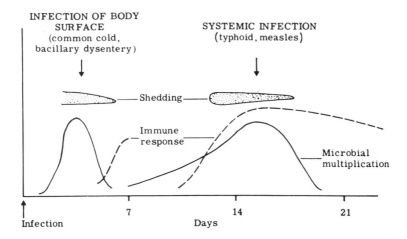

Fig. 25. Distinction between infections of body surfaces and systemic infections.

have circulating antibodies to yellow fever 75 years later. There had been no yellow fever since the time of the original epidemic. Similarly, evidence from isolated eskimo communities in Alaska show that antibody to poliomyelitis virus persists for 40 years in the absence of possible re-exposure. Perhaps microbial antigens persist somewhere in the body and continue to stimulate the formation of new antibody-producing cells, but the matter is not understood.*

As a general rule, the secretory IgA antibody response is short-lived compared with the serum IgG response.† Accordingly resistance to respiratory infection tends to be short-lived. Repeated infection with common cold or influenza viruses often means infection with an antigenically distinct strain of virus, but reinfections with respiratory syncytial virus or with the same strain of parainfluenza virus, for instance, are common. Re-infection of the respiratory tract or other mucosal surfaces is more likely to lead to signs of disease, because of the short incubation period of this type of infection. After re-infection with a respiratory virus there can be clinical disease within a day or two, before the immune response has been boosted and can control the infection. This is in contrast to reinfection with say measles or typhoid; these are generalized infections, and the long incubation period gives ample opportunity for the immune response to be boosted and control the infection long before the stage of clinical disease (Fig. 25).

* Large follicular dendritic cells scattered in lymphoid tissues are possible sites of persistence of antigens, which are retained for long periods on the cell surface. Lymphocytes circulating through lymphoid tissues encounter these cells which thus act as "antigen turnstiles".

† One factor is that although there are very large numbers of IgA-producing plasma cells in submucosal tissues, this immunoglobulin is exported to the outside world, whereas IgG accumulates in the blood as it is produced.

The newborn infant has acquired the antibodies of the mother via the placenta and is protected against most of the infections that she has experienced. There is also transfer of secretory IgA antibodies initially via the milk, human colostrum containing 20–40 mg ml^{-1} IgA.* This maternal "umbrella" of antibodies lasts for about six months in man, and the infant encounters many infectious agents while still partially protected. Under these circumstances the infectious agent multiplies, but only to a limited extent, stimulating an immune response without causing significant disease. The infant thus acquires active immunity while partially protected by maternal immunity. A very occasional mother has not encountered a common microorganism and therefore has no immunity to transfer to her offspring. Certain virus infections, such as herpes simplex, are especially severe in the totally unprotected small infant, causing systemic illness and often death. There are other major differences between the response to infectious agents of immature and adult individuals. They are due to age-related differences in the immune response, in the inflammatory response, in tissue susceptibility etc. and are dealt with more fully in Ch. 11. As the child encounters the great variety of natural infections total serum antibody levels rise, reaching adult levels by about five years of age. Immunological reactivity reaches peak levels in the adolescent or young adult, but falls off detectably in old individuals. This makes old people less resistant to primary infections, and less capable of keeping certain latent infections under control (see Ch. 10).

Protective action of antibodies

Antibodies are formed against a great variety of microbial components and products. The larger microorganisms have more components and products because they have more genes (see Table 12). The presence of antibody indicates present or past infection, but only some of the antibodies have a significant protective function. Protective antibodies generally combine with antigenic components on the surface of microorganisms and prevent them attaching to cells or body surfaces, prevent them from multiplying, and sometimes kill them. The antimicrobial actions of antibodies can be categorized as follows (in approximate order of importance):

(1) Antibodies promote phagocytosis and subsequent digestion of micro-organisms by acting as cytophilic antibodies or opsonins (see below).

---

*Milk also contains other protective factors such as lactoferrin (see p. 293), lactoperoxidase, lysozyme and ill-defined lipids and glycoproteins with an antiviral activity. Oligosaccharides or glycolipids in milk can bind to pathogenic bacteria by resembling the natural receptors for these bacteria (see pp. 20–21). In horses, cows, sheep etc. the uptake of colostrum immediately after birth is vital for protection against certain infections. For instance, calves deprived of colostrum are likely to die of *E. coli* septicaemia within a few day of birth.

Table 12. Sizes of genome of microorganisms

Microorganism		No. of genes[a]
Viruses	Polyoma virus	6
	Poliovirus	5
	Influenza virus	10
	Adenovirus	30
	Herpesvirus	160
	Poxvirus (vaccinia)	300
Chlamydias	Trachoma	800
Mycoplasmas	*Mycoplasma* spp.	900
Rickettsias	*Rickettsia prowazeki* (typhus)	1000
Bacteria	*Neisseria gonorrhoeae*	1000
	E. coli	3000
Protozoa	Malaria	5000–10 000

[a] Known, or calculated (as number of medium sized proteins that can be coded for) from molecular weight of nucleic acid.

(2) Antibodies combining with the surface of microorganisms may prevent their attachment to susceptible cells or susceptible mucosal surfaces (streptococci, gonococci, influenza virus) (see Table 2, pp. 20–21).

(3) Antibodies to microbial toxins or impedins (see p. 73) neutralize the effects of these materials.

(4) By combining with microbes or antigens and activating the complement sequence, antibodies induce inflammatory responses and bring fresh phagocytes and serum antibodies to the site of infection. This can have pathological as well as antimicrobial results (see Ch. 8).

(5) Antibodies combining with the surface of bacteria, enveloped viruses etc., may activate the complement sequence and cause lysis of the microorganism (e.g. *Vibrio cholerae*, *E. coli*, parainfluenza virus, *Mycoplasma pneumoniae*). Host cells bearing new antigens on their surface as a result of virus infection are lysed in the same way, often before virus replication is completed (see Ch. 9).

(6) Antibodies enable certain cells to kill infected host cells bearing viral or other foreign antigens on their surface. These so-called killer (K) cells act when IgG antibody is specifically attached to the target cell surface. Bacteria such as *Shigella* and meningococci can also be killed in this way. K cells are present in blood and lymphoid tissues and bear Fc receptors. Some are lymphocytes or monocytes, but polymorphs also act in this way. Antibody-dependent cell-mediated cytotoxicity (ADCC) of this type is more efficient per antibody molecule than complement-dependent cell killing and is therefore more likely to be relevant *in vivo*.

(7) Antibodies combining with the surface of microorganisms agglutinate them, reducing the number of separate infectious units and also, at least with the smaller microorganisms, making them more readily phagocytosed because the clump of particles is larger in size.

(8) Antibodies attaching to the surface of motile microorganisms may render them nonmotile, perhaps improving the opportunities for phagocytosis.

(9) Antibodies combining with extracellular microorganisms may inhibit their metabolism or growth (malaria, mycoplasmas).

The ways in which antibodies can be detected or assayed in the laboratory as shown in Table 13.

Table 13. Tests for antibodies formed against microorganisms

Name of test	Nature of antigen	Positive test result	Microorganism (examples)
Haemagglutination inhibition	Haemagglutinin, forming part of surface of virus particle	Inhibition of erythrocyte agglutination	Rubella Influenza
Haemagglutination	Microbial antigen absorbed to surface of erythrocyte	Antibody to microbial antigen agglutinates erythrocytes	Hepatitis B
Precipitation or agglutination	Antigen on surface of microorganism Soluble microbial antigen	Antibody causes visible pre-cipitation of microorganism or antigen	*Salmonella* (Widal test), *Brucella* Diphtheria toxin (Elek test)
Gel diffusion	Diffusible microbial antigen	Antibody reacts with antigen to form precipitation line in gel	Histoplasmosis, Hepatitis B
Complement fixation	Microbial antigen that reacts with antibody; resulting complex combines with ("fixes") complement	Complement depleted ("fixed")	Most micro-organisms
Latex test	Microbial antigen adsorbed to latex particle	Antibody to microbial antigen agglutinates latex particles	Hepatitis B

Table 13. (*Contd.*)

Name of test	Nature of antigen	Positive test result	Microorganism (examples)
Neutralization test	Viral surface antigen necessary for multiplication in experimental animal or cell culture	Antibody inhibits multiplication and prevents pathological lesions, death or cell damage	Most viruses
	Bacterial toxin	Biological effect of toxin inhibited	Diphtheria etc.
Immobilization test	Antigen on locomotor organ (flagellum, cilium)	Inhibition of mobility	*Treponema pallidum*
Immuno-fluorescence test (see pp. 88–89)	Antigen on micro-organism or antigen formed in infected cell	Fluorescein-labelled antibody seen on microorganism or in infected cell by UV micro-scopy	*Treponema pallidum*, Respiratory syncytial virus, Toxoplasmosis
Radioimmunoassay	Microbial antigen	Radiolabelled anti-body bound to microbial antigen	Hepatitis B
Enzyme-linked immunosorbent assay (ELISA)	Microbial antigen	Antibody linked to enzyme reacts with antigen. Specific binding revealed when enzyme causes colour change in substrate	Rubella etc.; widely used
Capsular swelling	Capsules on surface of bacteria	Swelling of capsule	Pneumococci, *Klebsiella*
Immune electron microscopy (used in research)	Antigen on surface of virus	Virus particles clumped by electron microscopy	Hepatitis B
Complement lysis (used in research)	Microbial surface antigen	Antibody plus complement lyses bacterium or enveloped virus	*Vibrio cholerae*, *E. coli*, Parainfluenza virus

Cell-Mediated Immune Response

The T cells that generate CMI responses are present in the lymphoid tissues, especially around the splenic arterioles and paracortical areas of lymph nodes; also in the blood and lymph. There is a constant and large-scale recirculation of lymphocytes through the body. About 90% of the recirculation takes place from blood to lymph nodes via the post capillary venules and then via lymphatics back to the blood (Fig. 26). The rest takes place by cells leaving capillaries in various parts of the body, moving through the tissues, entering lymphatics and passing through local lymph nodes. This last route is particularly important in the small intestine. The lymphocytes engaged in this recirculation are mostly (70–80%) T cells, and a given T cell circulates about once in 24 hours in a man, and once in two hours in a mouse. Each T cell carries on its surface antibody-like receptors specific for a certain antigen, and for every possible antigen there are a few specifically reactive T cells. The continual movement of T cells through tissues and lymph nodes ensures that antigens or microbes entering the body sooner or later come into contact with specifically reactive cells. The larger the number of specifically reactive cells, the earlier this will take place.

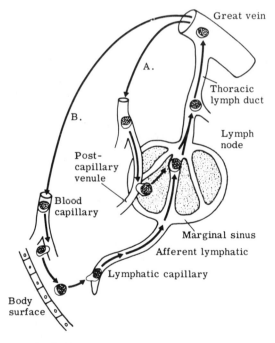

Fig. 26. Lymphocyte recirculation. Recirculating lymphocytes in man are mostly T lymphocytes; approximately 90% of recirculation is by Route A and 10% by Route B.

Different types of T cells carry out different functions and only recognize antigens in the appropriate setting. Those that recognize foreign antigen in association with MHC Class 2 (Ia) antigen on the surface of antigen-presenting cells (see above) respond by:

(1) Triggering specifically reactive B cells to differentiate, make antibody and divide. These are Th cells.
(2) Suppressing the response, thus helping to control it. These are Ts cells.

Both these types of T cell act during the induction of the immune response. Other T cells act during the expression of the immune response in the tissues of previously sensitized individuals. One type recognizes the foreign antigen only when it is associated with the MHC Class I antigens that are present on nearly all host cells. Following this specific recognition, the T cell destroys that particular host cell (see p. 235). These are cytotoxic T cells (Tc) and their powerful cytotoxic action is turned on only when they are in physical contact with the foreign antigen on a host cell—in other words when they recognize the foreign antigen in association with the universally present Class I antigens. If they responded to antigen by itself they could react with it when it was free in extracellular fluids, and their cytotoxic activity would be triggered off to no purpose. If they responded to antigen in association with host Ia (Class 2) antigen they would destroy the macrophages that are carrying out a useful function by presenting antigen to lymphocytes (see above).

Another set of T cells that also act during expression of the immune response, recognize the foreign antigen in association with either Class I or Class 2 MHC antigens. They respond by differentiating to form lymphoblasts, with a ribosome-rich cytoplasm equipped for protein synthesis, and then release active mediators called lymphokines. These are delayed-type hypersensitivity T cells (Tdth). The lymphokines induce a local inflammatory response, and attract leucocytes. Blood monocytes arriving at the site are activated (see below) and their movement away from the site is inhibited. One lymphokine with a direct antiviral effect in the susceptible cell is gamma interferon (see Fig. 34, p. 244). Gamma interferon also exerts an antimicrobial function by activating macrophages and natural killer (NK) cells.* Lymphokines thus function by focusing circulating leucocytes into the site where the immunologically specific encounter took place, locally preparing macrophages for their antimicrobial tasks, stimulating NK cells, and giving antiviral cover to nearby tissue cells by means of gamma interferon.

---

*Natural killer cells are found naturally, in normal individuals. They kill tumour cells and sometimes virus-infected cells without the need for antibody after recognizing ill-defined antigens on their surface and releasing cytotoxic proteins call *perforins*. But they also kill normal cells and their role in infectious diseases is still not firmly established. They are distinct from regular T or B cells or macrophages, and their activity is enhanced by interferon.

Different lymphokines are characterized by *in vitro* tests as macrophage migration inhibitory factor (MIF), macrophage aggregation factor, macrophage activating factor (gamma interferon) and various chemotactic factors. It is not known how many distinct substances are involved. Lymphokines are produced by other T cells (e.g. Tc) as well as by Tdth, and possibly each releases a different mixture of lymphokines. T_H cells, for instance, are a major source of interleukin-2 (Il-2, see Glossary), a lymphokine that is necessary for the proliferation (clonal expansion) of T cells referred to below.

Cooperative interactions between cells are a feature of all immune responses, and soluble mediators, including interleukins (see Glossary), helper and suppressor factors, play an essential part. The details are gradually becoming clearer.

Cell-mediated immune responses are detected and quantified by the methods listed in Table 14.

Table 14. Detection and assay of cell-mediated immunity

Response of sensitized lymphocytes to antigen	Test system
DNA synthesis and mitosis	Incoporation of tritiated thymidine into lymphocyte DNA
Liberation of lymphokines:	
migration inhibition factor (MIF)	Inhibition of migration of normal macrophages
macrophage aggregation factor (MAF)	Agglutination of suspended normal macrophages
macrophage activation factor (gamma interferon)	Increases macrophage resistance to infection with certain bacteria and viruses. Protects cultured cells against virus infection.
chemotactic factor(s)	Causes migration of macrophages and polymorphs through a millipore filter
skin reactive factor	Induces delayed hypersensitivity type skin reactions in normal guinea pig
lymphotoxin	Kills certain virus-infected and tumour cells. *In vivo* role not clear
Cytotoxicity	Destruction of cells bearing e.g. viral antigen on surface
Induction of inflammation and mononuclear infiltration into tissues	"Delayed" swelling and induration (dth response), after injection of antigen into skin
Antimicrobial activity (attributable to above activities)	Transfer 10^8 T lymphocytes into animal infected 1–2 days earlier (before onset of CMI response) and test for reduction in microbial titre in organs 24 h later

As part of the response T cells divide to produce a clone of cells of the same reactivity (clonal expansion), some of which will remain in the body for a longer period, giving the individual an increased ability to react with the same antigen. These are memory cells. It is not clear, however, which of the subsets of T cells undergo clonal expansion, and which ones become memory cells.*

Immune responses are initiated almost immediately after an infecting microorganism enters the body. Cell division is an important part of the CMI (as well as the antibody) response, and cell division and the seeding out of reactive cells to other parts of the body takes a few days. As the infection progresses and the antigen increases in amount, a significant cell-mediated response, in which the whole body is involved, becomes demonstrable. The delayed hypersensitivity reaction in the skin (see below) does not become positive until several weeks in infections such as tuberculosis, brucellosis and leishmaniasis, but after smallpox vaccination (vaccinia virus infection) it is positive within one week† (see Ch. 9). If, however, the individual has been previously exposed to the antigen so that there are larger numbers of sensitized cells in the body, the response takes a shorter time to develop, and there is a noticeable reaction at the site of infection or introduction of antigen within one to two days. In the standard *in vivo* test for the presence of cell-mediated immunity, antigen is introduced into the skin, and the inflammatory cellular response which evolves over the course of one to two days is measured by the increase in skin thickness or area of induration. This is called a delayed hypersensitivity reaction, distinguished from the immediate (2–4 h) reaction that is mediated by antibody. It is an illicited illustration of what is taking place at foci of infection throughout the body. The same response occurs wherever antigen is present, whether in brain, liver or skin, but the skin is a convenient and accessible site for the test.

CMI responses are generated in all infections but the relative magnitude of CMI and antibody responses shows great variation in different hosts and with different infectious agents. Examples of recognized CMI skin test reactions are listed in Table 15. The tuberculin test, for instance, is of some practical value in determining previous exposure to tuberculosis. Those with a positive response have at some time been infected or are at present infected with tuberculosis, with related mycobacteria, or with the attenuated mycobacteria in the BCG vaccine. Those with a negative response have never been infected, or have been infected but have recovered and elimi-

---

* Different types of T cells have different surface components, and most of these can now be identified by the use of monoclonal antibodies, and the T cell subsets distinguished.

† The CMI response can be demonstrated not only by skin testing, but also by the other tests listed in Table 14. T lymphocytes from the mouse spleen can be shown to have antiviral activity (Tc) within 4–5 days of experimental infection with certain viruses.

Table 15. Infectious diseases of man in which CMI is detectable by skin testing

Disease or organism	Name of antigen or test
Brucellosis	Brucellin
Candidiasis	Candidin
Leprosy	Lepromin
Lymphogranuloma inguinale	Frei test
Tuberculosis	PPD (tuberculin test)
Histoplasmosis	Histoplasmin
Trichophyton (ringworm, athlete's foot)	Trichophyton
Vaccinia virus	Vaccinia virus (reaction of immunity to smallpox vaccination)
Mumps	Mumps antigen

Most infections induce CMI responses, but skin tests have only been used clinically in a few infections, and can cause undesirable reactions.
Skin tests may be negative in patients with active disseminated infections (e.g. military tuberculosis, lepromatous leprosy, see Ch. 7).

nated bacteria from the body. The response may also be negative early after infection before CMI has had time to develop, or in acute disseminated infection when the CMI response is feeble.

The ability to generate a CMI response tends to appear later in development than the ability to produce antibodies. As measured by the capacity to reject skin grafts, foetal lambs can develop CMI by 12 weeks (gestation period 21 weeks) whereas IgM antibodies are formed by seven weeks. Information about CMI responses in the human foetus and infant is incomplete. Mammals are born at differing physiological ages but when corrections are made for physiological maturity, immunocompetence appears at about the same equivalent age in different mammals. As with antibody production, the CMI response tends to fall during senescence, probably because of a fall in the total number of immune reactive cells.

Macrophages and Polymorphs

Macrophages, because of their phagocytic prowess and their positioning in the body, are inevitably important in the uptake of invading microorganisms, and they have important functions as phagocytes whether or not an immune response has been generated. They are also inevitably involved in the initiation of immune response to infection, as described above. Macrophages control the rate of delivery and the type of antigen delivered, and thus have a controlling influence in the induction of immunity. As well as playing this part in the induction of the immune response, macrophages also help to give expression to the immune response at a later stage in the infection. In this they operate in close association with both antibodies and CMI (see below).

Polymorphs are also of extreme importance, operating in association with antibody and complement. They are present in the blood and bone marrow, and do not continuously monitor the tissues and fluids* of the body. They are, however, rapidly delivered to tissues as soon as inflammatory responses are initiated (see Ch. 3). They are short-lived; during an infection macrophages are always having to deal with dead polymorphs containing microorganisms in various stages of destruction and digestion. Both polymorphs and macrophages bear Fc and C3b receptors on their surfaces which promote the phagocytosis of immune complexes or microorganisms coated with antibody (see below). By preparing microorganisms for phagocytosis in this way, specific antibodies and complement act as opsonins. When a microorganism is coated with antibody it undergoes a different fate after phagocytosis. *Toxoplasma gondii*, for instance, normally manages to enter macrophages without triggering an oxidative metabolic burst (see p. 68) but this antimicrobial response does occur when the parasite is coated with antibody, and is presumably triggered by Fc-mediated phagocytosis.† In the case of viruses, antibody can prevent attachment and entry into susceptible cells and at the same time promote uptake and degradation by macrophages. When C3 is associated with antibody on the surface of a microorganism it often increases the degree of opsonization.‡ IgM antibodies attached to *Pseudomonas* or other Gram-negative bacilli may even require complement before there is opsonization. Sometimes, however, C3 is activated on the microbial surface by the alternate pathway (see below), and acts as an opsonin independently of antibody. This may be important early in pneumococcal infection, for instance, when there is not much antibody available. Opsonized phagocytosis is the principal method of control of infections with microorganisms such as the streptococcus, staphylococcus or encapsulated pneumococcus, the antibody response and complement acting in conjunction with phagocytic cells.

---

* Sometimes, however, circulating polymorphs are arrested in capillaries, especially in the lung, and can then phagocytose microorganisms present in the blood.

† Interestingly enough, with viruses like dengue that can infect macrophages, small amounts of antibody actually *enhance* infection of these cells, presumably by enhancing the uptake or altering the intracellular fate of the virus. The Fc receptor becomes a Trojan horse (see p. 215). Larger amounts of antibody prevent infection in the conventional fashion.

‡ Complement also often increases the virus-neutralizing action of antibody, presumably by adding to the number of molecules coating the virus particle and further preventing its attachment to susceptible cells.

Macrophages also help give expression to the CMI response, and this seems particularly important in the case of microorganisms such as mycobacteria, *Leishmania*, herpes viruses, brucellas, lymphogranuloma inguinale etc. that survive and multiply within phagocytes and other cells. When sensitized T cells encounter specific antigen they release a number of lymphokines, as described above, with profound effect on macrophages. Some induce inflammation and are chemotactic, bringing circulating macrophage precursors (monocytes) to the site of the reaction, and others inhibit their movement away from the site. Mere assembling of macrophages at a focus of infection is sometimes enough to control the infection, but especially for microorganisms that are not easily killed in macrophages something more than this is needed. Thus there are other lymphokines that "activate" macrophages, causing them to develop increased phagocytic and digestive powers. The increased phagocytosis can be demonstrated directly by the uptake of particles or microorganisms, and is also evident by increased attachment and spreading on a glass surface, in what can be regarded as a heroic attempt to phagocytose the entire vessel in which the macrophages are contained. The increased digestive powers are associated with increased lysosomes and lysosomal enzyme content, and there is also an increased ability to generate oxygen radicals (see p. 68). As a result of these changes macrophages show increased ability to destroy ingested microorganisms. For instance, in mice that have recently developed CMI to tuberculosis, macrophages are activated and have an increased ability to ingest and destroy tubercle bacilli. Indeed resistance to tuberculosis in man is largely attributable to the antibacterial activity of activated macrophages. Mouse macrophages activated in this way by tuberculosis also show increased ability to ingest and destroy certain unrelated intracellular bacteria such as *Listeria monocytogenes*, and protozoa such as *Leishmania* (see below). In other words the macrophage is activated by the lymphokine following an immunologically specific interaction between lymphocyte and microbial antigen, but expresses this reactivity nonspecifically against a wider range of microorganisms. Some of the lymphokines necessarily have a restricted local area of action, but activated macrophages are not confined to the immediate vicinity of the lymphocyte encounter with antigen. Macrophages elsewhere in the body are often affected, suggesting that the mediators spread throughout the body. Activation lasts only for a short time and is no longer detectable a week after termination of the infection. In persistent infections such as tuberculosis, macrophages can remain activated for longer periods because of the continued expression of the CMI response.

Macrophages are also activated during the course of certain virus infections, and can express this reactivity against unrelated microorganisms. For instance, when mice are infected with ectromelia (mousepox) virus and six days later injected intravenously with *Listeria*, the reticuloendothelial macrophages in the spleen show an increased ability to ingest and destroy the bacteria. Macrophages activated in virus infections may show increased resistance to the infecting virus, and sometimes they are also resistant to infection with unrelated viruses. Macrophage activation is important in protozoal infections, and specific antibody responses may add to the macrophage's antimicrobial capacity. In a resistant host, *Leishmania* parasites are destroyed after phagocytosis by activated macrophages and unrelated microorganisms such as *Listeria* are also killed.* Nonactivated macrophages, in contrast, generally support the growth of both *Leishmania* and *Listeria*. Normal macrophages support the growth of *Toxoplasma gondii* (see p. 83), but after activation during the infection they increase their H_2O_2 production (see p. 68) 25-fold and kill the parasite.

Complement

Complement consists of a complicated system of at least nine protein components (C1–C9) present in normal serum. It functions by mediating and amplifying immune reactions. The first component (C1) consists of three principal subfractions, C1q, C1r and C1s. It is activated in the classical complement pathway, after C1q combines with immunoglobulin in immune complexes (antibody bound to antigen).† The immune complex may be free in the tissues or located on a cell surface following the reaction of specific antibody with a cell-surface antigen. The activated first component is an enzyme system, and acts on the next component to form a larger number of molecules of the second component's enzyme. This in turn activates larger amounts of the next component, and so on, producing a cascade reaction (Fig. 27). A single molecule of activated C1 generates thousands of molecules of the later components and the final response is thus greatly

---

* Certain species of *Leishmania* are pathogenic for experimental animals such as guinea-pigs and mice. This is related to the fact that the infecting pathogenic species of *Leishmania* is not killed by activated macrophages from these hosts, although other (nonpathogenic) species of *Leishmania* are killed. Susceptibility to infection is thus associated with reduced ability of the activated macrophage to kill the infecting microorganism, but the basis for this is not known.

† Fc sites on the immunoglobulin are slightly altered as a result of the combination with antigen, and the altered Fc sites (near the hinge region, see p. 128) bind to the C1q fraction of C1. Each C1q must bind to at least two Fc sites and this means that there must be several IgG molecules close together on the immune complex. With IgM, several Fc sites are present on a single molecule, and IgM therefore activates complement much more efficiently. Although in Fig. 26 antibody is shown attached to the complex throughout the sequence, the amplification phenomenon leads to the formation of thousands of additional and separate molecules of the later components.

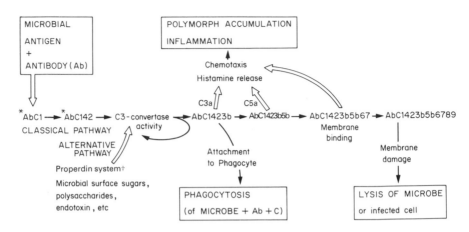

Fig. 27. Diagram to show complement activation sequence and antimicrobial actions. Unfortunately the components were numbered before this sequence of action was elucidated. † (see glossary).

amplified. The later complement components have various biological activities, including inflammation and cell destruction, so that an immunologically specific reaction at the molecular level can lead to a relatively gross response in the tissues.

After activation of the C1 components, C4 and then C2 are activated to form a C3-convertase, and this in turn acts upon C3 to generate C3a with chemotactic and histamine-releasing activity. The residual C3b becomes bound to the antigen–antibody complex, and the whole complex can now attach to C3b receptors present on macrophages and polymorphs.* C5 is the next component to be activated, forming C5a with additional chemotactic and histamine-releasing activity. C5b remains with the complex and binds with C6 and C7, and finally with C8 and C9. The membrane attack complex is formed when the last component (C9) is polymerized to form a tubule, and is inserted into it so as to traverse the cell membrane. This allows a net influx of Na^+ and water, resulting in death of the cell (e.g. red blood cell, see below).

Each activation must be terminated somehow, rather than snowball into generalized activation. The complement sequence is therefore controlled by a number of built-in safety devices in the form of inhibitors (regulatory

---

*The complex also attaches to C3b receptors on nonphagocytic cells (platelets and red cells) in some species, and this is called immune adherence. In the blood it can lead to aggregation and lysis of platelets with release of vasoactive amines (see p. 209).

proteins) and unstable links in the complement chain. The activated components have a short half-life and therefore cannot diffuse through the body and affect distant tissues.

A convertase can also be generated independently of antigen–antibody reactions and C142 formation. It can be generated by certain substances such as microbial polysaccharides and endotoxin, by IgA antibody in an immune complex, or as a result of activation of the properdin system (see Glossary). It is also formed by the products of C3 activation, giving a feedback amplification of the complement sequence. These are called alternative complement pathways. The fact that the complement sequence can be activated without the need for an antigen–antibody reaction may be important in certain infectious diseases. The peptidoglycan of the cell wall of staphylococci, or the polysaccharides on the surface of the pneumococcus, for instance, could activate the alternative pathway very early in infection before specific antibodies have been formed, leading to antibacterial effects as described below.*

Complement is capable of causing considerable inflammation and tissue damage, especially because of the amplification phenomenon. Once the sequence is activated there are four principal antimicrobial functions, each of which is enhanced when both classical and alternative pathways are involved. (Fig. 27):

(1) The inflammation induced at the site of reaction of antibodies with microbes or microbial antigens focuses leucocytes and plasma factors onto this site.
(2) The chemotactic factors attract polymorphs to the site.
(3) The C3b component bound to complexes attaches to C3b receptors on phagocytes and thus acts as an opsonin, promoting phagocytosis of microbes and microbial antigens.
(4) Where antibody has reacted with the surface of certain microorganisms (Gram-negative bacilli, enveloped viruses etc.) or with virus-infected cells, the later complement components are activated to form the membrane attack complex. Small "holes" 9–10 nm, in diameter appear in the wall of Gram-negative bacilli for instance, and lysozyme completes the destructive effect. Cells infected with budding viruses and bearing viral antigens on their surface (Fig. 33, p. 234) can be destroyed by complement after reaction with specific antibody, even at an early stage in the infectious process (see also Ch. 9).

---

* On the other hand *Babesia* activate the alternative pathway and depend on this for entry into susceptible erythrocytes, which bear C3b receptors.

The binding or fixing of complement to immune complexes forms the basis of the complement fixation test. In the test for antibody a known antigen is used in the reaction and vice versa. Complement is added to the reaction mixture, and if there has been a specific antigen–antibody interaction, this complement is fixed and is no longer detectable. The test for complement is by adding sheep red blood cells coated with specific antibody; if complement is present the cells are lysed, but if it has been used up (fixed) the cells are not lysed.

Conclusions Concerning the Immune Response to Microorganisms

Each T or B cell is committed to respond to a given group of closely related antigens. The initial encounter with antigen, whether in lymphoid tissues or elsewhere in the body is a small-scale microscopical event. The purpose of the response, especially when the antigen is from an infecting micro-organism, is to turn this microscopical event into a larger event as soon as possible, so that both antibody and CMI can be brought into action on a significant scale. Both types of immune reactive cell are small, and each must differentiate, generating the cytoplasmic machinery needed for synthesis of antibodies (B cell) or other proteins (T cell). The stimulated cell also gives rise to a dividing population of cells with the same specific immune reactivity, and the response is thus magnified.

The two arms of the immune response to microorganisms are contrasted in Fig. 28. Antibody-forming cells remain for the most part in lymphoid tissues, and antigens are brought to them via blood or lymph. The antibodies formed circulate through the body, acting at a distance from the producer cells that are situated in lymphoid tissues. Antibodies needed on mucosal surfaces must pass through an epithelial cell layer onto these surfaces, and they are produced by cells below these surfaces. Antibodies bathe tissues and mucosal surfaces where they can react with microbes and microbial antigens in a mostly useful antimicrobial fashion. At the site of the antigen–antibody interaction in tissues, complement is activated and inflammatory responses are generated so that antibodies, phagocytes and more immune reactive cells are delivered to the scene of action.

Cell-mediated immunity, in contrast, depends on the local action of individual sensitized cells. The body's population of sensitized T cells must therefore be circulated throughout the tissues of the body like antibody, and especially through the lymph nodes to which microbes and their antigens are brought from the tissues. In this way microbial antigens can be recognized wherever they are and the cell-mediated response initiated. The response, involving an accumulation of mostly lymphocytes and macrophages, can be

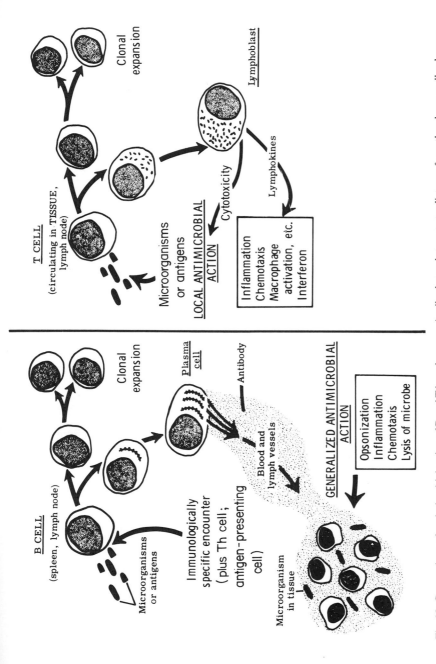

Fig. 28. Comparison of antimicrobial action of B and T lymphocytes. Antibody tends to act at a distance from the plasma cell, whereas CMI requires the local presence of the effector cell.

149

generated locally in the tissue and also more centrally in lymph nodes or spleen. Microbial antigens are most commonly presented to the immune system at the periphery of the body. Langerhans cells in the skin (see p. 123), submucosal lymphoid tissues and local lymph nodes are involved, and there is a tendency for CMI responses to predominate. At a later stage in the response central immune tissues in the spleen are also active. Sometimes, however, there is a reversal of this normal sequence, and antigens are presented directly to central immune tissues. There is then a tendency for the antibody response to be dominant. This is a generalization, but it may have some bearing on problems of tolerance and suppression (see Ch. 7) and on the subject of CMI versus antibody in recovery from infection (see Ch. 9).

Immune reactions are specifically triggered off by the T and B cells whose antigen-binding receptors function as prime movers. Macrophages and other antigen-presenting cells, by processing and presenting antigens, exercise a controlling influence at this stage, and are in close physical association with T and B cells. Macrophages, polymorphs and complement play an important part as effectors and amplifiers of the reaction in tissues.

The part played by antibody, CMI, polymorphs, macrophages and complement in recovery from microbial infections is discussed at greater length in Ch. 9.

References

Allison, A. C. (1978). Macrophage activation and non-specific immunity. *Int. Rev. Exp. Path.* **18**, 303.

Doherty, P. C. (1985). T cells and viral infections. *Brit. Med. Bull.* **41**, 7.

Frank, M. M. (1979). The complement system in host defence and inflammation. *Rev. Inf. Dis.* **1**, 483–501.

Greene, M. I. and Bach, B. A. (1979). The physiological regulation of immunity: differential regulatory contributions of peripheral and central lymphon compartments. *Cell Immunol.* **45**, 446–451.

Halstead, S. B. (1979). *In vivo* enhancement of dengue virus infection in rhesus monkeys by passively transferred antibody. *J. Inf. Dis.* **140**, 527–533.

Joiner, K. A., Brown, E. J. and Frank, M. M. (1984). Complement and bacteria: chemistry and biology in host defence. *Ann. Rev. Immunol.* **2**, 461.

Lowell, G. H. *et al.* (1980). Antibody-dependent cell-mediated antibacterial activity: K lymphocytes, monocytes and granulocytes are effective against Shigella. *J. Immunol.* **125**, 1278–1284.

McNabb, P. C. and Tomasi, T. B. (1981). Host defences at mucosal surfaces. *Ann. Rev. Microbiol.* **35**, 477–496.

Reiter, B. (1978). Review of the progress of dairy science: anti-microbial systems in milk. *J. Dairy Res.* **45**, 131–147.

Roitt, I., Brostoff, J. and Male, D. (1985). "Immunology". Gower Medical Publishing, London.

Unanue, E. R. (1984). Antigen-presenting function of the macrophage. *Ann. Rev. Immunol.* **2**, 395.

Winkelstein, J. A. (1973). Opsonins; their function, identity and clinical significance. *J. Paed.* **82**, 747–753.

7

Microbial Strategies in Relation to the Immune Response

The very existence of successful infectious agents indicates that host defences do not constitute an impenetrable barrier for microorganisms. Infections are common. There are more than 400 distinct microorganisms that infect man alone, and all of us by the time of death, have experienced at least 150 different infections. Many of these infections are asymptomatic but a disease sometimes appears before the microorganism has been controlled and eliminated. In many instances, discussed in Ch. 10, the infection is not eliminated but persists in the body. Persistence represents a failure of the host's antimicrobial forces—forces that can be regarded as having been designed to eliminate invading microorganisms from tissues. The infecting microorganism can then continue to cause pathological changes or continue to be shed from the body.

Once the epithelial surfaces have been penetrated, the major host defences are antibody, CMI, complement, phagocytic cells and interferon. These constitute a mighty pentad whose action is described in Chs 6 and 9. Generally speaking, if there is a way in which host defences can be successfully by-passed or overcome, then at least some microorganisms can be expected to have "discovered" this. Microorganisms evolve very rapidly in relation to their host, so that most of the feasible anti-host strategies are likely to have been tried out and exploited. The microbial devices for overcoming the phagocytic cell system and thus contributing to invasiveness, virulence or persistence have been discussed in Ch. 4. This chapter is largely devoted to an account of the microbial strategies that have been developed to overcome or by-pass the immune response. Strategies for interference with antibody defences are summarized in Table 18 (pp. 176–7).

Tolerance

Tolerance is an immunologically specific reduction in the immune response to a given antigen. As discussed here, it is due to a primary lack of responsiveness, rather than to an active suppression of immune response, which is dealt with on pp. 159–162. If there is a feeble host immune response to the relevant antigens of a microorganism, the process of infection is facilitated and the possibility of persistence increased. This does not involve a general failure of the host immune response of the type discussed in Ch. 9, but a particular weakness in relation to an antigen or antigens of a given microorganism.* Sometimes it is said that a particular microbial component is a "poor antigen", an observation that suggests tolerance to this antigen. All microorganisms except the smallest viruses have numerous antigens on their surfaces and if infection with a given microorganism is to be favoured then the immunological weakness must be in relation to the microbial antigens that are important for infectivity, invasiveness or persistence. Also, because in a given infection either antibody or CMI may be the most important antimicrobial force (see Ch. 9) there must be a weakness in that arm of the immune response to which the microorganism is most susceptible. Tolerance can involve either antibodies or CMI to some extent independently. For instance, CMI tolerance makes the host more susceptible to infections in which the CMI response is critical, and here a strong antibody response is either irrelevant or perhaps actually useful to the microorganism if it gets harmlessly coated with specific antibody and thus protected from the action of immune cells. Tolerance is rarely absolute, with no trace of an immune response to an antigen, but even slight specific weakness (or slowness) in a host may favour a microorganism. There are a variety of ways in which tolerance, defined in this way, can arise.

Genetic

Specific immune responses are undoubtedly controlled by genetic factors, and in several instances the genetic locus responsible for the immune

---

* Most tolerance is exerted at the level of the T cell, whether by failure to respond or following the generation of suppressor T cells. B cells, however, are susceptible to "tolerization" by antigen during their differentiation.

response to a given antigen has been identified. Many of the thousands of genes controlling specific immune responses are linked to those controlling the major histocompatibility antigens. This is so in the mouse, guinea-pig, rat and man. For instance, there are genes in mice that are responsible for the immune response to the antigens of murine leukaemia virus of the Gross strain. Strains of mice with the Rgv-1 ("Recovery from Gross virus") gene have a strong immune response to leukaemia virus and to cells transformed by or carrying leukaemia virus antigens. These mice, which also have the genetically linked histocompatibility antigen type H-2k, are resistant to the induction of leukaemia. Resistance is dominant and is mediated by Tc responses. Strains of mice without this gene and with different histocompatibility antigens such as H-2b, show poor resistance to this type of leukaemia. A second example also involves virus infections of mice. Mice of the C57 B1 strain are particularly resistant to the disease mousepox caused by ectromelia virus. Infection is lethal in other strains of mice, but C57 B1 mice, partly because they have a superior immune response to the virus, control and terminate the infection before it has gone too far. There is another virus infection of mice in which pathological changes and death are due entirely to the host CMI response to viral antigens, the viral infection *per se* being quite harmless. This is LCM virus (see Ch. 8 and Glossary), and interestingly enough here, too, mice of the C57 B1 strain are resistant to the disease, this time because their CMI response to LCM virus is particularly feeble.

Apart from these few examples, there is very little clear evidence that susceptibility to infectious disease is attributable to genetically determined weaknesses in the specific immune response to microbial antigens. In man, the strength of the immune response to streptococcal, tetanus and vaccinia virus antigens has been shown to be linked to histocompatibility (HLA) type (see pp. 277–8), so that it is probably controlled by specific immune response genes. Little more than this can be said. It is well established that susceptibility to autoimmune diseases is associated with certain histocompatibility types (see pp. 277–8), suggesting that the immune responses to autoantigens are controlled genetically. Genetically controlled immune tolerance clearly plays a part, perhaps sometimes an important part, in susceptibility to infectious disease. But it should be noted that genetic control of susceptibility may have nothing to do with immune responses (see pp. 275–7).

Prenatal infection

There is commonly a degree of tolerance to a microorganism when infection occurs during foetal or early postnatal life. At one time it was thought that any antigen present in the foetus during development of the immune system was regarded as "self", and that as a result there was no immune response to it. It is now clear that immune responses do occur under these circumstances, but they are often weak and fail to control an infection. For instance, rubella virus infects the human foetus, causing congenital malformations, and although the foetus receives rubella antibodies (IgG) from the mother and makes its own IgM antibody response to the infection, the CMI response is particularly poor, enabling the virus to persist during foetal life and for long periods after birth. In the mouse, LCM virus is transmitted vertically (see Glossary) via the egg, so that the foetus is infected from the earliest stages of development. The congenitally infected mouse nevertheless makes a feeble antibody response (and no CMI response) to the virus, but this fails to control the infection, and virus persists in most parts of the body for the entire life of the animal. In contrast to this, when adult mice are infected for the first time with LCM virus, they develop both antibody and a vigorous CMI response, and the CMI response becomes a pathogenic force that can lead to tissue damage and death (see Ch. 8).

Desensitization of immune cells by circulating antigens

Tolerance to a given microorganism can arise when large amounts of microbial antigen or antigen–antibody complexes are circulating in the body. For instance, patients suffering from disseminated coccidiomycosis or cryptococcosis, both fungal infections, show antibodies but little or no CMI response to the microorganisms. This is referred to as a state of anergy. It seems to be due to excessive amounts of circulating fungal antigen, and the CMI response to unrelated microorganisms is not affected. Those suffering from kala-azar (visceral leishmaniasis) or diffuse cutaneous leishmaniasis have a defective CMI response to the protozoal antigens, again associated with the presence of circulating leishmania antigens and resulting in systemic spread and chronicity of the infection. Antibody is formed, at least in kala-azar, a severe generalized form of leishmaniasis, but this is not enough by itself; if there is to be recovery and healing, a good CMI response is also necessary, enabling sensitized lymphocytes to destroy host cells infected with *Leishmania* microorganisms. A possible mechanism for tolerization (desensitization) of specifically reactive circulating T cells by antigen is as follows. When they are circulating through the body, T cells cannot make their usual intimate association with macrophages, B cells etc. There is no opportunity for the orderly generation of interleukins, lymphokines etc. that forms the basis for a normal immune response in lymphoid tissues. T cells can then be exposed to high concentrations of antigen rather than the small amounts normally offered to them by antigen-presenting cells. Under these circumstances helper T cells, although not damaged, lose their ability to respond to the specific antigen. They are "defused". In a similar way, developing B cells can be rendered immunologically impotent by direct exposure to antigen.

After infection with *Treponema pallidum* immobilizing and other anti-bodies (see Ch. 6) are formed* and there is an initial CMI response, as detected by marked lymphocyte transformation *in vitro* in the presence of treponemes. This initial response disappears as the bacteria multiply and spread through the body, and lymphocytes from patients with early secondary syphilis fail to respond *in vitro* to *Treponema pallidum*. Later in the secondary stage, weeks or months after infection, lymphocyte reactivity reappears, delayed skin reactions are demonstrable, granulomata appear in lymph nodes and the infectious process is finally brought under control. It is not known why lymphocytes from patients with early secondary syphilis fail to respond to the infecting bacteria. Antigen-specific suppression (see pp. 160–2) is a possibility, or alternatively, T cells are desensitized by circulating bacterial antigen or antigen–antibody complexes.

Molecular mimicry

If a microbial antigen is very similar to normal host antigens the immune response to this antigen may be weak, giving a degree of tolerance. Strong immune responses to normal host antigens are abnormal and potentially harmful. The mimicking of host antigens by microbial antigens is referred to as molecular mimicry. The hyaluronic acid capsule of streptococci, for instance, appears to be identical to a major component of mammalian connective tissue. The commonest resident bacteria of the normal mouse intestine are *Bacteroids*, and these share antigens with mouse intestine. Cross-reactions are seen, even with foetal mouse intestine, which absorbs antibacterial antibodies from serum. Mice are known to be generally rather unresponsive to *Bacteroides* antigens, and it is tempting to suggest that this facilitates establishment of these bacteria as life-long intestinal commensals (see Ch. 2). Generally, however, there is little evidence that molecular mimicry is a cause of poor immune responses. On the contrary, there is good evidence that antibodies formed against microorganisms sometimes cross-

---

* The antibodies that are formed are not protective, but little is known about opsonins in this infection. Could antigenic variation (see pp. 170–4) be a feature of this chronic infection? Nowadays the few patients who get syphilis are treated and immunologists have not had the opportunity to catch up with this disease, but the major antigens are now being defined, characterized by monoclonal antibodies, and produced by recombinant DNA technology.

react with host tissues and therefore cause disease. Two diseases that follow human streptococcal infection have this basis (see Ch. 8). Also, antigens in *Treponema pallidum* cross-react with components in normal tissues, and antigens in EB virus cross-react with human foetal thymus, but this does not prevent antibodies being formed and providing the basis for the Wasserman and the Paul Bunnell (heterophile antibody) tests, respectively.

Viruses such as influenza, measles and mumps mature by budding from the surface of infected cells, and viral antigens are incorporated into the host cell membrane (see Ch. 9 and Fig. 33, p. 234). The envelope that forms the outer membrane of the virus particle could therefore contain some of the host cell antigens. At first sight there would appear no better way of microorganisms acquiring host antigens. But in fact the possibilities are more limited, because when careful studies have been made all the proteins of the envelope have proved to be viral in origin. The envelope lipids, however, are derived from the host cell and their carbohydrate moieties serve as antigenic determinants. Does this make the immune response to the virus any weaker? On the contrary, the immune response reacts powerfully against the antigens on the infected cell, often destroying the cell and serving a useful antiviral purpose. Indeed, there are one or two infections in which antibodies react with normal uninfected host cells. For instance, in atypical pneumonia caused by *Mycoplasma pneumoniae*, antibodies to heart, lung, brain and red blood cells may be formed. The antibodies to red blood cells (called cold agglutinins) very occasionally cause haemolytic anaemia.

Molecular mimicry, in summary, sounds like a good idea from the point of view of the infecting microorganism, and there are observations suggesting that it occurs, but so far there is no very convincing evidence that it is in fact important. Indeed, there is the possibility that antigenic determinants of microbes could resemble those of the host purely by accident rather than by sinister microbial design. It was found that about one-third of 800 different monoclonal antibodies to defined virus antigens cross-reacted with normal host tissue components. Computer searches for shared amino acid sequences between viral polypeptides and host components such as myelin basic protein showed that shared stretches of 8–10 amino acids, which could give cross-reactive immune responses, were quite common. Only a few viral polypeptides and one or two host components have been tested, and cross-reactive responses would turn out to be very common indeed if other host components and the polypeptides of other viruses, chlamydia, bacteria etc. were examined. Although these phenomena are examples of molecular mimicry it would be unreasonable to suggest that they have any meaning in terms of microbial strategies. Rather the host, in responding to such an immense variety of different microbial antigens, is always in danger of responding accidentally, as it were, to its own tissues. The resulting autoimmune response, however, only rarely leads to harmful, immunopathological, results (see Ch. 8).

Conclusion

Usually, when there is a weak immune response to a microbial antigen, it is not known which of the above mechanisms is responsible. There is, for instance, a very weak antibody response to the microorganisms present in the normal intestinal tract of mice. These microorganisms have been present during the evolution of the host animal. They are symbiotic in the sense that they may supply nutrients to the host and tend to prevent infection with other more pathogenic microorganisms (see Ch. 2). Perhaps the immune response is poor because the bacteria share antigens with the mouse intestine, as mentioned above. Perhaps mice have a genetically determined immunological weakness as regards these microorganisms. Perhaps infection shortly after the birth has induced a large degree of tolerance. Perhaps large amounts of antigen are constantly absorbed from the intestine, desensitizing immune cells and inducing tolerance. At present we do not have enough evidence to decide between these possibilities. In man, the urinary tract is commonly infected with *E. coli*, and the frequency of different bacterial serotypes is in proportion to their frequency in the faecal flora. Strains rich in the polysaccharide K antigens, however, are more likely to invade the kidneys. Children with pyelonephritis due to *E. coli* show a correspondingly poor antibody response to these antigens, but the cause of the poor response is not known. Sometimes one suspects tolerance to a microorganism, but there is no evidence. For instance, when species of dermatophyte fungi of animal origin infect the skin of man, there is inflammation followed by healing and relative resistance to reinfection. But with species of fungi adapted to man there tends to be less inflammation, a more chronic infection and less resistance to reinfection. This sounds as if it could be due to a weak immune response to antigens of the human type of fungus.

Studies of autoimmunity have revealed that in normal people there are lymphocytes that respond to autoantigens. Autoimmune disease is avoided by suppressing these responses. This leads to the possibility that specific suppression is commoner than primary unresponsiveness. Indeed, the autoimmune phenomena seen in certain infectious diseases (see Ch. 8 and pp. 274–9) could be attributed to disturbance of these suppressor systems. Also, there are indications that in certain persistent infections a weak response to microbial antigens is due to antigen-specific suppression rather than to a shortage of responding cells. The following section deals with immunosuppression in infectious diseases.

Immunosuppression

General immunosuppression

A large variety of microorganisms cause immunosuppression in the infected host. This means that the host shows a depressed immune response to antigens unrelated to those of the infecting microorganism. Infectious agents that multiply in macrophages or lymphoid tissue (viruses, certain bacteria and protozoa) are especially likely to do this. For instance, during the acute stage of measles infection, patients with positive tuberculin skin tests become temporarily tuberculin-negative. Even after vaccination with live attenuated measles virus immune responses are depressed, and there is a reduction in cutaneous sensitivity to poison ivy,* lasting several weeks. Depressed CMI or antibody responses to unrelated antigens have also been described in people with mumps, EB virus and cytomegalovirus infections. Immunosuppression is a feature in mice infected with cytomegalovirus, LCM virus, murine leukaemia virus or *Toxoplasma gondii* and in cows infected with rinderpest virus. Patients with certain types of malaria, trypanosomiasis, leishmaniasis and lepromatous leprosy show reduced responses to various unrelated antigens and vaccines.†

At present we do not know how such a variety of microorganisms inhibit immune responses. Interference with the immune functions of macrophages and lymphocytes may be important. Alternatively, the reduced responses may be due to "antigenic competition" rather than actual suppression of responses by the infecting microorganisms. Antigenic competition might be expected when an urgent, generalized response to an invading micro-

---

*Poison ivy is a common plant on the east coast of North America. The leaves bear a substance (urushiol, a catechol derivative) of low molecular weight that sticks to the skin and in most people induces delayed hypersensitivity (CMI). On subsequent exposure the delayed hypersensitivity is expressed as contact dermatits. The lesions are localized to the site of contact with the leaf and consist of erythema, papules and vesicles, later becoming scaly and thickened.

†In the case of lepromatous leprosy the signs of immunological disturbance include impaired delayed-type hypersensitivity responses to unrelated antigens, a polyclonal activation of B cells (see p. 167) and in addition there is a specific unresponsiveness to *Mycobacterium leprae*. Suppressor T cells obtained from skin lesions have been shown to inhibit the response of other T cells specifically *M. leprae* antigens. The Ts are possibly induced by the terminal sugars on a leprosy-specific phenolic glycolipid.

Some of the above possibilities involve antigen-specific unresponsiveness rather than active immunosuppression, and another example of unresponsiveness is when the microorganism exploits "holes" in the immunological repertoire of the host. Immune responses to given antigens, as noted earlier, are controlled by immune response genes. Successful microorganisms therefore would tend to develop surface antigens that are poorly seen, poorly responded to by the host.

Interest in virus-induced immunosuppression received a great stimulus with the appearance of AIDS in 1979. In this disease the infecting virus (HIV, Human Immunodeficiency Virus) attaches to and infects both T helper cells and antigen-presenting cells. This results in serious loss of immune function. In severely affected patients the immune deficit allows a variety of persistent yet normally harmless infections (*Pneumocystis carinii*, cytomegalovirus, toxoplasmosis, candidiasis etc.) to become active, and these, together with various other infections, eventually prove fatal. The AIDS virus is responsible for the immunosuppression (and also for the independently evolving neurological disease), which gives the other microorganisms the opportunity to cause the lethal disease. The virus persists in the body, and patients remain infectious probably for life. Cat leukaemia virus (also a retrovirus) causes a similar condition in cats, and infected cats are more likely to die of secondary infection than of the leukaemia itself. Patients with AIDS develop poor neutralizing antibody and possibly poor cell-mediated immune responses to the infecting virus. This could be regarded as a useful result from the point of view of the virus, favouring persistence and transmission to fresh hosts, the more general and disastrous immunosuppression being an "unfortunate" side effect.

Absence of Suitable Target for Immune Response

There are various ways in which intracellular microorganisms can avoid exposing themselves to immune forces. They evade host immune responses as long as they stay inside infected cells, and allow at the most a low density of microbial antigen to form on the cell surface. This is what happens in dorsal root ganglion cells persistently infected with herpes simplex or varicella virus (see Ch. 10), in circulating lymphocytes infected with EB virus, and in most of the cells of a mouse infected with the persistent murine leukaemia virus. It is also seen in susceptible macrophages infected with *Brucella*, *Listeria* or leprosy bacilli. The macrophages support the growth of bacteria and at the same time give them protection from immune responses. Again, malaria parasites are present in liver cells during the exoerythrocytic stages of infection and during this silent latent period the parasite avoids stimulating or presenting a target for the immune response. Even when the malaria parasites are growing in red blood cells and causing the disease, their very presence inside the red blood cells protects them from circulating antibodies. The merozoites that emerge from infected red cells are only briefly exposed to antibodies before entering fresh uninfected cells. Some of the parasite components, however, may be present on the surface of the infected red cell, which then becomes a less protected site.

Some of the intracellular microorganisms that expose their antigens on the infected cell surface benefit from a host-mediated mechanism for disposal of those antigens. This involves antibody and depends on the phenomenon called capping. Substances can move in the fluid matrix comprising the cell membrane, and when microbial antigens on the cell surface react with specific antibody the antigen–antibody complex moves to one pole of the cell (capping). Here the complex is either shed, or taken into the cell by cytosis. The antibodies that should have prepared the infected cell for immune destruction are diverted from this purpose and used to rid the cell of microbial antigens, making it less susceptible to immune lysis. Capping probably occurs on brain cells infected with measles virus in SSPE (subacute sclerosing panencephalitis) and is a factor favouring persistence of the infection in this condition. In certain protozoa, capping by antibody can lead to the loss of the microbe's own surface antigens. It occurs with *Toxoplasma gondii* and with *Leishmania* but it's importance in resistance to host immune defences is unknown.

Intracellular microorganisms also escape the action of antibodies if they spread directly from cell to cell without entering the extracellular fluids. This is seen when herpes simplex virus or defective* measles virus spreads progressively from cell to cell in the presence of potent neutralizing antibody. Cells formed by division of an infected cell are also infected without virus entering extracellular fluid. For example, cells derived from the ovum of a mouse infected with leukaemia virus are all infected, whether or not virus is released from the cell, and in the newborn infant with rubella virus, a cell that was initially infected in the foetus has given rise to a group of infected progeny cells in spite of the presence of neutralizing antibodies. The ability to stay inside cells certainly contributes to the success of persistent intracellur microorganisms, without in most cases being the sole factor.

Microbial Presence in Bodily Sites Inaccessible to the Immune Response

Many viruses persist in the infected host and are shed to the exterior via the saliva (herpes simplex, cytomegalovirus, rabies in vampire bats), milk (cytomegalovirus in man, mammary tumour virus in mice) or urine

---

*As seen in subacute sclerosing panencephalitis (p. 129), the virus is defective in that replication is incomplete. Viral nucleic acids and proteins are produced, but few infectious particles are formed.

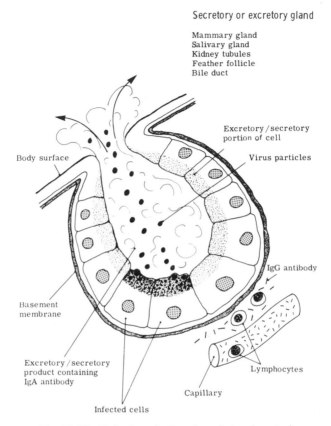

Secretory or excretory gland

Mammary gland
Salivary gland
Kidney tubules
Feather follicle
Bile duct

Excretory/secretory
portion of cell

Body surface

Virus particles

IgG antibody

Basement
membrane

Excretory/secretory
product containing
IgA antibody

Lymphocytes

Capillary

Infected cells

Fig. 29. Viral infection of cell surfaces facing the exterior.

(polyoma virus in mice). The surface of the infected cell can be said to face the external world as represented by the lumen of the salivary gland, mammary gland or kidney tubule (Fig. 29). As long as virus particles and viral antigens are only formed on the lumenal surface of the cell and there is little or no cell destruction, it is difficult for sensitized lymphocytes* or antibodies to reach the site and eliminate the infection. Secretory IgA antibodies could react with viral antigens on the infected cell surface, but the complement sequence would be unlikely to be activated and the cell would not be destroyed. IgA antibodies could also react with extracellular virus particles but would at the most render them noninfectious, again without

---

* Although Fig. 29 shows a continuous layer of epithelial cells, infiltrating lymphocytes with possible antimicrobial potential are a normal feature of certain epithelial surfaces (e.g. intestinal).

acting on the source of the infection. The same considerations apply to epidermal infection with human wart viruses, or to infection of the epidermis lining the chicken's feather follicle with Marek's disease virus (see Glossary). In the case of a wart, neither virus nor viral antigens are manufactured in significant quantities until the infected epidermal cell is keratinized and about to be released from the body, and is physically far removed from host immune forces.

Bacteria that are present and multiply in the lumen of glands, tubes and tubules also enjoy some freedom from immune forces. In rats persistently infected with *Leptospira*, for instance, the bacteria multiply in the lumen of kidney tubules and are shed in urine. If the urine enters water in a river or puddle it remains infectious and can cause leptospirosis in man. Commensal intestinal bacteria, unless they are very closely associated with the intestinal epithelium, enjoy similar freedom and it is therefore impossible to eliminate these bacteria by artificially inducing immune responses against them. Other bacteria, such as *Brucella abortus* in the cow, persistently infect mammary glands and are shed in the milk. In typhoid carriers, the bacteria colonize scarred avascular sections of the biliary or urinary tract and are thence shed, often in large quantities, into the faeces or urine. Bacteria may also lurk in biliary or renal stones, and in a similar way the staphylococci in the devascularized bone of patients with chronic osteomyelitis are protected from host defences.

Induction of Ineffective Antibodies

Many types of antibody molecule are formed against a given antigen, reacting with different antigenic determinants (epitopes) on the molecule. For instance, studies with monoclonal antibodies (see Glossary) have shown that there are more than 20 different antigenic determinants on the haemagglutinin that occupies most of the surface of influenza virus (see p. 15), although only four of them are important. Also, antibodies tend to have a range of avidities (see Glossary). If the antibodies formed against a given microorganism are of low avidity, or if they are mostly directed against unimportant antigenic determinants on the microorganism, then they will only have a weak antimicrobial action and there are likely to be difficulties in controlling infection with that particular microorganism. For instance, there are several persistent (life-long) virus infections of animals in which antibody is formed and reacts specifically with the surface of the infecting virus, but fails to render it noninfectious. The virus–antibody complexes are therefore infectious and they circulate in the blood. These viruses include LCM and leukaemia infections in mice, also Aleutian disease virus in mink.

In the latter disease (see Glossary) there is a stupendous immune response on the part of the infected animal, with a fivefold increase in total IgG levels and viral antibody titres of one in a hundred thousand. The antibody is not only of no antiviral value, but causes life-threatening immunopathological damage. Since there is also no effective CMI response to these infections, and since these viruses grow in host cells without harming them, the infections persist for life.

Ineffectual ("non-neutralizing") antibodies of this sort are particularly important if they combine with microbial antigen and block the action of any good quality antibodies that may also be present. Antibodies to LCM virus formed in infected mice are known to have this property. The antibodies formed in patients with syphilis (a persistent infection) are only very feebly antimicrobial. Although they combine with the surface of the treponemes and perhaps aid phagocytosis (act as opsonins), they cause little neutralization and, after 36 hours' treatment with antibody plus complement, most of the treponemes remain infectious.

It is not known how commonly ineffective antibodies are induced in other microbial infections, but it they are induced, the antimicrobial task of the host is certainly made more difficult. From a microorganism's point of view it would also be an advantage to be able to induce the host to make the wrong type of immune response. There is a tendency for the antibody and the CMI responses to given antigens to vary inversely, and if for a given infection the host's major antimicrobial force was the CMI response, the microorganism could with advantage induce the formation of a strong antibody response. Unfortunately there are no generally acceptable examples known at present. However, infections with Gram-negative bacteria such as *Salmonella typhi* are controlled by the CMI response, and it has been suggested that endotoxin (see Ch. 8), which acts as a general B cell (antibody) stimulator, directs the host response in favour of antibody rather than CMI, to the benefit of the infecting bacteria.

Persistent protozoal infections such as malaria and African trypanosomiasis are characterized by the formation of very large amounts of antibody. But most of this appears to have little or no protective value in the host, although it sometimes shows some *in vitro* inhibition of parasite motility, viability, multiplication or metabolism. Although some of these antibodies are directed against microbial antigens, most are truly nonspecific in the sense that they do not react at all with any microbial antigens.* Some react with host tissues, such as the heterophil antibodies (see Glossary) and

---

*Adults in West Africa chronically infected with malaria show seven times the normal (European) rate of IgG production, on a body weight basis. Much of this is associated with malaria infection because it is reduced by 30% after several years of prophylactic antimalarial therapy. Only 5% of the circulating IgG, however, is found to react with malarial antigens.

antibodies to DNA, Schwann cells and cardiac myofibrils, that are seen in the various types of trypanosomiasis, and this raises the question of autoimmune damage (see Ch. 8). Similar anti-host antibodies occur in certain virus infections such as those caused by EB and cytomegaloviruses. The basis for these irrelevant or excessive antibody responses is B cell proliferation induced by the infection, often referred to as polyclonal activation. This is seen in malaria, lepromatous leprosy, and also in infection with *Mycoplasma pneumoniae*, *Trypanosoma* species, EB virus and many other microorganisms. It would make sense if it reflected microbial interference with host immune responses (see Ch. 10) but its significance in these important infectious diseases is still shrouded in mystery.

Antibodies Mopped up by Soluble Microbial Antigens

The antimicrobial action of antibodies is to a large extent due to their attachment to the surface of microorganisms. Antibody on the microbial surface prevents entry into susceptible cells (viruses), promotes uptake by phagocytes, activates complement lysis of the microorganism etc., as discussed in Ch. 6. One strategy that microorganisms could use to defend themselves against the antibody weapon would be to liberate their surface components in soluble form into tissue fluids. These surface components would combine with and "neutralize" antibody before it reached the microorganism. Circulating T lymphocytyes could be desensitized in the same way (see above).

Soluble antigens are liberated into tissue fluids in most microbial infections, but it is not often that these are known to be surface antigens. Most normal tissue cells bud off tiny membrane-bound blebs of cytoplasm into surrounding fluids. Cells infected with budding viruses produce virus particles but they probably also liberate tiny blebs of cytoplasm whose limiting membrane contains viral antigens. The 20 nm particles present in the serum of patients and carriers with hepatitis B virus infection are produced in this way. There are up to 10^{13} particles (ml of serum)$^{-1}$.* Polysaccharide antigens from *Candida* contain mannan, and this material, which is present in the serum of patients suffering from candidiasis, inhibits lymphocyte proliferation in response to *Candida* antigens. Perhaps *Candida* polysaccharides are handled abnormally in these patients, allowing free mannan to stay in the circulation and interfere with CMI responses. In certain bacterial infections surface polysaccharides are liberated. Bacterial polysaccharides

---

* They are not infectious. Could they be regarded as a viral "device" to tolerize (pp. 155–6) host lymphocytes?

are detectable in the serum in pneumococcal pneumonia, and in the serum and cerebrospinal fluid in fulminating meningococcal meningitis. The surface polysaccharide of *Pseudomonas aeruginosa* is also released from multiplying bacteria *in vitro*, and presumably *in vivo*. Even endotoxin is released in small amounts into the surrounding fluid by Gram-negative bacteria. Antigens from *Trypanosoma cruzi*, *Candida albicans*, *Toxoplasma gondii*, *Plasmodium* spp. and *Babesia* spp. are present in serum during systemic infections. The phenomenon may prove to be a common one. But in spite of the theoretical advantages for the microorganism, it is not known whether the released surface components mop up enough antibody or inactivate enough T or B cells to be of significance in the infection.

Local Interference with Immune Forces

There are several ways in which microorganisms, without preventing the generation of immunity, interfere with the local antimicrobial action of immune forces. For instance, a few microorganisms induce the formation round themselves of a capsule or cyst. Cysts are formed in certain protozoal infections, but they occur inside cells, especially macrophages, and protect the microorganism from destruction by the host cell rather than from host immune forces. *Toxoplasma gondii*, for instance, infects man and a wide range of mammals and birds, forming cysts inside macrophages in the central nervous system, muscle and lung.* Shielded by the tough wall of the cyst, the microorganism multiplies without provoking a host reaction, and thousands of parasites may be present in a single cyst in the chronic stage of the disease. Cysts that restrict the access of antibody and phagocytic or immune cells are best seen with helminth parasites. The dog tapeworm, for instance, lives in the alimentary canal of dogs, and enormous numbers of eggs are present in faeces. When a human being ingests these eggs, the parasite develops and travels from the intestine to reach the lung or liver, where a hydatid cyst is formed. This consists of larval worms inside a firm capsule made up of parasite and host components. The cyst gradually grows larger, in spite of the antibody and cell-mediated immune response of the host, often reaching the size of a coconut, and may cause serious disease. The natural hosts for the cysts are grazing animals such as sheep, which ingest the eggs; after the sheep had been killed and eaten by a predatory carnivore such as the dog, the larval worms in the cyst grow to form adult worms in the intestine.

Virulent staphylococci produce a coagulase and this acts on plasma components at the site of infection and leads to the deposition of a layer of

---

* *Toxoplasma gondii* is primarily a parasite of members of the cat family, in whom it infects intestinal epithelium and is shed in faeces. Human infection is worldwide, and common in the UK, but nearly always symptomless.

host fibrin around the bacteria. It is possible that this restricts the local access of host cells, and that the bacteria are also "disguised" immunologically, so that they are less readily identified as targets for immune responses. There are other examples from bacterial infections. The K antigens on the surface of *E. coli* are closely associated with the pathogenicity of these bacteria. They can mediate attachment of *E. coli* to intestinal epithelial cells (p. 20), and certain K antigens can increase the ability of *E. coli* to grow in the kidney or other sites. First, the K antigen is a polysaccharide and makes phagocytosis a more difficult task for host cells (see Ch. 4). Also, some of them are poor immunogens, possibly resembling host polysaccharides. Finally, the K antigen interferes with the alternative pathway of complement activation, so that the bacteria escape this early (see p. 147) antibacterial defence mechanism.

One theoretically simple strategy for bacteria would be to produce an enzyme that destroys antibody, and it has been shown that pathogenic strains of the gonococcus, a human pathogen, liberate a protease that specifically cleaves human IgA antibody. The protease acts at the site of a Pro–Thr peptide bond in the hinge region of the heavy chain of the IgA molecule (see Fig. 24, p. 128). The significance of this enzyme *in vivo* is not yet clear because antigen-combining sites on the cleaved fragments would remain intact, but such enzymes are obviously likely to be important, and might help account for the apparent indifference of the gonococcus to the host's antibody response. A similar enzyme is produced by the meningococcus, a frequent resident in the nasopharynx, by many strains of *Haemophilus influenzae* and *Streptococcus pneumoniae*, and also by *Streptococcus sanguis*, one of the common commensal bacteria of the mouth. In each case the bacteria producing the protease are normally exposed to secretory IgA antibody. The staphylococci provide a more plausible example of the local interference with the action of antibody by bacteria. Virulent staphylococci have a factor called protein A in the cell wall which is excreted extracellularly, and this inhibits the phagocytosis of antibody-coated bacteria by attaching to the Fc portion of the antibody molecule. *Pseudomonas aeruginosa* produces an elastase that inactivates the C3b and C5a components of complement and thus tends to inhibit opsonization and the generation of chemotactic and other inflammatory responses. Perhaps this contributes to invasiveness,* *Pseudomonas* infections tend to show minimal inflammatory responses. Factors that inhibit the action of complement or opsonizing antibodies are perhaps also produced by other bacteria, but even when such factors are discovered and defined it is generally difficult to decide how important they are in the actual process of infection.

---

*The *Pseudomonas* elastase also inactivates lysozyme and cleaves type I collagen. As with many other bacterial products, its role in pathogenicity may be clarified when elastase-negative strains are produced by genetic engineering and tested for virulence.

Gram-negative bacteria have a very complex cell wall, consisting primarily of a membrane-like arrangement of phospholipids, lipopolysaccharide (endotoxin, see Ch. 8 and Fig. 14) and protein. In virulent strains of bacteria, the polysaccharide chains project from the general bacterial surface, carrying on their tips the important O antigens of the cell wall. The O antigens are the key targets for the action of host antibody and complement, but when this reaction takes place on the end of the polysaccharide chains, a significant distance external to the general bacterial cell surface, complement fails to have its normal lytic effect. Such bacterial strains are virulent because of this resistance to host immune forces. Their colonies happen to have a smooth appearance on agar surfaces and they are therefore called "smooth" strains. If the projecting polysaccharide chains are shortened or removed, antibody reacts with O antigens on the general bacterial surface or very close to it, and complement can then lyse the bacteria. Strains without the projecting polysaccharides are therefore nonvirulent and they have a "rough" colonial morphology. Gram-negative bacteria therefore can be thought of as protecting themselves from the damaging consequences of antibody and complement reactions by having antigens that project a short distance out from the bacterial cell surface.

Certain bacteria activate complement via the alternative pathway (without antibody) and this promotes opsonization and thus increases host resistance early in infection (see p. 147). Group A streptococci would do so were it not for their special outer covering. These bacteria are poorly opsonized by complement alone but, when the M protein on the pili is gently removed with trypsin to expose peptidoglycan, the alternative pathway is activated, the bacteria bind complement and are then efficiently opsonized and phagocytosed. Encapsulated strains of *Staphylococcus aureus* activate the alternative pathway and bind complement, but C3 is somehow hidden by capsular material and the bacteria are not opsonized.

Viruses of the herpes group (herpes simplex, varicella zoster and cytomegalovirus) induce virus-coded Fc receptors on the surface of infected cells. This could be useful for the virus by binding IgG nonspecifically to the cell surface and thus protecting it from immune lysis. Fc receptors are present on staphylococci (protein A, see p. 169), on certain types of streptococci and on trypanosomes, and could protect these microorganisms in a similar fashion. The Fc and C3 receptors present on the various forms of *Schistosoma mansoni* conceivably aid the survival of this large parasite in the host.

Antigenic Variation

One way in which microorganisms can avoid the antimicrobial consequences of the immune response is by periodically changing their antigens. This happens in a few bacterial and protozoal infections where it is an important factor promoting their persistence in the body. The spirochaetal micro-organism *Borrelia recurrentis* is transmitted from person to person by the body louse and causes relapsing fever. After infection the bacteria multiply and cause a febrile illness, until the onset of the immune response a week or so later. Bacteria then disappear from the blood because of antibody-mediated lysis or agglutination, and the fever falls. But antigenically distinct mutant bacteria then arise in the infected individual so that 4–10 days later bacteria reappear in blood and there is another febrile episode, until this in turn is terminated by the appearance of a new set of specific antibodies. Ensuing attacks become progressively less severe, but there may be up to ten of them before final recovery. The disease is called relapsing fever because of the repeated febrile episodes, each caused by a newly emerging antigenic variant of the infecting bacterium.

Some protozoa have a similar antigenic versatility. Sleeping sickness is a disease of man in Africa caused by parasitic protozoa of the *Trypanosoma brucei* group, and is spread by biting (tsetse) flies. The infection spreads systemically to the lymph nodes and blood and is characterized by recurrent fever and headache. In the later stages the central nervous system is involved to give chronic meningoencephalitis, occasionally with the condition of lethargy from which the disease gets its name.* The surface coat of the trypanosome is 12–15 mm thick, and is composed of carbohydrate and a glycoprotein of mol. wt. 65 000. During the infection, an antigenically new coat is produced spontaneously in about 1 in 10 000 trypanosomes, to give a series of antigenic variants. These arise by changes in gene expression rather than by mutation, and a single clone of trypanosomes can express hundreds of variants. The systemic stage of the infection consists of a series of parasitaemic waves, each wave being antigenically different from preceding and successive waves. During this time the immune system is constantly trying to catch up, as it were, with the trypanosomes. A large part (about 10%) of the genome of the trypanosome is taken up with the different surface coat genes, but this is a worthwhile investment for the parasite, allowing it to stay for long periods in the blood, and also offering a dismal outlook for a vaccine.

Parasitic worms have even greater opportunities for this type of hide-and-seek with the immune response. Schistosomiasis is a common disease of man in Egypt and elsewhere in Africa, caused by trematodes (flukes) of the genus *Schistosoma*. There is a larval stage of the parasite in the blood, and the adult worm lives in the veins around the bladder and rectum, causing frequent, painful and bloody urination. The adult worm liberates antigens into the blood, and although the antibodies formed are effective against new larval

---

*But many patients are said to suffer from insomnia.

invaders, they have no effect on the adult because it is safely covered with a layer of host antigens. This ensures that the adult worms remain few in number, and prevents overcrowding in the host.

Antigen variation in *Neisseria gonorrhoeae* contributes to the pathogenicity of this resourceful parasite. During the initial stages of infection, adherence to epithelial cells of the cervix or urethra is mediated by pili (see p. 20), but equally efficient attachment to phagocytes would be undesirable. Hence rapid switching on and off of the genes controlling pili are necessary at different stages of the infection. Changes are also seen in the expression of the outer-membrane proteins of the bacteria. Finely tuned control of expression of the genes for pili and outer-membrane proteins, giving changes in adherence to different host cells, in resistance to cervical proteolytic enzymes, in cytotoxicity etc., are presumably necessary for successful infection, spread through the body, growth and shedding of these bacteria.

The different strains of gonococci circulating in the community also show great antigenic variation in pili and in outer-membrane proteins, which helps account for the multiple attacks of gonorrhoea that can occur in an individual (see p. 43 footnote). *Pilin*, the protein subunit of the pili, consists of constant, variable and hypervariable regions (analogous with immunoglobulin molecules) and genetic rearrangements and recombinations occurring in the repertoire of pilin genes forms the basis for the antigenic variation.

The above microorganisms are complex enough to be capable of undergoing a series of antigenic variations during the course of a single infection. An occasional virus (visna in goats, equine infectious anaemia in horses and HIV in man) show antigenic variation within a given infected individual. For most viruses antigenic variation occurs outside the initially infected animals, so that re-infection with a fresh antigenic variant can occur at a later stage.* With infections limited to mucosal surfaces, resistance to infection is often of limited duration (see Ch. 6) and there is a strong selective advantage for virus strains with altered antigenic characters. The time between initial infection and shedding is only a few days, and an antigenically altered virus variant can infect, replicate, and be shed from the body before a significant local secondary immune response is generated. In contrast to this, re-infection with resheding of viruses such as rubella, measles, mumps or smallpox, which cause systemic infection, is less likely. The incubation period is two to

---

* Variants of a different sort arise when the microorganism infects geographically separated populations of the host species. In each population there is the opportunity for antigenic or other variants to appear. For instance, Asian strains of tubercle bacillus and rabies virus can be distinguished from European strains by phage typing and by monoclonal antibody studies. Geographical differences in herpes viruses would doubtless be revealed by "fingerprinting" of viral DNA.

three times as long as in a respiratory virus infection, and the secondary immune response has time to come into action and prevent the spread of infection through the body. The growth of virus in the skin and respiratory tract that occurs late in the incubation period is therefore prevented, and there is no shedding of virus to the exterior. For reasons such as these antigenic variation is a feature of virus infections limited to the respiratory and perhaps the alimentary tracts, whereas viruses that cause systemic disease such as rubella, measles, mumps or smallpox tend to be of uniform character (monotypic) antigenically.

The significance of antigenic variation is well illustrated by influenza viruses. Influenza B virus is limited to the respiratory tract and evolves as it spreads through communities, showing repeated small antigenic changes over the years. This is called immunological drift. A given individual can be reinfected later in life by an antigenic variant that has been gradually generated in other groups of individuals. Human rhinoviruses and foot and mouth disease virus are also evolving rapidly and show a similar antigenic drift. Established strains of influenza A, however, show more drastic antigenic changes in addition to immunological drift. New pandemic strains of influenza A virus emerge periodically to infect man, after the production of major antigenic changes, probably by genetic recombination between human and animal virus strains. It is thought that the animal virus "reservoir" consists of populations of susceptible birds which are known to harbour their own strains of influenza A virus infecting especially the intestinal tract. Recombinants are readily formed because the influenza virus genome is segmented, consisting of eight RNA fragments. The major antigenic change involves one or both of the surface components of the virus, either haemagglutinin (H) or neuraminidase (N). Very occasionally the recombinant virus shows major antigenic differences from previous human influenza A virus strains, having H or N antigens of bird origin, and is at the same time capable of infecting and being efficiently transmitted in man. Initial infection of man with the new strain perhaps takes place in parts of the world where people live in close association with domestic birds. The world's population, with no previous immunological experience of such a virus, is completely susceptible. Pandemic strains of influenza A virus have arisen periodically in this century to give major global outbreaks in 1918, 1946, 1957 (Asian 'flu) and 1968 (Hong Kong 'flu). The new variant spreads from one continent to another, in 1918 at the speed of ships and trains, but nowadays at the speed of jet aircraft. Pandemic strains are designated according to the H or N antigens (see Table 17).

As a viral adaptation for the overcoming of host immunity, antigenic variation is more likely to be important in longer lived species such as the horse or man where there is a need for multiple re-infection during an

Table 17. Pandemic strains of influenza virus

Time of pandemic	Designation of strain
1889–1890	H_2N_2?
1918–1919	$H_{sw1}N_1$?
1946	H_1N_1
1957–1958	H_2N_2 ("Asian")
1968–1969	H_3N_2 ("Hong Kong")
1987?	?

H = Haemagglutinin; N = neuraminidase.
H_{sw1} = H possibly derived from pig influenza virus.

individual's life time if the virus is to remain in circulation, and if the virus does not have the ability to become latent (Ch. 10). In shorter lived animals such as mice or rabbits, on the other hand, populations renew themselves rapidly and fresh sets of uninfected individuals appear fast enough to maintain the infectious cycle. Human respiratory viruses are among the most successful animal viruses in the world. Many show regular antigenic variation and, because of assured increases in human numbers and density, this group of viruses are perhaps entering their golden age, with an almost unlimited supply of susceptible hosts in the foreseeable future, and poor chances of control by vaccination (see Vaccines, Addendum).

The bacteria responsible for superficial infections also tend to show something similar to immunological drift, with the appearance of new variants or subtypes that can re-infect the individual. Staphylococci and streptococci, for instance, exist in a great variety of antigenic types, and this, although it may have some other biological significance, can perhaps be regarded as antigenic drift. Among the intestinal bacteria, *E. coli* shows a similar antigenic variety but it is not clear that this has the immunological significance suggested. Just as with virus infections, the bacteria that cause sytemic infections are relatively conservative, antigenically speaking, and tend to be monotypic in type, as for instance with plague, tuberculosis, syphilis, typhoid etc.

Microorganisms that Avoid Induction of an Immune Response

There is an intriguing group of virus-sized microorganisms of uncertain nature that multiply, persist and spread in the infected host, giving pathological changes only after very lengthy incubation periods consisting of a large fraction of the host's life span. The microorganism multiplies in the brain and causes a neurological disease that is always fatal (if the host lives long enough). These "slow" infections are scrapie (sheep), transmissible mink encephalopathy (mink) and Kuru and Creutzfeld-Jacob disease in man; they comprise the "transmissible viral dementias" (see Ch. 10). In the best studied of these, scrapie, not the slightest flicker of an immune response has been detected and the infection neither induces nor is susceptible to the action of interferon. These microorganisms therefore multiply in an unrestricted and inexorable fashion in the host. Multiplication is in close association with cell membranes, but neither the structure nor the method of intracellular multiplication of these organisms is understood, and it is not known whether the genome is RNA or DNA. A promising scrapie-specific protein, isolated from infected tissues and now identified and sequenced, turns out to be coded for by the host cell. They are difficult to study, and even to identify. Conceivably some immunological wizard will one day demonstrate a specific immune response but meanwhile we can ask why there appears to be none. It may be no accident that scrapie, like other persistent infections, first multiplies in the spleen of a mouse, where it has the opportunity to manipulate host immune responses to its own advantage (see Table 16).

Their presence is inferred when a characteristic disease with characteristic pathology appears after injection of test material into animals, and the incubation period is long. Multiplication is slow, with a doubling time of a week or more (see Table 20). The most rapidly detectable member of the group is scrapie when injected intracerebrally into hamsters, the disease appearing within 4 months; Kuru injected into monkeys may take several years. Infection cannot be detected serologically because there is no immune response. It seems likely there are more of these microorganisms waiting to be discovered, but they pose formidable problems for the investigator.

Reduced Interferon Induction or Responsiveness

Interferon production is not strictly an immunological phenomenon, but it is considered here because it does seem to involve recognition of foreign macromolecules by the cell (see Ch. 9) and because immune tolerance to microorganisms sometimes goes with interferon tolerance (see Table 18).

Viruses are generally sensitive to interferon and they can evade this host defence mechanism if they fail to induce interferon in the host or if they are resistant to the action of interferon. There are a few persistent virus infections in which this is the case. Mice persistently infected with LCM or leukaemia virus do not produce detectable interferon in spite of the continued multiplication of virus. This is also true of mouse cells infected *in vitro* with these viruses, although virus multiplication is readily inhibited when

Table 18. Microbial interference with or avoidance of immune defences

Type of interference/avoidance		Mechanism	Example	Status
Induction of	Ineffective antibody	Antibody of poor specificity or affinity fails to neutralize or opsonize	LCM virus *Treponema pallidum*	+ +
	Blocking antibody	Ineffective antibody bound to microbe blocks action of "good" antibody or immune cells	Disseminated gonorrhoea?	±
	Enhancing antibody	Antibody bound to microbe enhances infection of phagocyte	Dengue	++
	No antibody	No detectable antibody	Scrapie	++
Destruction of antibody		Liberation of IgA protease	Gonococcus *Haemophilus influenzae* Streptococci	+ + +
Antigenic variation		Microbial antigens vary within individual host	Trypanosomiasis Relapsing fever	++ ++
		Microbial antigens vary within host population	Influenza Streptococci	++ +

Mechanism	Description	Examples	
Infection in bodily site inaccessible to antibody	Persistent infection of glands etc. inaccessible to circulating antibody and immune cells (see Fig. 29)	Cytomegalovirus Rabies virus Mareks disease virus	++
"Silent" infection of host cell without making it vulnerable to immune lysis	Failure to display microbial antigen on infected cell surface	Herpes simplex ⎱persistence EB virus ⎰ Malaria in erythrocyte	++ ?
	Loss of microbial antigen by capping	Measles	+
Fc receptors present on microbe or induced on infected host cell	IgG antibodies nonspecifically bind to microbe or infected cell and block immune lysis/opsonization, etc.	Staphylococci (protein A) Certain streptococci Herpes simplex Cytomegalovirus	+ + ? ?
Induction of antigen-specific immune suppression	Microbial invasion of lymphoid tissue leads to suppressor T cell induction or clonal deletion of T cells or tolerization of T or B cells	LCM virus Lepromatous leprosy Hepatitis B	+ ? ?
Antibodies mopped up by microbial antigens	Microbial surface antigens in extracellular fluids combine with and "divert" antibodies	Hepatitis B Pneumococcal infection	? ?
Molecular mimicry	Microbial antigens mimic host antigens, leading to poor antibody response	*Mycoplasma pneumoniae*	−

interferon is added. The infected mice form interferon normally when infected with other viruses, so the defect is specifically in relation to these particular viruses. Mink infected with Aleutian Disease virus fail to respond with interferon production, although they give normal responses to other interferon inducers. Here there is an additional feature, because the infecting virus appears to be insensitive to the action of interferon. Presumably the cells of mice have difficulty in recognizing LCM or leukaemia virus nucleic acid as foreign, but nothing is known about this. Some persistent viruses, such as human adenoviruses tend to be insensitive to interferon, and perhaps others are poor inducers of interferon. If it were possible for viruses to induce less interferon or become insensitive to its action, some of them would be expected to have done so. This could obviously have significance in viral infection and persistence, but too little is known to draw any general conclusions.

References

Baucke, R. B. and Spear, P. G. (1979). Membrane proteins specified by herpes simplex virus. V. Identification of an Fc-binding glycoprotein. *J. Virology* **32**, 779–789.

Costerton, J. W. *et al.* (1974). Structure and function of the cell envelope of Gram-negative bacteria. *Bact. Rev.* **38**, 87–110.

Dwyer, D. M. (1976). Antibody-induced modulation of *Leishmani donovani* surface membrane antigens. *J. Immunol.* **117**, 2081.

Foo, M. C. and Lee, A. (1974). Antigenic cross reaction between mouse intestine and a member of the autochthonous microflora. *Infect. Immunity* **9**, 1066–1069.

Male, C. J. (1979). Immunoglobulin A protease production by *Haemophilus influenza* and *Streptococcus pneumoniae*. *Infect. Immunity* **26**, 254–261.

Levy, J. A., Kaminsky L. S., Morrow W. J. W. *et al.* (1985). Infection by the retrovirus associated with the acquired immunodeficiency syndrome. *Ann Int. Med.* **103**, 694–9.

Sparling, P. F., Cannon, J. G. and So, M. (1986). Phase and antigenic variation of pili and outer-membrane protein II of *Neisseria gonorrhoeae*. *J. Inf. Dis.* **153**, 196.

Mims, C. A. (1986). Interactions of viruses with the immune system. *Clin. Exp. Immunol.* **66**, 1–16.

Fujinami, R. S. and Oldstone, M. B. A. (1985). Amino acid homology between the encephalitogenic site of myelin basic protein and virus: mechanisms for autoimmunity. *Science* **230**, 1043.

McDevitt, H. O. *et al.* (1974). Histocompatibility-linked genetic control of specific immune responses to viral infection. *Transplant. Rev.* **19**, 209–225.

Pererson, P. K. *et al.* (1979). Inhibition of the alternative complement pathway opsonization by Group A streptococcal M protein. *J. Inf. Dis.* **139**, 575–585.

Sasazuki, D. *et al.* (1978). Association between an HLA haplotype and low responsiveness to tetanus toxoid in man. *Nature, Lond.* **272**, 359.

Schild, G. C. (Ed.) (1979). "Influenza". Br. Med. Bull. Vol. 35.

Toossi, Z., Kleinhenz, M. E., and Ellner, J. J. (1986). Defective interleukin-2 production and responsiveness in human tuberculosis. *J. Exp. Med.* **163**, 1162.

8

Mechanisms of Cell and Tissue Damage

The impact on the host of microbial damage depends very much on the tissue involved. Damage to muscle in the shoulder or stomach wall, for instance, may not be serious, but in the heart the very existence of the host depends on a strong muscle contraction continuing to occur every second or so, and here the effect of minor functional changes may be catastrophic. The central nervous system is particularly vulnerable to slight damage. The passage of nerve impulses requires normal function in the neuronal cell membrane, and viruses especially have important effects on cell membranes. Also a degree of cellular or tissue oedema that is tolerable in most tissues may have serious consequences if it occurs in the brain, enclosed in that more or less rigid box, the skull. Therefore encephalitis and meningitis tend to cause more severe illness than might be expected from the histological changes themselves. Oedema is a serious matter also in the lung. Oedema fluid or inflammatory cell exudates appear first in the space between the alveolar capillary and the alveolar wall, decreasing the efficiency of gaseous exchanges. Respiratory function is more drastically impaired when fluid or cells accumulate in the alveolar air space.* The effect of tissue damage is much less in the case of organs such as the liver, pancreas or kidney, which have considerable functional reserves. More than two-thirds of the liver must be removed before there are signs of liver dysfunction.

---

* In the normal lung, bronchioles and alveoli have an immense capacity to absorb surplus fluid, as indicated by the observation that 21 litres of fluid can be given intratracheally to a horse over the course of 3.5 h with no ill effect. There are nearly 10^9 alveoli in man, richly supplied with lymphatics, and with a combined absorptive area of 90 m^2.

Cell damage has profound effects if it is the endothelial cells of small blood vessels that are involved. The resulting circulatory changes may lead to anoxia or necrosis in the tissues supplied by these vessels. Here too, the site of vascular lesions may be critical, effects on organs such as the brain or heart having a greater impact on the host, as discussed above. Rickettsiae characteristically grow in vascular endothelium, and this is an important mechanism of disease production. By a combination of direct and immunopathological factors there is endothelial swelling, thrombosis, infarcts, haemorrhage and tissue anoxia. This is especially notable in the skin, and forms the basis for the striking rashes seen in typhus and the spotted fevers. These skin rashes, although important for the physician, are less important for the patient than similar vascular lesions in the central nervous system or heart. It is damage to cerebral vessels that accounts for the cerebral disturbances in typhus; involvement of pulmonary vessels causes pneumonitis, and involvement of myocardial vessels causes myocardial oedema. In Q fever, rickettsias sometimes localize in the endocardium, and this causes serious complications.

Sometimes an infectious agent damages an organ, and loss of function in this organ leads to a series of secondary disease features. The signs of liver dysfunction are an accepted result of infections of the liver, just as paralysis or coma is an accepted result of infection of the central nervous system. Diabetes may turn out to be caused by infection of the islets of Langerhans in the pancreas. Coxsackie and other virus infections of the islets of Langerhans can certainly cause diabetes in experimental animals, and coxsackieviruses have been associated with juvenile diabetes in man.

There are many diseases of unknown aetiology for which an infectious origin has been suggested. Sometimes it is fairly well established that an infectious agent can at least be one of the causes of the disease, but in most instances it is no more than a hypothesis, with little or no good evidence. For conditions as common and as serious as multiple sclerosis, cancer and rheumatoid arthritis it would be of immense importance if a microorganism were incriminated, since this would give the opportunity to prevent the disease by vaccination. Accordingly, there is a temptation to accept or publicize new reports even though the evidence is weak or the observations poorly controlled. As if to warn us about this and remind us of possibilities from environmental toxins, Parkinson's disease, a chronic neurological condition in which there is loss of neurons in a sharply defined region of the brain (substantia nigra), can be caused by exposure to the chemical MPTP. Since the aetiology of such diseases raises interesting problems in pathogenesis, the present state of affairs is summarized in Table 19, which includes some of the human diseases whose infectious origin is probable, possible, conceivable, or inconceivable.

Table 19. Microorganisms as causes of human diseases of unknown aetiology

Disease	Features	Microorganism	Pathogenic mechanism	Comments	Status of infectious aetiology
Juvenile diabetes	Onset early in life; sensitive to insulin	Coxsackie B viruses	Infection and damage of islets of Langerhan; secondary immune phenomena	Accounts for some cases How many?	+
		Mumps virus		No direct evidence	±
		Rubella virus		Late result congenital rubella	+
Crohn's disease	Granulomatous inflammation intestine	Mycobacteria Viruses	Not clear; secondary immune phenomena	} No good evidence	−
Ulcerative colitis	Inflammation of colon	Viruses	Not clear; secondary immune phenomena	No good evidence	−
Multiple sclerosis	Demyelinating disease of central nervous system. Waxes and wanes.	Viruses (measles, distemper, parainfluenza, coronavirus)	Viral damage to oligodendrocytes, or triggering of auto-immune damage	No direct evidence	−
Rheumatoid arthritis	Chronic inflammation and damage to joints	Mycoplasmas	?	Cause arthritis in animals but no evidence for man	−
		Viruses (EB, rubella)	?	No evidence	−
Paget's disease of bone	Localized deformation of bone	Measles virus	Persistent infection of osteoclasts		±

(Continued)

Table 19. (*Cont.*)

Disease	Features	Microorganism	Pathogenic mechanism	Comments	Status of infectious aetiology
Ankylosing spondylitis	Chronic arthritis of spine	*Klebsiella* spp.	Immune response to bacterial antigen cross reacts with joint antigen, giving auto-immune damage	Strong association with HLA B27 genotype	+
Alzheimer's disease	Presenile (<55 yrs) dementia	Member of Kuru, Creutzfeld-Jakob group	Infectious agent replicates slowly in brain, destroying cells	Some cases?	±
Senile dementia	Loss of neurons; very common at 65+ years	"Slow virus"?		No evidence	−
Old age	Not a disease but early death offers reliable prophylaxis; Degenerative changes	?	?	No evidence. Universal infection plus very long incubation period could give onset of "disease" with ageing	−
Cancer Carcinomas Nasopharyngeal carcinoma		EB virus	Transformation epithelial cell; plus cocarcinogen in food?	Susceptibility gene in Chinese people	+
Cervical carcinoma		Papillomaviruses	Transformation epithelial cell	Associated with sexual promiscuity	+

Carcinoma of liver	Hepatitis B virus	Transformation of hepatic cell	Liver cancer especially common in those with persistent hepatitis B infection[a]	+
Skin cancer (basal cell carcinoma)	Papillomaviruses	UV light as cocarcinogen	Evidence in animals but so far not in humans	+
Lymphomas Burkitt's lymphoma	EB virus	Transformation B lymphocyte plus cofactor (? malaria)	Evidence compelling but not conclusive	+
Hodgkin's disease	EB virus	Transformation B lymphocyte	No direct evidence	−
Leukaemias	Retroviruses	Transformation white cell precursor	Cause leukaemia in animals, and certain T cell leukaemias in humans (HTLV 1 and 2)	+

[a] In a study of 22 797 civil servants in Taiwan, 1.2% of hepatitis B carriers developed liver cancer compared with 0.005% of noncarriers.

Causal connections between infection and disease states are particularly difficult to establish when the disease appears a long time after infection. It was not too difficult to prove and accept that the encephalitis that occasionally occurs during or immediately after measles was due to measles virus. But it was hard to accept that a type of encephalitis (subacute sclerosing panencephalitis or SSPE) occurring up to ten years after apparently complete recovery from measles was also due to measles virus, and this was only established after careful studies and the eventual difficult isolation of measles virus from brain cells. "Slow" infections, in which the first signs of disease appear a long time after infection, are now an accepted part of our outlook. The disease Kuru occurs in New Guinea, and is transmitted from person to person by cannibalism. The incubation period of the disease in man appears to be 12–15 years, and it is caused by a subviral infectious agent that grows in the brain. This was established when the same disease appeared in monkeys several years after the injection of material from the brain of Kuru patients. A similar microorganism called scrapie infects mice, sheep and other animals, and also has an incubation period representing a large portion of the life span of the host. In both Kuru and SSPE the microorganism was eventually shown to be present in the brains of patients. If in a slow infection the microorganism that initiated the pathological process is no longer present by the time the disease becomes manifest, then the problem of establishing a causal relationship will be much greater. This may possibly turn out to be true for diseases like multiple sclerosis and rheumatoid arthritis. The types of virus infections that cause cancer are generally of the slow type, as illustrated by liver cancer in humans and leukaemia in mice, cats, humans and cattle. Cancer or leukaemia appears as a late and occasional sequel to infection. The virus, its antigens, or its nucleic acid "fingerprints" are detectable in malignant cells.

One important factor that often controls the speed of an infectious process and the type of host response, is the rate of multiplication of a microorganism*. Different infectious agents show doubling times varying from 20 minutes to a week, and some of these are listed in Table 20. Often the rate of multiplication in the infected host, in the presence of antimicrobial and other limiting factors and when many bacteria are obliged to multiply inside phagocytic cells, is much less than the optimal rate in artificial culture. Clearly a microorganism with a doubling time of a day or two will tend to cause a more slowly evolving infection and disease than one that doubles in an hour or less.

This chapter deals with demonstrable cell and tissue damage or dysfunc-

---

*Every infection is a RACE between the spread and multiplication of the microbe and the generation of an antimicrobial response by the host. A day or two's delay in this response may let the microbe reach the critical levels of growth that give tissue damage and disease.

Table 20. Growth rates of microorganisms expressed as doubling times

Microorganisms	Situation	Mean doubling time
Most viruses	In cell	<1 h
E. coli, staphylococci, streptococci etc.	In vitro	20 min
Salmonella typhimurium	Mouse spleen	5–12 h
	In vitro	30 min
Tubercle bacillus	In vitro	24 h
Malaria (Plasmodium falciparum)	Erythrocyte or hepatic cell	8 h
Fungi Candida albicans	In vitro (37°C)	30 min
Dermatophytes	In vitro (28°C)	1–24 h
Treponema pallidum	In vivo (rabbit)[a]	30 h
Scrapie group	Mouse brain[a]	4–7 days
Leprosy bacillus	In vivo[a]	2 weeks

[a] Canot be cultivated in vitro.

tion in infectious diseases. But one of the earliest indications of illness is malaise, "not feeling very well". This is distinct from fever or a specific complaint such as a sore throat and although it is difficult to define and impossible to measure, we all know the feeling. It can precede the onset of more specific signs and symptoms, or accompany them. Sometimes it is the only indication that an infection is taking place. Almost nothing is known of the basis for this feeling. "Toxins", of course, have been invoked, and the earliest response to pyrogens (see pp. 245–7) before body temperature has actually risen, may play a part. Interferons may have something to do with it because pure preparations of human α or β interferons cause malaise and often headaches and muscle aches after injection into normal individuals. If interferon is eventually recognized as an important antimicrobial force, we may have to regard these side effects as unfortunate but acceptable. Soluble mediators of immune and inflammatory responses, such as interleukin 1 (see Glossary) may also play a part. In some infectious diseases weakness and debility are prominent during convalescence. This can be especially notable following influenza and hepatitis, but its basis is as mysterious as in the case of malaise.

Infection with no Cell or Tissue Damage

The infections that matter are those causing pathological changes and disease. Before giving an account of the mechanisms by which these changes are produced, it is important to remember that many infectious agents cause little or no damage in the host. Indeed, it is of some advantage to the microorganism to cause minimal host damage, as discussed in Ch. 1. Virus infections as often as not fall into this category. Thus, although infection with rabies or measles viruses nearly always causes disease, there are many enterovirus, reovirus and myxovirus infections that are regularly asymptomatic. Even viruses that are named for their association with disease (poliomyelitis, influenza, Japanese B encephalitis) often give an antibody response as the only sign of infection in the host. Tissue damage is too slight to cause detectable illness. There is also a tendency for persistent viruses to cause no more than minor or delayed cellular damage during their persistence in the body, even if the same virus has a more cytopathic effect during an acute infection, e.g. adenoviruses, herpes simplex (see Ch. 10). A few viruses are remarkable because they cause no pathological changes at all in the cell, even during a productive infection in which infectious virus particles are produced. For instance, mouse cells infected with LCM or leukaemia virus show no pathological changes. A mouse congenitally infected with LCM virus shows a high degree of immune tolerance, and all tissues in the body are infected. Throughout the life of the animal virus and viral antigens are produced in the cerebellum, liver, retina etc. without discernible effect on cell function. But sometimes there are important functional changes in infected cells which lead to a pathological result. For example, the virus infects growth hormone-producing cells in the anterior pituitary. Although the cells appear perfectly healthy, the output of growth hormone is reduced, and as a result of this suckling mice fail to gain weight normally and are runted.

When bacteria invade tissues, they almost inevitably cause some damage, and this is also true for fungi, protozoa and rickettsiae. The extent of direct damage, however, is sometimes slight. This is true for *Treponema pallidum*, perhaps because the lipopolysaccharide–protein components that might have induced inflammatory responses, are not exposed on the surface of the bacteria. It produces no toxins, does not cause fever, and attaches to cells *in vitro* without harmful effects. Leprosy and tubercle bacilli eventually damage and kill the macrophages in which they replicate, but pathological changes are to a large extent caused by indirect mechanisms (see below). In patients with untreated lepromatous leprosy, the bacteria in the skin invade blood vessels, and large number of bacteria, many of them free, may be found in the blood. In spite of the continued presence of up to 10^5 bacteria (ml of blood)$^{-1}$ there are no signs or symptoms of septicaemia or toxaemia. *Mycobacterium leprae* can be regarded as a very successful parasite that induces very little host response in these patients, even when the blood stream is invaded. The resident bacteria inhabiting the skin and intestines of man and animals do not invade tissues and are normally harmless; indeed, as discussed in Ch. 1, they may benefit the host. Bacteria such as meningococci and pneumococci, whose name implies pathogenicity, spend most of their time as harmless inhabitants of the normal human nasopharynx; only occasionally do they have the opportunity to invade tissues and give rise to meningitis or pneumonia.

Direct Damage by Microorganisms

Cell and tissue damage is sometimes due to the direct local action of the microorganism. When poliovirus, for instance, grows in cells it causes an early shutdown of RNA, protein and DNA synthesis in the host cell. Within a few hours there is an inevitable cytopathic effect and the cell dies. In the affected host, if enough motor neurons in the spinal cord are infected, damaged and destroyed, the corresponding muscles cannot function and the patient develops paralytic poliomyelitis. Another example of direct viral damage is seen in the common cold when caused by the rhinovirus group of picornaviruses. Rhinoviruses infect nasal epithelial cells, and at an early stage the cells round up, fall off the mucosal surface and are carried away, often with their cilia still beating, in a stream of fluid induced by the infection. This leaves areas of raw mucosa, with the exposed underlying tissues inflamed, oedematous, and susceptible to infection by the normally harmless resident bacteria. Many other viruses, including other picornaviruses, poxviruses and herpes viruses, cause a shutdown in macromolecular synthesis and directly damage the infected cell in the same way. Viral proteins accumulating in the cell during replication possibly have a toxic effect and contribute to cell damage. Cell membranes are generally the site of the initial damage, and interference with membrane function causes a leakage of cell material through the cell surfaces to the exterior; when lysosomes are affected and lysosomal enzymes leak into the cytoplasm, the cell undergoes autolytic destruction. Lysosomes have been referred to as "suicide bags" to draw attention to this aspect of cell necrosis.

The lesions in cells infected with viruses are generally nonspecific, very like those induced in cells by the toxins of diphtheria bacilli and streptococci, or by physical and chemical agents. The most common and potentially reversible change, the oedema seen as "cloudy swelling" by routine histology, is associated with membrane permeability changes. Changes in the endoplasmic reticulum, mitochondria and polyribosomes are seen by electron microscopy at this stage. Later the nuclear chromatin moves to the edge of the nucleus ("margination" of chromatin) and becomes condensed (pycnosis), but the cell has already died by this time. There are two more characteristic types of morphological change produced by certain viruses, and these were recognized by histologists more than 50 years ago. The first are inclusion bodies, parts of the cell with altered staining behaviour which develop during infection. They often represent either cell organelles or virus factories in which viral components are being synthesized and assembled. Herpes group viruses form intranuclear inclusions, rabies and pox viruses intracytoplasmic inclusions, and measles virus both intranuclear and intra-cytoplasmic inclusions. The second characteristic morphological change caused by viruses is the formation of multinucleate giant cells. This is a result of cell fusion, and occurs for instance in measles and certain herpes virus infections. Sendai virus (a paramyxovirus) has a powerful viral "fusion" protein which fuses plasma membranes of neighbouring cells *in vitro*, to form multinucleate cells.

Before leaving the subject of direct damage by viruses, one supreme example will be given. Here the direct damage is of such a magnitude that the susceptible host dies a mere six hours after infection. Rift Valley Fever virus, an arthropod-borne virus infecting cattle, sheep and man in Africa, is injected in very large doses intravenously into mice. The injected virus passes straight through the Kupffer cells and endothelial cells lining liver sinusoids (see Ch. 5) and infects nearly all hepatic cells. Hepatic cells show nuclear inclusions within an hour, and necrosis by four hours. As the single cycle of growth in hepatic cells is completed, massive liver necrosis takes place, and mice die only six hours after initial infection. The host defences in the form of local lymph nodes, local tissue phagocytes etc. are completely overcome by the intravenous route of injection, and by the inability of Kupffer cells to prevent infection of hepatic cells. Direct damage by the replicating virus destroys hepatic cells long before immune or interferon responses have an opportunity to control the infection. This is the summit of virulence. The experimental situation is artificial but it illustrates direct and lethal damage to host tissues after all host defence mechanisms have been overwhelmed.

Most viruses, rickettsiae and chlamydia damage the cells in which they replicate, and it is possible that some of this damage is due to the action of toxic microbial products. This action, however, is confined to the infected cell, and toxic microbial products are not liberated to damage other cells. Mycoplasma (see Table 32, p. 298) can grow in special cell-free media, but in the infected individual they generally multiply while attached to the surface of host cells. As studied in culture and on the respiratory epithelium they "burrow" down between cells, inhibit the beat of cilia and cause cell necrosis and detachment. The mechanism is not clear. If a complete "lawn" of mycoplasma covers the surface of the host cell, some effect on the health of the cell is to be expected, but it is possible that toxic materials are produced or are present on the surface of the mycoplasma.

Dental caries provides an interesting example of direct pathological action. Colonization of the tooth surface by *Streptococcus mutans* leads to plaque formation, and the bacteria held in the plaque utilize dietary sugar and produce acid (see p. 24). Locally produced acid decalcifies the tooth to give caries. Caries, arguably the commonest infectious disease of Western man, might logically be controlled by removing plaque, withholding dietary sugar, or vaccinating against *Streptococcus mutans*.

Bacteria generally damage the cells in which they replicate, and these are mostly phagocytic cells (see Ch. 4). *Listeria, Brucella* and *Mycobacteria* are specialists at intracellular growth, and the infected phagocyte is slowly destroyed as increasing numbers of bacteria are produced in it. Bacteria such as staphylococci and streptococci grow primarily in extracellular fluids, but they are ingested by phagocytic cells, and virulent strains of bacteria in particular have the ability to destroy the phagocyte in which they find themselves, even growing in the phagocytes, as described in Ch. 4. Many bacteria cause extensive tissue damage by the liberation of toxins into extracellular fluids. Various toxins have been identified and characterized. Most act locally, but a few cause pathological changes after spreading systemically through the body.

Microbial Toxins

Bacterial toxins are broadly divided into those that are liberated from multiplying bacteria (exotoxins) and those that are associated with the cell wall and are released after death of the bacterium (endotoxins). The substances liberated, however, are not necessarily toxic, and not all bacterial cell walls are particularly toxic.

Exotoxins

Most exotoxins are produced by Gram-positive bacteria. They are proteins and a few of them have been identified as specific enzymes. When liberated locally they can cause local cell and tissue damage and those that damage phagocytic cells and are therefore particularly useful to the microorganism have been described in Ch. 4. Those that promote the spread of bacteria in tissues have been referred to in Ch. 5. If enough of the toxins produced in tissues enter the blood, or when multiplying bacteria themselves enter the blood (anthrax), there are generalized toxic effects. Important exotoxins are listed in Table 21 and the best studied examples will be described.

Clostridium perfringens (welchii) is the organism most commonly associated with gas gangrene. It is strictly anaerobic, and occurs as a normal inhabitant in the large intestines of man and animals; its spores are ubiquit-

Table 21. Exotoxins[a]

Microorganism	Toxin	Action	Significance *in vivo*
Clostridium perfringens	α Toxin	Phospholipase (action on cell membrane)	Cell necrosis, haemolysis, toxaemia
Clostridium tetani	Toxin	Blocks action of inhibitory neurons	Overaction of motor neurons, muscle spasm, lockjaw
Corynebacterium diphtheriae	Toxin	Inhibits cell protein synthesis	Epithelial necrosis, heart damage, nerve paralysis
Shigella dysenteriae	Enterotoxin (neurotoxin)	Induces fluid loss and local cell death in intestine; vascular endothelial damage in brain	Diarrhoea, neurological disturbances
Vibrio cholerae	Toxin (choleragen)	Activates adenylate cyclase, and raises cAMP level in cells	Acts on intestinal epithelial cell; water and electrolyte loss into intestine
Bacillus anthracis	Toxic complex	Three factors form a toxic complex and cause increased vascular permeability	Oedema and haemorrhage (primary lesion); circulatory failure (systemic disease)

Organism	Toxin	Action	Effect
Clostridium botulinum	Toxin	Blocks release of acetylcholine	Neurotoxic signs, paralyses
Bordetella pertussis	Toxin	Ciliary damage	?
Streptococcus pyogenes	Erythrogenic toxin	Vasodilation	Causes scarlet fever rash
	Leucocidin	Kill phagocytes	Antiphagocytic
	Streptolysins		
	Streptokinase	Lyses fibrin	Promote spread of bacteria in tissues?
	Hyaluronidase	Liquifies connective tisse matrix	
Staphylococcus aureus	α Haemolysin	Cytotoxic; action on cell membranes	Necrosis at site of infection; systemic toxicity
	Leucocidin	Kills phagocytes	Antiphagocytic
	Enterotoxin	Action on gut nerve endings	Nausea, vomiting, diarrhoea (food poisoning)
	Exfoliating toxin	Splits epidermis	Scalded skin syndrome
Legionella pneumophilia	Toxin	Damages cells	Contributes to extrapulmonary disturbances in legionnaire's disease?

[a] Exotoxins are proteins liberated from bacteria; highly antigenic; convertible into immunogenic toxoids.

ous in soil, dust and air. *Clostridium perfringens* does not multiply in healthy tissues, but grows rapidly when it reaches devitalized and therefore anaerobic tissues. This could be after contamination of a natural wound with soil or dust, particularly on battlefields or in automobile accidents, or after contamination of a surgical operation site with clostridia from the patient's own bowels or skin. After abortions, particularly in the old days before antibiotics, intestinal clostridia often gained access to necrotic or devitalized tissues in the uterus and set up life-threatening infections. Invasion of the blood was common and soon resulted in death, the clostridia localizing and growing in internal organs such as the liver after death. *Clostridium perfringens* has various enzymes that enable it to break down cell membranes and connective tissue materials, including collagen. These facilitate spread of the infection along tissue planes. Most of the enzymes are toxic to host cells and tissues. Five designated types of *Clostridium perfringens* are distinguished (A–E) according to the various combinations of toxins they produce. Alpha toxin is the most important one, causing tissue necrosis on injection into the skin of laboratory animals. It is an enzyme, phospholipase (lecithinase), and kills cells by damaging the cell membrane. It readily attacks the membrane of red blood cells, causing haemolysis, and is sometimes responsible for large-scale intravascular haemolysis in infected patients. There are more than ten other named toxins (beta, gamma, delta, epsilon etc.); some have lethal or necrotizing actions and others are less pathogenic. Cultures of virulent strains of *Clostridium perfringens* kill guinea-pigs within 24 h after subcutaneous or intramuscular injection, causing inflammation, oedema and the production of gas and tissue necrosis at the site of infection. In the infected patient, absorption of toxins into the circulation causes toxaemia and shock. The exact sequence of events and the role of each of the defined toxins is not clear, but the amount of alpha toxin formed is generally associated with virulence. The bacteria produce a capsule *in vivo* so that phagocytosis is impaired (see Ch. 4).

There are other pathogenic clostridia that cause gas gangrene and produce similar toxins. Infected tissues show inflammation, oedema and necrosis, not necessarily with the formation of gas, and the illness can be mild or very severe according to the extent of bacterial spread and the nature and quantity of toxins that are formed and absorbed. Since the bacteria grow and produce their toxins only in devitalized tissues, the most important form of treatment is to remove the devitalized tissues. Clostridia are strictly anaerobic, and exposure of the patient to hyperbaric oxygen (pure oxygen at 2–3 atmospheres in a pressure chamber) has been found useful in addition to chemotherapy.

Another bacterial exotoxin that undoubtedly plays a part in disease is the exfoliating toxin of *Staphylococcus aureus*. This is produced by certain strains of *Staphylococcus aureus*, and is controlled by a plasmid. It causes exfoliation of the skin of infected children, a clinical condition known as the "scalded-skin syndrome". The condition is not common and is mentioned because the toxin has been purified, its action has been studied (on the naked skin of newborn mice), and it has an accepted pathological significance. It has a molecular weight of 23 500, and acts by cleaving the epidermis at the stratum granulosum and forming bullae.

The versatility of staphylococci is further illustrated by the toxic shock syndrome, seen characteristically in menstruating women whose tampons harbour multiplying staphylococci. It is due to a defined 22 000 mol. wt. toxin called toxic-shock-syndrome toxin 1 (TSST1).

Exotoxins formed in the intestine

An important group of locally acting exotoxins are produced by certain bacteria infecting the intestinal tract, and these toxins are actually responsible for the disease. *Vibrio cholerae* multiplies in the lumen of the small intestine and does not invade tissues. Helped by its motility it attaches to intestinal epithelium (see Table 2, p. 20) and releases a toxin (enterotoxin) that reacts rapidly with a ganglioside receptor on epithelial cells and makes a specific attachment. The enterotoxin is a protein of mol. wt. 90 000, and like many other toxins consists of a portion that binds to the susceptible cell (in this case, to any vertebrate cell!) and a portion that is responsible for the toxic action. It does not damage the cell, but activates adenylate cyclase and thereby raises the intracellular level of cyclic adenosine monophosphate (cAMP). As a result of this, water and electrolytes are lost through the intact epithelial cells into the small intestine. As the multiplying bacteria increase in numbers and more and more epithelial cells are affected, the absorptive capacity of the colon is overwhelmed and there is a profuse watery diarrhoea, as much as 1 litre h^{-1} in severe cases.* The massive loss of isotonic fluid with excess of sodium bicarbonate and potassium leads to hypovolemic shock, acidosis and haemoconcentration. Anuria develops, and the collapsed, lethargic patient may die in 12–24 h. Lives are saved by replacing the lost water and salts. The effect of toxin on an intestinal epithelial cell is long lasting, but the patient recovers as affected cells are shed and replaced in the normal fashion. The infection is particularly severe in children, who easily develop low levels of plasma potassium.

*The toxic action can be demonstrated by injecting bacteria-free culture fluid into tied off segments of a rabbit's (or infant mouse) small intestine. The intestinal segments begin to secrete fluid within 0.5 h, and fluid accumulation is maximal by 12 h.

Certain strains of *E. coli* produce a similar and antigenically related enterotoxin which attaches to different receptors on the intestinal epithelium. These strains of bacteria themselves make specific attachments enabling them to colonize intestinal epithelium so that the enterotoxin can be adsorbed and act locally. Some of them produce an additional enterotoxin that activates guanylate cyclase and makes a further contribution to fluid loss and pathogenicity. These enterotoxigenic *E. coli* (ETEC) are common causes of diarrhoea in visitors to developing countries. *E. coli* strains such as O 55, O 111 etc. are particularly pathogenic in infants, causing a cholera-like illness (infantile gastroenteritis).

Some of the pathogenic intestinal bacteria penetrate the intestinal epithelial cells after attachment. *Shigella dysenteriae* attaches specifically to colonic epithelium and enters the cell after locally dissolving the cell membrane. An enterotoxin is produced in the infected cell, which dies, and small eroded areas (ulcers) appear on the mucosa. The enterotoxin has an action on small blood vessels, and blood-stained fluids, mucus and pus exudes from the ulcers to give the bloody diarrhoea of classical bacillary dysentery. If enough enterotoxin is adsorbed from the intestines, there are vascular changes in the brain and spinal cord that give rise to the neurotoxic manifestations seen in severe (*Shigella dysenteriae*) dysentery. Presumably the endotoxin of *Shigella dysenteriae* (see below) also makes a contribution to the local lesions and to the disease. There is little if any bacterial invasion of subepithelial tissues. Pathogenicity depends on entry into epithelial cells and strains of *Shigella* that are unable to penetrate epithelial cells are nonpathogenic. There are great variations in virulence within the shigellas, *Shigella dysenteriae* causing more severe dysentery and *Shigella sonnei* a very mild disease. Some of the pathogenic *E. coli* strains behave in a similar manner to the shigellas, penetrating intestinal epithelial cells. Strains of *E. coli*, in fact, have a broad spectrum of biological properties and pathogenicity, from the harmless commensal to the serious pathogen, and overlap with *Vibrio cholerae*, *Salmonella* and *Shigella*. Indeed, antigenic relationships between these bacteria and *E. coli* have been described. *E. coli* strain 0124, for instance, causing an outbreak of *Shigella*-like illness, was found to have identical somatic antigens to *Shigella dysenteriae* strain 3. Perhaps the pathogenic strains have been formed by the transfer of plasmids* from the more pathogenic bacteria to *E. coli*. The different types of intestinal infections are compared in Table 22.

Intestinal infections more recently identified in man include the viral diarrhoeas, whose pathogenesis is discussed on pp. 220–3, and *Campylobac-*

---

* A plasmid is a small extrachromosomal piece of genetic material in a bacterium, replicating autonomously in the cytoplasm. It may carry 50–100 genes. Plasmids are common in Gram-negative bacilli, and also occur in staphylococci.

Table 22. Types of intestinal infection

Type of infection	Microorganism	Disease
Bacteria attach to epithelium of small intestine, rarely penetrate, and cause disease (diarrhoea) by forming an enterotoxin which induces fluid loss from epithelial cells.	*Vibrio cholerae* *E. coli* (certain strains)	Cholera Infantile gastroenteritis (certain types) or mild cholera-like disease in adults (travellers' diarrhoea) Calf diarrhoea
Microorganism attaches to and penetrates epithelium of large intestine (*Shigella*) or ileum (*Salmonella*), causing disease by killing epithelial cells (some form an exotoxin) and inducing diarrhoea. Subepithelial penetration uncommon.	*Shigella* spp. *Salmonella* (certain species)[a] *E. coli* (certain strains) *Campylobacter jejuni* Human diarrhoea viruses *Eimeria* spp. *Entamoeba histolytica*	Bacillary dysentery Salmonellosis ⎱ Coliform enteritis or ⎰ dysentery Piglet diarrhoea Enteritis in man[b] Gastroenteritis Coccidiosis in domestic animals (may cause diarrhoea and blood loss) Amoebic dysentery
Bacteria attach to and penetrate epithelium of small intestine. Also invade subepithelial tissues, sometimes (typhoid) spreading systemically.	*Salmonella typhi* and *paratyphi* *Salmonella* (certain species) *E. coli* (certain strains)	Enteric fever (typhoid) Salmonellosis (severe form) Calf enteritis

[a] There are more than 1000 serotypes of *Salmonella*, distinct from *Salmonella typhi* and *Salmonella paratyphi*. They are primarily parasites of animals, ranging from pythons to elephants, and their importance for man is their great tendency to colonize domestic animals. Pigs and poultry are commonly affected, and human disease follows the consumption of contaminated meat or eggs. The pathophysiology of Salmonellosis, and the role of toxins, is not clear.

[b] Other campylobacters cause sepsis, abortion, enteritis in animals.

ter jejuni infections. The latter are bacteria present in wild birds, chickens and in the faeces of up to 10% of healthy cows in the UK. Milk becomes contaminated and those who drink raw (unpasteurized) infected milk develop diarrhoea, sometimes with dysentery (blood and pus in the stools) and fever. The incubation period is 2–7 days and diarrhoea occurs after bacterial replication in the upper small intestine (jejeunum).* So far an enterotoxin has not been detected and it seems likely that the bacteria invade mucosal cells.

A final group of intestinal pathogens not only penetrates epithelial cells, but also invades subepithelial tissues, sometimes multiplying in the phago-cytes that engulf them. In man this group includes *Salmonella typhi* and *paratyphi*, which invade and cause a characteristic systemic disease (typhoid or enteric fever) and a very occasional invasive species of *Salmonella* of animal origin. The role of toxins in these diseases is discussed below.

One other toxin that causes intestinal disturbances is the enterotoxin formed by certain strains of *Staphylococcus aureus*. Staphylococci are not normal intestinal inhabitants, but when the toxin is ingested in food in which staphylococci have been growing profusely it causes nausea, vomiting and diarrhoea within 6 h (staphylococcal food poisoning). This toxin is absorbed from the intestine and acts directly on nerve endings in the intestine with eventual stimulation of the vomiting centre in the central nervous system. Food poisoning is a loosely used term, but generally refers to the illness that comes on within a day or so after the ingestion of contaminated food. The food may be contaminated with plant poisons, fungal poisons (e.g. "mush-room" poisoning due to *Amanita phalloides*)† fish poisons, heavy metals etc. or with certain bacteria. Bacterial food poisoning is caused either by preformed toxins, as in staphylococcal food poisoning, or by large numbers of bacteria which undergo at the most a limited amount of multiplication in the intestine before causing disease. The pathogenesis in this second type of bacterial food poisoning is not clear, but presumably toxins are produced which act locally and often systemically. Pathological changes are minimal. Examples of food poisoning are given in Table 23.

Exotoxins acting systemically

There is an important group of bacterial toxins that act at a distance from the site of bacterial infection and in this way give rise to the manifestations of disease. These diseases are diphtheria, tetanus and scarlet fever. In diphtheria, bacteria multiply on the epithelial surfaces of the body (nose, throat, skin) but do not penetrate deeply into underlying tissues. A powerful

---

*Related bacteria live in mucus-filled crypts in the intestine of most animals. For instance *Campylobacter pyloridis* in the human stomach, which makes its way through the mucus by corkscrew movements, sometimes causes gastritis.

†Ingestion of scombroid fish (mackerel etc.) containing large amounts of histamine or similar substances leads to headache, flushing, nausea and vomiting within an hour.

Table 23. Types of food poisoning

Features	Examples	Pathogenesis	Incubation period
Preformed toxin in food	*Staphylococcus aureus*	Enterotoxin acts on nerve endings in intestine	1–6 h
	Clostridium botulinum	Powerful neurotoxin absorbed from intestine	12–36 h
	Bacillus cereus	Emetic toxin with early or late effects (typically in fried rice)	1–20 h
Large numbers (>10^6) bacteria in food	*Clostridium perfringens* type A	Limited multiplication and production of enterotoxin during spore formation	10–20 h
	Vibro parahaemolyticus	Multiplication in intestine (acquired from seafoods)	1–2 days
	Salmonella spp.	Limited multiplication; ill-defined local and systemic effects. Some epithelial damage	1–2 days

toxin is formed, which is absorbed from the infected site and has important actions, especially on the heart and nervous system. The toxin, a protein of molecular weight 62 000, consists of two parts; one responsible for adsorption to the cell and the other an enzyme that inhibits protein synthesis in the cell by inactivating elongation factor (a protein required for the translocation step of protein synthesis). One molecule of toxin per cell is effective, and a single bacillus can produce 5000 molecules an hour. The heart and peripheral nerves are particularly susceptible, perhaps because the synthesis of some specific protein is affected, and this leads to myocarditis and neuritis. The infection on the body surface causes necrosis of mucosal cells with an inflammatory exudate and the formation of a thick "membrane" and if the infection spreads into the larynx there may be respiratory obstruction. The toxin probably assists colonization of the throat or skin by killing epithelial cells and polymorphs.

Tetanus occurs in man and animals when *Clostridium tetani* grows in an infected wound and produces its toxin. The bacterial spores, ubiquitous in faeces and soil, require a reduced oxygen tension for germination and this is provided locally in the wound by foreign bodies (splinters, fragments of earth or clothing) or by tissue necrosis as seen in most wounds, the uterus after septic abortion, or the umbilical stump of the new-born.* The site of infection may be a contaminated splinter just as well as an automobile or battle injury. The toxin (mol. wt. 150 000) is a highly potent protein which passes up the axon of the peripheral nerve fibres, reaching motor neurons and diffusing locally through the central nervous system. It also reaches the central nervous system by travelling up other peripheral nerves following blood-borne dissemination of the toxin through the body. The heavy chain of the molecule binds to a ganglioside receptor on neurons and the light chain is toxic, acting like strychnine by interfering with the normal control of anterior horn cell activity. The motor nerves in the brain stem are short and therefore the cranial nerves are among the first to be affected, causing spasms of eye muscles and jaw (lock-jaw). There is also an increase in tonus of muscles round the site of infection, followed by tonic spasms. In generalized tetanus there is interference with respiratory movements, and without skilled treatment the mortality rate is about 50%. All strains of *Clostridium tetani* produce the same toxin. A related bacterium (*Clostridium botulinum*) causes botulism.† This organism, a widespread saprophyte present in soil and vegetable materials, is not infectious. It contaminates food, particularly inadequately preserved meat or vegetables, and produces a powerful neurotoxin. The toxin is destroyed at 80°C after 30 min and is one of the most toxic substances known, 1 g being enough to kill 10^{10} mice. There are seven antigenically distinct toxins produced by different strains of bacteria. It is absorbed from the intestine and acts on the peripheral nervous system, interfering with the release of acetylcholine at cholinergic synapses and the neuromuscular junction. Somewhere between 12 and 36 hours after ingestion there are clinical signs suggesting an acute neurological disorder, with vertigo, cranial nerve palsies and finally death a few days later with respiratory failure.‡

The final example of a toxin that acts at a distance from the site of infection is seen in the disease scarlet fever. It is one of the many conditions caused by streptococcal infection (see below) and may accompany a streptococcal sore throat or occasionally a streptococcal wound infection. There is a

---

* In developing countries about 10^6 newborn children die of tetanus each year.

† Botulus (Latin) = sausage. In 1793 a large sausage was eaten by 13 people in Wildbad in Germany; all became ill, and six died. The disease was subsequently referred to as botulism.

‡ In recent years a less typical form of botulism has been described in small infants. The spores, present in honey applied to rubber teats, appear to colonize the gut, so that the toxin is produced *in vivo* after ingestion.

generalized erythematous rash together with fever and a sore throat. The rash is due to an erythrogenic toxin produced by certain strains of *Streptococcus pyogenes*. The toxin is a protein of mol. wt. 29 000 and is liberated by bacteria that are themselves infected with a certain temperate bacteriophage. As little as 0.001 ng of the toxin will produce local erythema when injected into the skin of a sensitive person. It is also a powerful lymphocyte mitogen, but the significance of this is not clear. Although there are many antigenically distinct types of *Streptococcus pyogenes*, there is only one erythrogenic toxin. Repeated attacks of streptococcal sore throat are therefore possible, but the production of specific antibody to the toxin ensures that there is only one attack of scarlet fever. The only significance of the rash of scarlet fever is that it accompanies a streptococcal infection, and at one time death was a common sequel because of streptococcal septicaemia, puerperal sepsis or malignant endocarditis. Improvements in nutrition, social and environmental conditions and the development of antibiotics have made streptococcal infections less severe, and hence the significance of the rash has been greatly reduced.

There is one systemic bacterial infection in which an exotoxin causes disease and death. Locally formed bacterial exotoxins can give systemic disease if adequate amounts enter the blood, but exotoxaemia can also result from the multiplication of bacteria in the blood stream. Bacteraemia is a regular occurrence in anthrax, and for many years the pathogenesis of anthrax was not clear, but Professor Harry Smith and his colleagues showed that disease and death is caused by bacterial toxins. Anthrax is a disease of animals, particularly sheep and cattle, and to a lesser extent man, caused by infection with *Bacillus anthracis*. Infection takes place following the ingestion of spores, the inhalation of spores or by the entry of spores through abraided skin. The spores germinate and then the bacteria form an exotoxin that increases vascular permeability and gives rise to local oedema and haemorrhage. Infection of the skin in man leads to the formation of a lesion (malignant pustule) consisting of a necrotic centre surrounded by vesicles, blood-stained fluid and a zone of oedema and induration. In severe infections there is septicaemia with toxic signs and the effect of the exotoxin on the vascular system leads to loss of fluid into tissues, with widespread oedema and eventually death. The exotoxin consists of three components; a chelating agent and two proteins that act synergistically to increase vascular permeability. This exotoxin is largely responsible for the local lesions, and enters the circulation to account for the toxicity, oedema and death. The bacteria have a capsular polypeptide composed of D-glutamic acid, and this substance, found only in virulent strains, inhibits opsonization and phagocytosis (see Ch. 4). Anthrax in man occurs mainly in those whose work brings them into contact with infected animals. It is not a common disease in the UK, and the usual source therefore is from imported bones, hides, skins, bristles, wool and hair, or imported fertilizers made from the blood and bones of infected animals. The spores are resistant to chemical disinfectants and heat.

The exotoxins described above are the fairly well-defined ones, with an accepted role in the causation of disease. There are doubtless other microbial infections in which exotoxins play an important part, but these exotoxins have been less clearly defined and incriminated. An exotoxin produced by *Pseudomonas aeruginosa*, for instance, is very similar to the diphtheria toxin (see above), inhibiting protein synthesis, and is cytotoxic for polymorphs and lethal for experimental animals. *Haemophilus influenzae*, although it has no true exotoxin, produces histamine, and this may contribute to the inflammation and reduced airflow seen in lung infection. The lymphocytosis-promoting factor is the main toxic component of *Bordetella pertussis*, causing also hypoglycaemia and histamine sensitization. It acts on the adenylate cyclase system in cells, but its exact role in the disease whooping cough is still not clear.

As more and more toxins (and other microbial molecules) are described, there will be more that are "looking for a role" in virulence and pathogenicity. Recombinant DNA technology promises to provide firmer answers to such problems. A gene coding for a given toxin can be deleted from a virulent microbial strain or introduced into a non-virulent strain, and the effect on virulence determined. The cholera toxin gene, for instance, has been cloned in *E. coli*, altered by mutation, and then reintroduced into virulent *V. cholerae* to give toxin-negative *V. cholerae*. The fact that the new strain replicates in the intestine without causing disease does not tell us anything we did not know about pathogenicity, but is important for vaccines. Recombinant DNA approaches to virulence are also discussed on p. 320.

Even if the microbial gene conferring virulence is identified, it is a further big step to characterize the gene product and its mode of action. Ignorance of host responses and pathophysiological events add to the problem. Also, although investigators long for a simple, preferably single, explanation, virulence and pathogenicity are likely to prove multifactorial. The classic clarity of botulism, diphtheria and tetanus (see above), or the supreme reductionist simplicity of sickle-cell anaemia (see p. 275) are misleading precedents. Indeed microbes are on general principles unlikely to owe their success to or rely on single pathogenic mechanisms. This would make life easier for the investigator, but not for the microbe. The vertebrate host presents an immensely complicated challenge to which there is not likely to be a single successful answer. A single virulence determinant in any case provides the host with a simpler counter-strategy.

Fungal exotoxins

Many fungi contain substances that are harmful when taken by mouth, and there are two diseases that result from the ingestion of food containing preformed fungal toxins. As with *Clostridium botulinum*, the disease is caused without the need for infection. *Aspergillus flavus* infects ground nuts (monkey nuts) and produces a very powerful toxin (aflatoxin). Contaminated (badly stored) ground nuts used to prepare animal feeds caused the death of thousands of turkeys and pigs in the UK in 1960 and the survivors of intoxication nearly all developed liver cancer. Human disease has not yet been associated with this toxin. *Claviceps purpurae* is a rust fungus affecting rye, and it produces toxins (ergotamine especially) that give rise to ergot poisoning when contaminated grain is eaten. Mushrooms and toadstools have long been recognized as sources of poisons and hallucinogens.

Endotoxins

Endotoxins form part of the outer layer of the bacterial cell wall. Small quantities of endotoxins may be released in soluble form during bacterial growth, but for the most part they remain associated with the cell wall until the death and disintegration of bacteria. They are less toxic than exotoxins, and unlike most exotoxins they are heat stable and cannot be converted into toxoids (see Glossary). The word endotoxin generally refers to the complex phospholipid–polysaccharide–protein macromolecules associated with the cell wall of Gram-negative bacteria such as *Salmonella*, *Shigella*, *Escherichia* etc. and *Neisseria*. The lipopolysaccharide (LPS) is the important component, and the protein has therefore been somewhat neglected. Recent work indicates that the lipopolysaccharide of *Neisseria gonorrhoea*, which is excreted in "blebs" from the outer membrane of bacteria, is responsible for damage to epithelial cells. The LPS of *Pseudomonas aeruginosa* is less toxic than the LPS from other Gram-negative bacilli, and some Gram-negative bacteria, for instance *Brucella*, have a more or less nontoxic LPS. There are a few "endotoxins" such as those in the cell wall of *Yersinia pestis* and *Bordetella pertussis* that have different properties, consisting of protein rather than LPS, and the importance of the cell wall in streptococcal infections is referred to on p. 204.*

* Lipopolysaccharides from rickettsiae, trypanosomes and spirochaetes have similar properties to those of Gram-negative bacteria but their role in pathogenesis is unknown. The peptidoglycan (mucopeptide) components in cell walls of Gram-positive bacteria are quite different (p. 70). They consist of chains of alternating *N*-acetylglucosamine and *N*-acetylmuramic acid cross-linked through short peptide side chains, and comprise 50% of the cell wall, forming a scaffold and giving it shape and rigidity. In contrast to the teichoic acid component of the Gram-positive cell wall they have certain endotoxin-like activities, including the ability to cause fever (see pp. 245–7) and activate complement.

The LPS of Gram-negative bacteria consists of three components, a core polysaccharide common to many Gram-negative bacteria, an O specific polysaccharide which confers virulence and serological specificity on the macromolecule, and a lipid A component mainly responsible for toxicity (see Fig. 14). The LPS is an important virulence factor and small changes in the O antigen, involving no more than changes in the sugar sequences in side chains of the molecule, result in major changes in virulence. The importance of the polysaccharide chain for virulence, and the significance of smooth–rough variations are discussed on p. 170. Various toxic phenomena caused by LPS have been described, but the part played by these phenomena in Gram-negative infections is far from clear. LPS causes the release of vasoactive substances, activates the alternate pathway of the complement cascade, and also activates factor XII (Hageman factor), the first step of the coagulation cascade, which sometimes results in disseminated intravascular coagulation (see p. 215). There is an effect on the circulation, leading ultimately to vascular collapse. The vascular regions most affected differ from species to species; in man and sheep the main changes are found in the lungs. LPS has powerful immunological actions, which is surely no accident; as well as activating the complement system, it induces Il-1 production and is a potent B cell mitogen. Endotoxins are also pyrogenic, and man is one of the most sensitive of all species to this action. A dose of 2 ng per kg of body weight injected intravenously into man causes the release of an endogenous pyrogen (Interleukin-1, see Glossary) from macrophages which acts on the hypothalamus to give an elevation of body temperature within an hour. It is possible that the pyrogenic action of LPS helps to generate fever in Gram-negative bacterial infections, but there is evidence against this in typhoid fever, and bacteria with no known pyrogenic activity can give rise to equally good fevers (see also pp. 245–7).

Very large numbers of Gram-negative bacteria are normally present in the intestines (see Ch. 2), their continued death and exit in the faeces being balanced by multiplication in the lumen. There is a continuous, inevitable low-grade absorption of endotoxin from the intestine.* Absorbed (endogenous) endotoxin enters the portal circulation and is taken up and degraded by reticuloendothelial cells, mainly Kupffer cells in the liver. Continuous exposure to endotoxin probably has profound effects on the immune system and on the histology of the intestinal mucosa, stimulating development of the immune system in the immature individual, but there are no obvious pathogenic consequences. Normal people have low levels of antibody to

---

* In addition, various antigens are absorbed in small quantities from the intestine, and in normal individuals antibodies are formed against various food proteins and to some extent against resident intestinal bacteria (see Ch. 2). Kupffer cells remove any antigen–antibody complexes formed locally in the intestine and prevent them from entering the systemic circulation.

endotoxin as a result of this continuous exposure. The sick individual may be much more susceptible to endogenous endotoxin, perhaps because of defects in removal by Kupffer cells.

After trauma or after genito-urinary instrumentation endotoxin is detectable in peripheral blood by the *Limulus* test,* but this leads to no particular signs or symptoms. When large amounts of endotoxin enter the blood there are profound effects on blood vessels with peripheral vascular pooling, a drastic fall in blood pressure, collapse and sometimes death. Thus, if enough endotoxin enters the blood during massive Gram-negative bacterial sepsis, the vasomotor action of endotoxin becomes important and shock intervenes.† In experimental animals endotoxin also causes vasodilation and haemorrhage into the intestinal mucosa, and sometimes haemorrhage into the placenta with abortion, but these actions do not appear to be important in Gram-negative bacterial infections.

To summarize, endotoxin, although studied so carefully and for so long, has not yet been shown to play a vital part as a toxin in the pathogenesis of any infectious disease. Indeed, in spite of its effects on various host defence systems including polymorphs, lymphocytes, macrophages, complement, and on endothelial cells and platelets, its overall role in infection is still not clear. It can, however, cause shock when Gram-negative bacteria invade the blood and, quite separately, the characteristics of the O-antigen polysaccharide are important in determining virulence (see p. 170).

Indirect Damage via Inflammation

In infectious diseases there is nearly always a certain amount of direct microbial damage to host tissues, as discussed above. Host cells are destroyed or blood vessels injured as a direct result of the action of microbes or their toxins. Blood vessel injuries account for much of the disease picture in rickettsial infections (see above). Inflammatory materials are liberated from necrotic cells, whatever the cause of the necrosis. Also many bacteria themselves liberate inflammatory products and certain viruses cause living infected cells to release inflammatory mediators. Therefore it is not always clear how much of the inflammation is directly microbial rather than host in origin. But inevitably the host (see Ch. 3) generates inflammatory and other

---

* A sensitive test for endotoxin based on the ability of endotoxin to induce gelation of a lysate obtained from the blood cells of the horseshoe crab, *Limulus polyphemus*.

† It must be remembered that endotoxin is only one of the pathways to shock in infectious diseases. Shock is also seen for instance in leptospiral and rickettsial infections, in gas gangrene, and in sepsis due to Gram-positive bacteria (see above).

tissue responses and these responses sometimes account for the greater part of the tissue changes. Pathological changes can then be regarded as occurring indirectly as a result of these responses to the infection. Inflammation causes redness, swelling, pain and sometimes loss of function of the affected part (see Ch. 6) and is generally a major cause of the signs and symptoms of disease. Indirect damage attributable to the host immune response is discussed separately below. In most diseases direct and indirect types of damage both make a contribution to pathological changes but in a given disease one or the other may be the most important.

In a staphylococcal abscess the bacteria produce inflammatory materials but they also kill infiltrating polymorphs whose lysosomal enzymes are thereby liberated and induce further inflammation. This type of indirect nonimmunological damage is sometimes important in streptococcal infections. Virulent streptococci produce various toxins that damage phagocytes, and also bear on their surfaces substances that impede phagocytosis (see Ch. 4). Nevertheless, with the help of antibody, all streptococci are eventually phagocytosed and killed and the infection terminated. Unlike the staphylococci, however, killed group A streptococci pose a digestive problem for phagocytic cells. The peptidoglycan component of the streptococcal cell wall is very resistant to digestion by lysosomal enzymes. When streptococci are injected into the skin of a rabbit, for instance, streptococcal peptidoglycans persist in macrophages for as long as 146 days. Hence macrophages laden with indigestible streptococcal cell walls tend to accumulate in sites of infection. Lysosomal enzymes, including collagenase, leak from these macrophages, causing local destruction of collagen fibres and the connective tissue matrix. Macrophages secrete many other substances some of which may contribute to cell and tissue damage (see also p. 72). Many macrophages eventually die or form giant cells, sometimes giving rise to granulomatous lesions (see pp. 240–1). In this way persistent streptococcal materials sometimes cause chronic inflammatory lesions in the infected host. An additional immunopathological contribution to the lesions is to be expected if the host is sensitized to peptidoglycan components. Other pathogenic microorganisms that are digested with difficulty by phagocytes include *Listeria*, *Shigella*, *Candida albicans* and of course mycobacteria, but the importance of this in the pathogenesis of disease is not generally clear.

Indirect Damage via the Immune Response (Immunopathology)

The expression of the immune response necessarily involves a certain amount of inflammation, cell infiltration, lymph node swelling, even tissue destruction, as described in Ch. 6. Such changes caused by the immune response are classed as immunopathological. Sometimes they are very severe, leading to serious disease or death, but at other times they play a minimal part in the pathogenesis of disease. With the possible exception of certain vertically transmitted virus infections and the transmissible viral dementias (see Ch. 10), there are signs of an immune response in all infections. Therefore it is to be expected that there will nearly always be some contribution of the immune response to pathological changes.* Often the immunological contribution is small, but sometimes it forms a major part of the disease. For instance, in tuberculosis the pathological picture is dominated by the operation of a strong and persistent CMI response to the invading bacillus. In the classical tubercle a central zone of bacilli with large mononuclears and giant cells, often with some necrosis, is surrounded by fibroblasts and lymphocytes. Mononuclear infiltrations, giant cells and granulomatous lesions (see Ch. 6) are characteristic pathological features of tuberculosis. There are no recognized toxins formed by tubercle bacilli, and there seems to be no single antigen or other component that accounts for virulence. Bacterial glycolipids (e.g. "cord factor"), resistance to H_2O_2 (see pp. 68–9), ability to utilize host Fe (see p. 293) have been correlated with pathogenicity, and inhibition of phagosome–lysosome fusion in macrophages (see p. 83) by release of unidentified bacterial components would also contribute to pathogenicity. However, none of these factors is by itself absolutely necessary for virulence, which in such a complex, ancient parasite is likely to be multifactorial (see p. 200). As a gene library for *M. tuberculosis* is slowly built up there will be opportunities for clearer definition of virulence determinants. When macrophages are killed by intracellular mycobacteria the lysosomal enzymes and other materials released from the degenerating cell contribute to chronic inflammation as in the case of the streptococcal lesions referred to above.

The mere enlargement of lymphoid organs during infectious diseases is a morphological change that can often be regarded as pathological. The lymph node swelling seen in glandular fever, for instance, is an immunopathological feature of the disease, and the same can be said of the striking enlargement of the spleen caused by chronic malaria and other infections in the condition known as tropical splenomegaly.

As often as not the relative importance of direct microbial damage as opposed to immune and nonimmune inflammatory reactions have not yet been determined, but the picture is clearer in most of the examples given below.

---

* A number of different microbial antigens are produced during most infections (see Ch. 6) and the possible immunological reactions are therefore numerous. For instance, at least 18 types of circulating malarial antigen are found in heavily infected individuals.

In one important human disease, pathological changes are certainly immunopathological in nature, but not enough is known about it to classify the type of reaction (see Table 24). This disease is rheumatic fever, which follows group A streptococcal infections of the throat. It is the commonest form of heart disease in many developing countries. Antibodies formed against a streptococcal cell wall or membrane component also react with the patient's heart muscle or valves, and myocarditis develops a few weeks later. Many strains of streptococci have antigens that cross-react with heart, and repeated infections with different streptococci cause recurrent attacks of rheumatic fever. There is genetic predisposition to the disease, based either on a particular antigen present in the heart of the patient or on a particular

Table 24. Immunopathologial reactions and infectious diseases

Reaction	Mechanism	Result	Example from infectious disease
Type 1 Anaphylactic	Antigen + IgE antibody attached to mast cells → histamine etc. release	Anaphylactic shock Bronchospasm Local inflammation	Contribution to certain rashes?
Type 2 Cytotoxic	Antibody + antigen on cell surface → complement or K cell activation	Lysis of cell bearing microbial antigens	Liver cell necrosis in hepatitis B?
Type 3 Immune complex	Antibody + extra-cellular antigen → complex	*Extravascular complex* Inflammation ± tissue damage *Intravascular complex* Complex deposition in glomeruli, joints, small skin vessels, choroid plexus → glomerulonephritis, vasculitis etc.	Edge of smallpox vaccination site? Allergic alveolitis Glomerulonephritis in LCM virus infection (mice) or malaria (man) Prodromal rashes Fever
Type 4 Cell-mediated (delayed)	Sensitized T lymphocyte reacts with antigen; lymphokines liberated	*Extracellular antigen* Inflammation, mononuclear accumulation, macrophage activation Tissue damage *Antigen on tissue cell* T-lymphocyte lyses cell	Acute LCM virus disease in mice. Certain virus rashes Tuberculosis, leprosy (granulomas) ?

type of antibody response. Chorea, a disease of the central nervous system, is a rare complication of streptococcal infection and antistreptococcal antibodies have been shown to react with neurons in the caudate and subthalamic nuclei of the brain.

A number of microorganisms have antigens similar to host tissue components (p. 157) so that in the course of responding immunologically to such infections the host is vulnerable to autoimmune damage (see ankylosing spondylitis, p. 182). The antibodies to host components such as DNA, IgG, myofibrils, erythrocytes etc. that are seen in trypanosomiasis, *Mycoplasma pneumoniae*, and EB virus infections appear to result from polyclonal activation of B cells (see p. 167). It is not clear how important these autoimmune responses are in pathogenesis, but they reflect fundamental disturbances in immunoregulation.

Four types of immunopathology can be distinguished according to the classification of allergic reactions by Coombs and Gell, and microbial immunopathology will be described under these headings (see Table 24).

Type 1. Anaphylactic reactions

These depend on the reactions of antigens with reaginic (IgE) antibodies attached to mast cells, resulting in the release of histamine, leukotrienes (see p. 57) and heparin from mast cells, and the activation of serotonin and plasma kinins. If the antigen–antibody interaction takes place on a large enough scale in the tissues, the histamine that is released can give rise to anaphylactic shock, the exact features depending on the sensitivity and particular reaction of the species of animal to histamine. Guinea-pigs suffer from bronchospasm and asphyxia, and in man there are similar symptoms, sometimes with a fall in blood pressure and shock. This type of immunopathology, although accounting for anaphylactic reactions to horse serum or to penicillin, is not important in infectious diseases. When the antigen–IgE antibody interaction takes place at the body surface there are local inflammatory events, giving rise to urticaria in the skin, and hayfever or asthma in the respiratory tract. This local type of anaphylaxis may play a part in the pathogenesis of virus infections of the upper respiratory tract (e.g. common cold, respiratory syncytial virus infections of infants), or in skin rashes in infectious diseases.

Type 2. Cytolytic or cytotoxic reactions

Reactions of this type occur when antibody combines with antigen on the surface of a tissue cell, activates the complement sequence or triggers K cell action (see p. 135), with destruction of the cell. As discussed in Ch. 6, the same reaction on the surface of a microorganism constitutes an important part of antimicrobial defences, often leading to the destruction of the microorganism. Cells infected with viruses and bearing viral antigens on their surface are destroyed in a similar way.

Clearly the antibody-mediated destruction of infected cells means tissue damage, and it perhaps accounts for some of the liver necrosis in hepatitis B, for instance, and probably in yellow fever. Infected cells can also be destroyed by sensitized lymphocytes or NK cells (see below).

In certain infections antibodies are formed against host erythrocytes and these cells are particularly sensitive to lysis. Some of the haemolysis in malaria is caused in this way. In pneumonia due to *Mycoplasma pneumoniae* (atypical pneumonia), antibodies (cold agglutinins) are formed against normal human group O erythrocytes. Haemolytic anaemia is occasionally seen, and there is reticulocytosis (see Glossary) in 64% of patients. The lesions in the lungs are perhaps based on cell-mediated immunopathological reactions.

Type 3. Immune complex reactions

The combination of antibody with antigen is an important event, initiating inflammatory phenomena that are inevitably involved in the expression of the immune response. In the infected host, these inflammatory phenomena are most of the time of great antimicrobial value (see Ch. 6). But they are nevertheless immunopathological features of the infection, and immune complex reactions sometimes do a great deal of damage in the infected individual. The mechanisms by which antigen–antibody reactions cause inflammation and tissue damage are outlined in Fig. 30. IgA immune complexes are less harmful. Antigens absorbed from the intestine can combine locally with IgA antibody and the complex then enters the blood, to be filtered out in the liver and excreted harmlessly in bile (see p. 130).

When the antigen–antibody reaction takes place in extravascular tissues, there is inflammation and oedema with infiltration of polymorphs. If soluble antigen is injected intradermally into an individual with large amounts of circulating IgG antibody, the antigen–antibody reaction takes place in the walls of skin blood vessels, and causes an inflammatory response. The extravasating polymorphs degenerate and their lysosomal enzymes cause extensive vascular damage. This is the classical Arthus response. Antigen–antibody reactions in tissues are not usually as serious as this, and milder inflammatory sequelae are more common, as in the case of allergic alveolitis (see below), or the red zone seen round the borders of a smallpox vaccination

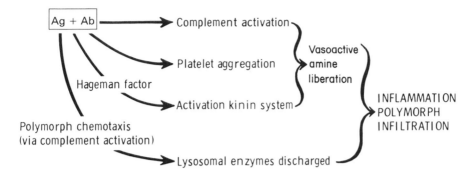

Fig. 30. Mechanisms of inflammation and tissue damage induced by antigen–antibody reactions.

site after seven or eight days. In the latter example circulating antibodies pass through vessel walls, meet smallpox virus antigen in the dermal tissues and an inflammatory response is generated. A similar mild response can be induced experimentally to cause a reaction known as cutaneous anaphylaxis (see Glossary), the test antigen being injected into the skin and reacting with blood-borne antibody. The resulting inflammation is detected by the visible local leakage of plasma proteins from blood vessels, circulating plasma proteins having been coloured by the intravenous injection of Evans blue.

Glomerulonephritis and vasculitis

When the antigen–antibody reaction takes place in the blood to give circulating immune complexes, the sequelae depend to a large extent on size and on the relative proportions of antigen and antibody. If there is a large excess of antibody, each antigen molecule is covered with antibody and is removed rapidly by reticuloendothelial cells, which have receptors for the Fc portion of the antibody molecule (see Ch. 4). When equal amounts of antigen and antibody combine, lattice structures are formed, and these form large aggregates whose size ensures that they are also rapidly removed by reticuloendothelial cells. If, however, complexes are formed in antigen excess, the poorly coated antigen molecules are not removed by reticuloendothelial cells. They continue to circulate in the blood and have the opportunity to localize in small blood vessels elsewhere in the body. The mechanism is not clear, but complexes are deposited in the glomeruli of the kidneys, the choroid plexuses, joints and ciliary body of the eye. Factors may include local high blood pressure and turbulent flow (glomeruli), or filtering function of vessels involved (choroid plexus, ciliary body). In the glomeruli the complexes pass through the endothelial windows (Fig. 31) and come to

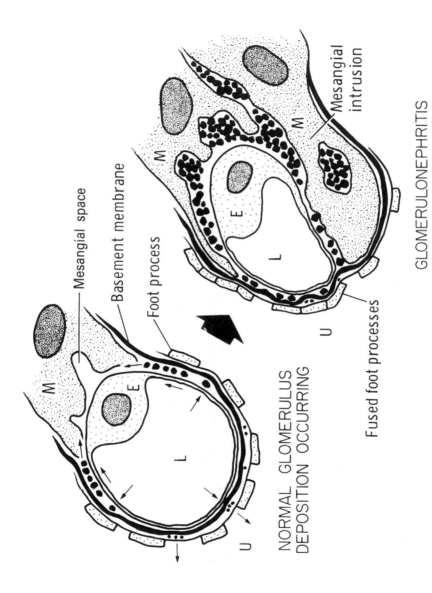

Mesangial space

Basement membrane

Foot process

M

E

L

U

NORMAL GLOMERULUS
DEPOSITION OCCURRING

Mesangial
intrusion

M

M

E

L

U

Fused foot processes

GLOMERULONEPHRITIS

Fig. 31. Immune complex glomerulonephritis. Arrows indicate the movement of immune complex deposits, some moving through to the urine and others (larger deposits) being retained. M = mesangial cell; U = urinary space; L = lumen of glomerular capillary; E = endothelial cell (contains 100 nm pores).

lie beneath the basement membrane. The smallest sized complexes pass through the basement membrane and seem to enter the urine. This is probably the normal mechanism of disposal of such complexes from the body.

Immune complexes are formed in many, perhaps most, acute infectious diseases. Microbial antigens commonly circulate in the blood in viral, bacterial, fungal, protozoal, rickettsial etc. infections. When the immune response has been generated and the first trickle of specific antibody enters the blood, immune complexes are formed in antigen excess. This is generally a transitional stage, soon giving rise to antibody excess, as more and more antibody enters the blood and the infection is terminated. Sometimes the localization of immune complexes and complement in kidney glomeruli is associated with a local inflammatory response.* There is an infiltration of polymorphs, swelling of the glomerular basement membrane, loss of albumin, even red blood cells, in the urine and the patient has acute glomerulonephritis. This is seen following streptococcal infections, mainly in children (see below). As complexes cease to be formed the changes are reversed, and complete recovery is the rule. Repeated attacks or persistent deposition of complexes leads to irreversible damage, often with proliferation of epithelial cells following the seepage of fibrin into the urinary space. Under certain circumstances complexes continue to be formed in the blood and deposited subendothelially for long periods. This happens in certain persistent microbial infections in which microbial antigens are continuously released into the blood but antibody responses are only minimal or of poor quality (see below). Complexes are deposited in glomeruli over the course of weeks, months or even years. The normal mechanisms for removal are inadequate. The deposits, particularly larger complexes containing high molecular weight antigens or antibodies (IgM) are held up at the basement membrane and accumulate in the subendothelial space together with the complement components. As deposition continues, they gradually move through to the mesangial space (Fig. 31) where they form larger aggregates. Mesangial cells, one of whose functions is to deal with such materials, enlarge, multiply and extend into the subepithelial space. If these changes are gradual there are no inflammatory changes, but the structure of the basement membrane alters, allowing proteins to leak through into the urine. Later the filtering function of the glomerulus becomes progressively impaired. In the first place the glomerular capillary is narrowed by the mesangial cell intrusion. Also, the filtering area is itself blocked by the mesangial cell intrusion, by the accumulation of complexes (Fig. 31), and by

---

*See also footnote p. 212; Cells in kidney glomeruli, in joint synovium and in choroid plexuses bear Fc or C3b receptors. This would favour localization in these tissues.

alterations in the structure of the basement membrane. The foot processes of epithelial cells tend to fuse and further interfere with filtration. The pathological processes continue, some glomeruli ceasing to produce urine, and the individual has chronic glomerulonephritis.

Circulating immune complex deposition in joints leads to joint swelling and inflammation but in choroid plexuses there are no apparent pathological sequelae. Circulating immune complexes are also deposited in the walls of small blood vessels in the skin and elsewhere, where they may induce inflammatory changes.* The prodromal rashes seen in exanthematous virus infections and in hepatitis B are probably caused in this way. If the vascular changes are more marked they give rise to the condition called erythema nodosum, in which there are tender red nodules in the skin, with deposits of antigen, antibody and complement in vessel walls. Erythema nodosum is seen following streptococcal infections and during the treatment of patients with leprosy. When small arteries are severely affected, for instance in some patients with hepatitis B, this gives rise to periarteritis nodosa.

Immune complex glomerulonephritis occurs as an indirect immuno-pathological sequel to a variety of infections. First there are certain virus infections of animals. The antibodies formed in virus infections generally neutralize any free virus particles, thus terminating the infection (see Ch. 6), but the infection must persist if antigen is to continue to be released into the blood and immune complexes formed over long periods. Non-neutralizing antibodies help promote virus persistence because they combine specifically with virus particles, fail to render them noninfectious, and at the same time block the action of any good neutralizing antibodies that may be present. Immune complexes in antigen excess are formed in the blood when the peristent virus or its antigens circulates in the plasma and reacts with antibody which is present in relatively small amounts. Virus infections with these characteristics are included in Table 25. In each instance complexes are deposited in kidney glomeruli and sometimes in other blood vessels as described above. In some there are few if any pathological changes (LDH) and leukaemia viruses in mice) probably because there is a slow rate of immune complex deposition, whereas in others glomerulo-nephritis (LCM virus in mice, ADV in mink) or vasculitis (ADV in mink) is severe.

A persistent virus infection that induces a feeble immune response forms an ideal background for the development of immune complex

---

* It is not clear how inflammation is caused. Complement activation would presumably take place while complexes were circulating in the blood. Perhaps the complexes bind more antibody after they have localized, or alternatively it is possible that free antigen circulates in the first place, localizes, and later binds antibody to generate mediators of inflammation.

Table 25. The deposition of circulating immune complexes in infectious diseases

Microbe	Host	Kidney deposits	Glomerulo- nephritis	Vascular deposits
Murine leukaemia virus	Mouse	+	±	−
Feline leukaemia virus	Cat	+	±	−
Lactic dehydrogenase virus (LDV)	Mouse	+	±	−
Lymphocytic choriomeningitis virus (LCM)	Mouse	+ +	+	±
Aleutian disease virus (ADV)	Mink	+ +	+	+ +
Equine infectious anaemia virus	Horse	+	+	+
Hepatitis B virus	Man	+	−	+
Streptococcus pyogenes	Man	+	+	−
Malaria (nephrotic syndrome)	Man	+	+	−
Treponema pallidum (nephrotic syndrome in secondary syphilis)	Man	+	+	?
Unknown causative agents of chronic glomerulonephritis	Man	+ +	+ +	−

glomerulonephritis, but there are no known viral examples in man. There are one or two other microorganisms that occasionally cause this type of glomerulonephritis, and it is seen for instance in chronic quartan malaria and sometimes in subacute bacterial endocarditis. In both these examples microbial antigens circulate in the blood for long periods. But immune complex deposition does not necessarily lead to the development of glomerulonephritis and immune complexes are detectable in the glomeruli of most normal mice and monkeys. Even in persistent virus infections the rate of deposition may be too slow to cause pathological changes, as with LDH and leukaemia virus infections of mice (see Table 25). During the acute stage of hepatitis B in man, when antibodies are first formed against excess circulating viral antigen (hepatitis B surface antigen), immune complexes are formed and deposited in glomeruli. But the deposition is short-lived and there is no glomerulonephritis. Persistent carriers of the antigen do not generally develop glomerulonephritis, because their antibody is usually directed against the "core" antigen of the virus particle, rather than against the large amounts of circulating hepatitis B surface antigen.

Kidney failure in man is commonly due to chronic glomerulonephritis, and this is known to be mostly of the immune complex type, but the antigens, if they are microbial, have not yet been identified.

Immune complex glomerulonephritis occurs in man as an important complication of streptococcal infection, but this is usually acute in nature with inflammation in glomeruli, as referred to above. Antibodies formed against an unknown component of the streptococcus react with circulating streptococcal antigen, perhaps also with a circulating host antigen, and immune complexes are deposited in glomeruli. Streptococcal antibodies cross reacting with the glomerular basement membrane may contribute to the picture. Deposition of complexes continues after the infection is terminated, and glomerulonephritis develops a week or two later. The streptococcal infection may be of the throat or skin, and *Streptococcus pyogenes* types 12 and 49 are frequently involved.

Allergic alveolitis

When certain antigens are inhaled by sensitized individuals and the antigen reaches the terminal divisions of the lung, there is a local antigen–antibody reaction with formation of immune complexes. The resulting inflammation and cell infiltration causes wheezing and respiratory distress, and the condition is called allergic alveolitis. Persistent inhalation of the specific antigen leads to chronic pathological changes with fibrosis and respiratory disease. Exposure to the antigen must be by inhalation; when the same antigen is injected intradermally, there is an Arthus type reaction (see p. 208).

There are a number of microorganisms that cause allergic alveolitis. Most of these are fungi. A disease called farmers lung occurs in farm workers repeatedly exposed to mouldy hay containing the actinomycete *Micromonospora faeni*. Cows suffer from the same condition. A fungus contaminating the bark of the maple tree cause a similar disease (maple bark stripper's disease) in workers in the USA employed in the extraction of maple syrup. The mild respiratory symptoms occasionally reported after respiratory exposure of sensitized individuals to tuberculosis or smallpox doubtless have the same immunopathological basis.

Other immune complex effects

In addition to their local effects, antigen–antibody complexes generate systemic reactions. For instance, the fever that occurs at the end of the incubation period of many virus infections is probably attributable to a large-scale interaction of antibodies with viral antigen, although extensive CMI reactions can also cause fever. The febrile response is mediated by endogenous pyrogen (interleukin-1) liberated from polymorphs and macrophages, as described on p. 245. Perhaps the characteristic subjective sensations of illness and some of the "toxic" features of virus diseases are also caused by immune reactions.

Systemic immune complex reactions taking place during infectious diseases very occasionally give rise to a serious condition known as disseminated intravascular coagulation. This is seen sometimes in severe generalized infections such as Gram-negative septicaemia, meningococcal septicaemia, plague, yellow fever and other haemorrhagic arthropod-borne virus diseases. Immune complex reactions activate the enzymes of the coagulation cascade (see Fig. 28), leading to histamine release and increased vascular permeability. Fibrin is formed and is deposited in blood vessels in the kidneys, lungs, adrenals and pituitary. This causes multiple thromboses with infarcts, and there are also scattered haemorrhages because of the depletion of platelets, prothrombin, fibrinogen etc. Systemic immune complex reactions were once thought to form the basis for dengue haemorrhagic fever. This disease is seen in parts of the world where dengue is endemic, individuals immune to one type of dengue becoming infected with a related strain of virus. They are not protected against the second virus, although it shows immunological cross-reactions with the first one. Indeed the dengue-specific antibodies *enhance* infection of susceptible mononuclear cells, so that larger amounts of viral antigen are produced (see p. 143). It was thought that after virus replication, viral antigens in the blood reacted massively with antibody to cause an often lethal disease with haemorrhages, shock and vascular collapse. However, it has proved difficult to demonstrate this pathophysiological sequence, and the role of circulating immune complexes and platelet depletion remains unclear. Perhaps in this and in some of the other viral haemorrhagic fevers the virus multiplies in capillary endothelial cells and thus causes the disease.

Immune complex immunopathology is probable in various other infectious diseases. For instance, the occurrence of fever, polyarthritis, skin rashes and kidney damage (proteinuria) in meningococcal meningitis and gonococcal septicaemia indicates immune complex deposition. Circulating immune complexes are present in these conditions. Certain African arthropod-borne viruses with exotic names (Chikungunya, O'nyong-nyong) cause illnesses characterized by fever, arthralgia and itchy rashes, and this too sounds as if it is immune complex in origin. Immune complexes perhaps play a part in the oedema and vasculitis of trypanosomiasis and in the rashes of secondary syphilis.

Sensitive immunological techniques are available for the detection of circulating complexes and for the analysis of the antigens and antibodies in deposited complexes. The full application of these techniques will perhaps solve the problem of the aetiology of chronic glomerulonephritis in man.

Type 4. Cell-mediated reactions

The mere expression of a CMI response involves inflammation, lymphocyte infiltration, macrophage accumulation and macrophage activation as described in Ch. 6, and can therefore by itself cause pathological changes. The CMI response to infection dominates the pathological picture in tuberculosis, with mononuclear infiltration, degeneration of parasitized macrophages, and the formation of giant cells as central features. These features of the tissue response result in the formation of granulomas (see Glossary) which reflect chronic infection and accompanying inflammation. There is a ding-dong battle as the host attempts to contain and control infection with a microorganism that is hard to eliminate. The granulomas represent chronic CMI responses to antigens released locally. Various other chronic microbial and parasitic diseases have granulomas as characteristic pathological features. These include chlamydial (lymphogranuloma inguinale), bacterial (syphilis, leprosy, actinomycosis), and fungal infections (coccidiomysosis). Antigens that are disposed of with difficulty in the body are more likely to be important inducers of granulomas. Thus, although mannan is the dominant antigen of *Candida albicans*, glucan is more resistant to breakdown in macrophages and is responsible for chronic inflammatory responses.

The lymphocytes and macrophages that accumulate in CMI responses also cause pathological changes by destroying host cells. Cells infected with viruses and bearing viral antigens on their surface are targets for CMI responses as described in Chs 6 and 9. Infected cells, even if they are perfectly healthy, are destroyed by the direct action of sensitized T lymphocytes, which are demonstrable in many viral infections. In spite of the fact that the *in vitro* test system so clearly displays the immunopathological potential of cytotoxic T cells, this is not easy to evaluate in the infected host. It may contribute to the tissue damage seen, for instance, in hepatitis B infection and in many herpes and pox virus infections. Antigens from *Trypanosoma cruzi* are known to be adsorbed to uninfected host cells, raising the possibility of autoimmune damage in Chagas' disease, caused by this bacterium.* It is also becoming clear that cells infected with certain

---

*Chagas' disease, common in Brazil, affects 12 million people, and is transmitted by blood-sucking bugs. After spreading through the body during the acute infection, the parasitaemia falls to a low level and there is no clinical disease. Years later a poorly understood chronic disease appears, involving heart and intestinal tract, which contain only small numbers of the parasite but show a loss of autonomic ganglion cells. An autoimmune mechanism is possible (see p. 157), because a monoclonal antibody to *T. cruzi* has been obtained that cross-reacts with mammalian neurons.

protozoa (e.g. *Theileria parva* in bovine lymphocytes; see p. 161) have parasite antigens on their surface and are susceptible to this type of destruction. Little is known about intracellular bacteria.

The most clearly worked out example of type 4 (CMI) immunopathology is seen in LCM virus infection of adult mice. When virus is injected intracerebrally into adult mice it grows in the meninges, ependyma and choroid plexus epithelium, but the infected cells do not show the slightest sign of damage or dysfunction. After 7–10 days, however, the mouse develops severe meningitis with submeningeal and subependymal oedema, and dies. The illness can be completely prevented by adequate immunosuppression, and the lesions are attributable to the mouse's own vigorous CMI reaction to infected cells. These cells have LCM virus antigens on their surface and sensitized T cells, after entering the cerebrospinal fluid and encountering the infected cells, generate the inflammatory response and interference with normal neural function that cause the disease. The same cells destroy infected tissue cells *in vitro*, but tissue destruction is not a feature of the neurological disease. It may be noted that the brain is uniquely vulnerable to inflammation and oedema, as pointed out earlier in this chapter. The infected mouse shows the same type of lesions in scattered foci of infection in the liver and elsewhere, but they are not a cause of sickness or death. LCM infection of mice is a classical example of immunopathology in which death itself is entirely due to the cell-mediated immune response of the infected individual. This response, although apparently irrelevant and harmful, is nevertheless an "attempt" to do the right thing. It has been shown that immune T cells effectively inhibit viral growth in infected organs. However, a response that in most extraneural sites would be useful and appropriate turns out to be self-destructive when it takes place in the central nervous system.

One human virus infection in which a strong CMI contribution to pathology seems probable is measles. Children with thymic aplasia show a general failure to develop T lymphocytes and cell-mediated immunity, but have normal antibody responses to most antigens. They suffer a fatal disease if they are infected with measles virus. Instead of the limited extent of virus growth and disease seen in the respiratory tract in normal children, there is inexorable multiplication of virus in the lung, in spite of antibody formation, giving rise to giant cell pneumonia. This indicates that the CMI response is essential for the control of virus growth. In addition there is a total absence of the typical measles rash, and this further indicates that the CMI response is also essential for the production of the skin lesions. There is evidence that cell-mediated immune responses also make a contribution to the rashes in pox virus infections.

Other Indirect Mechanisms of Damage

Stress, haemorrhage, placental infection and tumours

Sometimes in infectious diseases there are prominent pathological changes which are not attributable to the direct action of microbes or their toxins, nor to inflammation or immunopathology. The stress changes mediated by adrenal cortical hormones come into this category. Stress is a general term used to describe various noxious influences, and includes cold, heat, starvation, injury, psychological stress and infection. An infectious disease is an important stress, and corticosteroids are secreted in large amounts in severe infections (see also Ch. 11). They generally tend to inhibit the development of pathological changes, but also have pronounced effects on lymphoid tissues, causing thymic involution and lymphocyte destruction. These can be regarded as pathological changes caused by stress. It was the very small size of the thymus gland as seen in children dying with various diseases, especially infectious diseases, that for many years contributed to the neglect of this important organ, and delayed appreciation of its vital role in the development of the immune system.

Pathological changes are sometimes caused in an even more indirect way as in the following example. Yellow fever is a virus infection transmitted by mosquitoes and in its severest form is characterized by devastating liver lesions. There is massive mid-zonal liver necrosis following the extensive growth of virus in liver cells, resulting in the jaundice that gives the disease its name. Destruction of the liver also leads to a decrease in the rate of formation of the blood coagulation factor, prothrombin, and infected human beings or monkeys show prolonged coagulation and bleeding times. Haemorrhagic phenomena are therefore characteristic of severe yellow fever, including haemorrhage into the stomach and intestine. In the stomach the appearance of blood is altered by acid, and the vomiting of altered blood gave yellow fever another of its names, "black vomit disease". Haemorrhagic phenomena in infectious diseases can be due to direct microbial damage to blood vessels, as in certain rickettsial infections (see p. 114) or in the virus infection responsible for haemorrhagic disease of deer. They may also be due to immunological damage to vessels as in the Arthus response or immune complex vasculitis, to any type of severe inflammation, and to the indirect mechanism illustrated above. Finally there are a few infectious diseases in which platelets are depleted, sometimes as a result of their combination with immune complexes plus complement, giving thrombocytopenia and a haemorrhagic tendency (see also disseminated intravascular coagulation, p. 215). Thrombocytopenic purpura is occasionally seen in congenital rubella and in certain other severe generalized infections.

Infection during pregnancy can lead to foetal damage or death not just because the foetus is infected (see pp. 249–250), but also because of infection and damage to the placenta. This is another type of indirect pathological action. Placental damage may contribute to foetal death during rubella and cytomegalovirus infections in pregnant women.

Certain viruses undoubtedly cause tumours (leukaemia viruses, human papillomaviruses, several herpes viruses in animals) and this is to be regarded as a late pathological consequence of infection. As was discussed in Ch. 7, the tumour virus genome can be integrated into the host cell genome whether a tumour is produced or not, so that the virus becomes a part of the genetic constitution of the host. Sometimes the host cell is transformed by the virus and converted into a tumour cell, the virus either introducing a transforming gene into the cell or activating expression of a pre-existing cellular gene. The transforming genes of DNA tumour viruses generally code for T antigens which are necessary for transformation, and the transforming genes of RNA tumour viruses are known as *onc* genes.* Transformation has been extensively studied *in vitro*, and the features of the transformed cell described (changed surface and social activity, freedom from the usual growth restraints).

Dual infections

Simultaneous infection with two different microorganisms would be expected to occur at times, merely by chance, especially in children. On the other hand, a given infection generates antimicrobial responses such as interferon production and macrophage activation which would make a second infection less likely. Dual infections are commonest when local defences have been damaged by the first invader. The pathological results are made much more severe because there is a second infectious agent present. This can be considered as another mechanism of pathogenicity. Classical instances involve the respiratory tract. The destruction of ciliated epithelium in the lung by viruses such as influenza or measles allows normally nonpathogenic resident bacteria of the nose and throat, such as the pneumococcus or *Haemophilus influenzae*, to invade the lung and cause secondary pneumonia. If these bacteria enter the lung under normal circumstances, they are destroyed by alveolar macrophages or removed by the mucociliary escalator. In at least one instance the initial virus infection

---

* *Onc* genes (oncogenes) are also present in host cells, where they play a role in normal growth and differentiation, often coding for recognized growth factors (e.g. human platelet-derived growth factor). They can be activated and the cell transformed when tumour viruses with the necessary "promoters" are brought into the cell. The *onc* genes of the RNA tumour viruses themselves originate from cellular oncogenes which were taken up into the genome of infecting viruses during their evolutionary history.

appears to act by interfering with the function of alveolar macrophages. Mice infected with parainfluenza 1 (Sendai) virus show greatly increased susceptibility to infection with *Haemophilus influenzae*, and this is largely due to the fact that alveolar macrophages infected with virus show a poor ability to phagocytose and kill the bacteria. Specialized respiratory pathogens such as influenza, measles, parainfluenza or rhinoviruses damage the nasopharyngeal mucosa and can lead in the same way to secondary bacterial infection, with nasal catarrh, sinusitis, otitis media or mastoiditis. The normal microbial flora of the mouth, nasopharynx or intestine are always ready to cause trouble if host resistance is lowered, but under normal circumstances they hinder rather than help other infecting microorganisms (see Ch. 2).

As a final example of dual infections, microorganisms that cause immunosuppression can activate certain pre-existing chronic infections. In measles, for instance, there is a temporary general depression of CMI; tuberculin-positive individuals become tuberculin negative, and in patients with tuberculosis the disease is exacerbated. In AIDS (see p. 162) the infecting virus activates a variety of pre-existing persistent infections.

Diarrhoea

Diarrhoea deserves a separate section, which is summarized in Table 26. We know very little about its pathogenesis, in spite of the fact that it is one of the commonest types of illness in developing countries and a major cause of death in childhood. Particularly in infants, who have a very high turnover of water relative to their size, the loss of fluid and salt soon leads to life-threatening illness. It is estimated that in developing countries diarrhoea is responsible for 5–10 million deaths per year in children under 5 years old. In villages in West Africa and Guatemala the average 2–3 year old child has diarrhoea for about two months in each year. Diarrhoea also interacts with malnutrition and can cause stunted growth, defective immune responses and susceptibility to other infections (see pp. 284–6). Diarrhoea is also a common affliction of travellers from developed countries, and business deals, athletic successes and holiday pleasures can be forfeited on the toilet seats of foreign lands. The most reliable prophylaxis is to "cook it, peel it, or forget it". A large proportion of these episodes are due to enteropathogenic strains of *E. coli*.

Diarrhoea means the passage of liquid faeces,* or faeces that take the shape of the receptacle rather than have their own shape. This could arise

---

*Liquid faeces are not abnormal in all species. The domestic cow experiences life-long diarrhoea, but presumably does not suffer from it.

Table 26. Production of diarrhoea by microorganisms shed in faeces

Infectious agent	Diarrhoea	Site of replication	Comments
Rotaviruses	+	Intestinal epithelium; tips of villi	Impaired absorption; lactase deficiency → lactose intolerance?
Intestinal adenoviruses	+	Intestinal epithelium	
Intestinal coronaviruses[a]	+	Intestinal epithelium	Lactose intolerance
Norwalk virus group	+	Intestinal epithelium	
Avian influenza viruses	−	Intestinal epithelium	
Hepatitis A	−	Liver	Biliary excretion of virus into intestine
Certain cocksackie viruses, polioviruses	−	Striated muscle Intestinal lymphoid tissue	Biliary excretion of virus into intestine?
Cholera	+	Intestinal lumen	Well-defined toxin causes diarrhoea
Campylobacter jejeuni	+	Intestinal epithelium	Mucosal damage and inflammation. Toxin not demonstrated
Shigella	+	Intestinal epithelium	Mucosal damage and inflammation contribute to diarrhoea
Salmonella typhi	±	Intestinal lymphoid tissue, liver, biliary tract	Biliary excretion of bacteria into intestine
Giardia lamblia	±	Attached to intestinal epithelium	Diarrhoea mechanism not understood
Entamoeba histolytica	+	Invasion of intestinal epithelium	Mucosal damage and inflammation contribute to diarrhoea

[a] Described for pigs, foals, calves, sheep, dogs, mice, man and turkeys; maximum susceptibility in the first few weeks of life. Lactose intolerance does not account for diarrhoea in birds.

because of increased rate of propulsion by intestinal muscles, giving less time for reabsorption of water in the large bowel, or because there was an increase in the amount of fluid held or produced in the intestine. In most types of infectious diarrhoea the exact mechanism is not known. Diarrhoea on the one hand can be regarded as a microbial device for promoting the shedding and spreading of the infection in the community, or on the other hand as a host device to hasten expulsion of the infectious agent. Diarrhoea is a superb mechanism for the dissemination of infected faeces (see p. 41) and there is no doubt that strains of microbes are selected for their diarrhoea-producing powers. The advantages to the host of prompt expulsion of the infectious agent was illustrated when volunteers infected with *Shigella flexneri* were given Lomotil, a drug that inhibits peristalsis. They were more likely to develop fever and had more difficulty in eliminating the pathogen.

   The pathogenesis of diarrhoea is understood in the case of cholera, where the biochemical mechanisms are clear (see p. 193), and the mechanisms of diarrhoea due to enterotoxigenic *E. coli* are now being elucidated. These diarrhoeas, like the diarrhoeas caused by rotaviruses (see below), are watery, without inflammation, and involve the small intestine with alterations in the balance between absorption and secretion. The mechanisms are less well defined for diarrhoea caused by *Shigella*, but these bacteria penetrate intestinal epithelial cells and produce a toxin (mol. wt. 64 000) consisting, as so often, of a portion that binds to the cell membrane and a toxic portion which in this case inhibits protein synthesis. The toxin kills host cells, giving rise to mucosal ulcers and inflammation and this, together with an additional action on enterocyte secretion, accounts for the diarrhoea. Toxin-producing strains, however, do not cause disease unless they also have invasive powers and can colonize the host intestinal mucosa. Invasive powers appear to be due to a 38 000 mol. wt. protein, conserved among shigella, and coded for by a defined DNA fragment of a large plasmid (see p. 194 footnote) carried by pathogenic strains. The word dysentery is used to describe shigella diarrhoea, and this refers to the mucus and blood passed in faeces as a result of the ulcers and inflammation. Dysentery is also caused by *Entamoeba histolytica*. Once they have invaded the mucosa, the amoebae kill enterocytes and phagocytes and in some way increase intestinal secretion. However, 80–90% of infections are symptomless, with a complex interplay of host and parasite factors determining mucosal invasion. The pathophysiology of diarrhoea in Salmonellosis and in Campylobacter infections is less clear, and the role of enterotoxins, inflammatory responses etc. uncertain. For many diarrhoeas we need to know more about immune and inflammatory responses in the intestine, and about differential effects on the tips of villi (absorptive sites), as opposed to the crypts (secretory sites). Also mechanisms may well be multifactorial, rather than due to single defined toxins.

   In the above conditions the bacteria multiply in the intestine and are then shed in large amounts in the faeces. Diarrhoea follows local multiplication. Typhoid differs from these infections because here the intestinal mucosa is merely a site of entry into the body, without being a major site of multiplication. *Salmonella typhi* is shed into the faeces, but reaches the intestine largely by way of the bile, having multiplied in the biliary tract, liver and elsewhere. Diarrhoea, although it may be induced as a result of bacterial multiplication in submucosal lymphoid follicles, is not an essential part of the pathogenesis of this infection.

A similar distinction between local replication in the intestine and replication elsewhere in the body can be made for certain virus infections in which the pathogen is shed into the faeces. For hepatitis A virus in man, for reoviruses and probably for many enteroviruses, the intestinal mucosa is no more than a route of entry into the body. Entry may occur at certain specific sites. Peyer's patches are scattered collections of lymphoid tissue below the epithelium in the small intestine. The overlying epithelium is specialized and readily takes up certain antigens and particles from the lumen. These are then delivered rapidly to underlying mononuclear cells and thence to gut-associated lymphoid tissues or GALT (see p. 22) where immune responses are generated. Viruses in the gut are likely to be taken passively into the body through these sites, unless they have mechanisms for attaching specifically to intestinal epithelium elsewhere. Viruses that avoid destruction then have the opportunity to multiply and spread via lymphatics to cause systemic infection. After replication in the liver (hepatitis A) there is "excretion" of large amounts of virus into the bile and thus to the intestine and faeces. Intestinal viruses are resistant to destruction by bile. Viruses that have replicated elsewhere and are circulating free in the blood can be taken up by the liver and excreted into the bile in the same way (see p. 108). These viruses, although shed in faeces, do not replicate extensively in intestinal epithelial cells and do not cause diarrhoea.

In contrast, the rotaviruses are known to invade intestinal epithelial cells and cause diarrhoea in man, foals, dogs, pigs, mice etc. Extensive multiplication takes place and very large amounts of virus (10^{11} particles g^{-1}) are shed in faeces. The tips of villi especially are affected, leading to reduced absorption of fluid from the lumen. There is also an interesting indirect mechanism which might help account for the diarrhoea. Intestinal epithelial cells normally produce lactose-digesting enzymes (disaccharidases), and as more and more of these cells are destroyed or functionally impaired, ingested lactose accumulates in the gut. The lactose itself causes an osmotic flux of fluid into the intestine, and it is also fermented by intestinal bacteria to give additional products with osmotic activity. The increased water and salts in the intestinal lumen cause diarrhoea. Lactose intolerance is also referred to on p. 31. Other viruses such as the intestinal adenoviruses and coronaviruses also replicate in intestinal epithelial cells and cause diarrhoea. Similar pathogenic mechanisms may be involved.

References

Bizzini, B. (1979). Tetanus toxin. *Microbiol. Rev.* **43**, 224–240.

Buchmeir, M. J. *et al.* (1980). The virology and immunology of lymphocytic choriomeningitis virus infection. *Adv. Immunol.* **30**, 275–331.

Cash, R. A. *et al.* (1974). Response of man to infection with *Vibrio cholerae*. I. Clinical, serologic and bacteriologic responses to a known inoculum. *J. Inf. Dis.* **129**, 45.

Casali, P. and Oldstone, M. B. A. (1983). Immune complexes in viral infection. *Curr. Topics Microb. Immunol.* **104.**

Ciba Foundation Symposium No. 112 (1985). "Microbial Toxins and Diarrhoeal Diseases". Pitman, London.

Dale, J. B. and Beachey, E. H. (1985). Epitopes of streptococcal M proteins shared with cardiac myosin. *J. Exp. Med.* **162**, 583–591.

Easmon, C. S. F. and Adlam, C. (eds) (1983). "Staphylococci and staphylococcal infections." Academic Press, London.

Field, M. (1979). Modes of action of enterotoxins from *Vibrio cholerae* and *Escherichia coli. Rev. Inf. Dis.* **1**, 918.

Fitzgerald, T. J. (1981). Pathogenesis and immunology of *Treponema pallidum. Ann. Rev. Microbiol.* **35**, 29–54.

Greenwood, B. M. and Whittle, H. C. (1980). The pathogenesis of sleeping sickness. *Trans. R. Soc. Trop. Med. Hyg.* **74**, 716–725.

Hamilton, P. J. *et al.* (1977). Disseminated intravascular coagulation: a review. *J. Clin. Path.* **31**, 609–619.

Hazell, S. L. *et al.* (1986). *Campylobacter pyloridis* and gastritis: association with intercellular spaces and adaptation to an environment of mucus as important factors in colonization of the gastric epithelium. *J. Inf. Dis.* **153**, 658–663.

Hornick, R. B. *et al.* (1970). Typhoid fever: pathogenesis and immunologic control. *New Engl. J. Med.* **283**, 739.

Kass, E. H. and Wolff, S. M. (Ed) (1973). Bacterial lipopolysaccharides: chemistry, biology and clinical significance of endotoxins. *J. Inf. Dis.* Suppl. **128.**

Levine, M. M., Kaper, J. B., Black, R. E. and Clements, M. L. (1983). New knowledge on pathogenesis of bacterial enteric infections as applied to vaccine development. *Microb. Rev.* **47**, 510–550.

Mata, L. *et al.* (1978). "Diarrhoeal diseases: a leading world health problem", pp. 1–14. 43rd Nobel Symposium, Stockholm.

McGee, Z. A. *et al.* (1981). Pathogenic mechanism of *Neisseria gonorrhoeae*: observations on damage to human fallopian tubes in organ cultures by gonococci of colony Type 1 or Type 4. *J. Inf. Dis.* **143**, 413–422, 432–439.

Middlebrook, J. L. and Dorland, R. B. (1984). Bacterial toxins: cellular mechanisms of action. *Microb. Rev.* **48**, 199–221.

Mims, C. A. (1957). Rift Valley Fever virus in mice VI: Histological changes in the liver in relation to virus multiplication. *Aust. J. Exp. Biol. Med. Sci.* **35**, 595.

Mims, C. A. (1985). Viral aetiology of diseases of obscure origin. *Brit. Med. Bull.* **41**, 63–69.

Morrison, D. C. and Yulevich, R. J. (1978). The effect of bacterial endotoxins on host mediation systems. *Am. J. Pathol.* **93**, 527–617.

Raudin, J. I. (1986). Pathogenesis of diseases caused by *Entamoeba histolytica*: studies of adherence, secreted toxins and contact-dependent cytolysis. *Rev. Inf. Dis.* **8**, 247–260.

Read, S. E. and Zabriskie, J. B. (Ed.) (1980). "Streptococcal Disease and the Immune Response". Academic Press, New York.

Rodriguez, M., von Wedel, R. J., Garrett, R. S. *et al.* (1983). Pituitary dwarfism in mice persistently infected with lymphocytic choriomeningitis virus. *Lab. Investig.* **49**, 48.

Simpson, L. L. (1979). The action of botulinus toxin. *Rev. Inf. Dis.* **1**, 656.

Ter Meulen, V. and Hall, W. W. (1978). Slow virus infections of the nervous system: virological, immunological and pathogenetic considerations. *J. Gen. Virol.* **41**, 1–25.

Watanabe, H. and Nakamaru, A. (1986). Identification of *Shigella sonnei.* Form I plasmid genes necessary for cell invasion and their conservation among shigella species and enteroinvasive *Escherichia coli. Infect. Immunity* **53**, 352–358.

Welliver, R. C. *et al.* (1981). The development of respiratory syncytial virus-specific IgE and the release of histamine in naso-pharyngeal secretions after infection. *New Engl. J. Med.* **305**, 841–845.

Williams, R. C. (1981). Immune complexes in human diseases. *Ann. Rev. Med.* **32**, 13–28.

9

Recovery from Infection

If there is to be recovery from an infection it is first necessary that the multiplication of the infectious agent is brought under control. The microbe must decrease in numbers and cease to spread through the body or cause progressive damage. This is accomplished by immunological and other factors whose action is now to be described. The average multiplication rate of various microorganisms in the infected host as shown by doubling-times (Table 20, p. 185) is nearly always longer than in artificial culture under optimal conditions. This in itself reflects the operation of antimicrobial forces. In the process of recovery from an infectious disease, damaged tissues must of course be repaired and reconstituted. Sometimes the microorganism is completely destroyed and tissues sterilized, but often this fails to take place and the microorganism persists in the body, in some instances continuing to cause minor pathological changes. The individual is nevertheless said to have recovered from the acute infection and is usually resistant to re-infection with the same microorganism. Persistent infections are dealt with in Ch. 10.

Immunological Factors in Recovery

The mechanisms of recovery from a primary infection are not necessarily the same as those responsible for resistance to re-infection (see below). For instance antibody to measles is of prime importance in resistance to re-infection and susceptible children can be passively protected by the antibody present in pooled normal human serum. But, compared with CMI, antibody

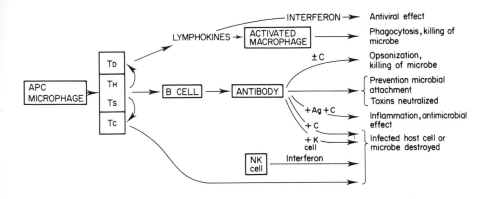

APC = antigen-presenting cell
Ag = antigen
C = complement
K cell = Killer cell (Antibody-Dependent-Cellular Cytotoxicity)

Fig. 32. Immune responses in infection.

plays only a small part in the recovery from initial infection with measles virus.

Antibody, CMI, complement, phagocytes and interferon are involved in the response to nearly all infections and without any doubt are together responsible for recovery. They constitute a mighty antimicrobial pentad, whose action is illustrated diagramatically in Fig. 32. In only a few instances, however, have the different components of this mighty pentad been dissected out and separately evaluated. All components normally operate together and to some extent the attempt to make separate evaluations is rather like deciding on the relative importance of 2, 3 and 4 in producing the product 24. For instance, polymorphs play a vital role in recovery from many bacterial infections but they necessarily operate in conjunction with antibody and complement. Macrophages play a vital role both in the induction and in the expression of CMI responses (see below). There are naturally occurring diseases in which one component is deficient or absent, and sometimes a component can be eliminated experimentally. More commonly the deficiency diseases are mixed in type, and experimentally it is often impossible to eliminate one component without also affecting the others. There has been some clarification and definition of the factors involved in recovery in the case of virus infections.

One major difficulty in assessing the importance of immune responses is that nearly all microorganisms are very complex, with large numbers of antigens. Various tests for antibody and CMI are carried out, but it is not often possible to test the response to a defined antigen, or to know precisely which antigens are important for infection and pathogenicity.

Antibody

The different types of antibody and the ways in which they have an antimicrobial action are listed in Ch. 6. Antibody actions against micro-organisms are further discussed at the end of this chapter under "Resistance to Re-infection".

In some infections antibody plays a major part in the process of recovery (see Table 28). For instance, viruses producing systemic disease, with a plasma viraemia (see p. 103), are controlled primarily by circulating antibody. This seems to be so in yellow fever or poliomyelitis virus infections. Children with severe hypogammaglobulinaemia are unable to form antibodies to poliovirus, and are about 10 000 times more likely than normal individuals to develop paralytic disease (which is generally of a chronic type) after live virus vaccination.* They have normal CMI and interferon responses, normal phagocytic cells and complement, but specific antibody must be produced if virus multiplication is to be inhibited. Poliovirus must attach to specific receptors on the surface of susceptible cells in the monkey or the human host; that is why mouse or rabbit cells, lacking these receptors, cannot be infected. When antibodies coat the surface of virus particles, attachment to receptors on susceptible cells is prevented so that infection cannot take place. The importance of specific attachments to cell surfaces is well established for other viruses also, and antibodies that combine with the virus surface often block attachment and thus prevent infection of cells. Sometimes attachment is not blocked, but the antibody nevertheless interferes with virus entry into the cell or with subsequent replication of virus. Antibody also promotes the uptake and digestion of virus by phagocytic cells, so that the virus–antibody complex is finally taken up and disposed of. Antibodies neutralizing virus infectivity are called neutralizing antibodies. Antibodies also act against viruses by clumping them, by destroying them with the help of complement, or by inducing inflammatory responses following their interaction with viral antigens (see Ch. 6).

---

* Agammaglobulinaemics are also susceptible to pneumococcal infections. Theoretically opsonization of these bacteria should occur after activation of the alternate pathway (see p. 147), but antibody appears to be needed for optimal uptake and killing by phagocytes. Antibody may also be needed for lysis of virus-infected host cells after alternative pathway activation (see p. 241).

Various bacteria have been shown to make specific attachments to epithelial surfaces and here secretory IgA antibodies are significant. IgA antibodies are formed in most infections of mucosal surfaces whether bacterial, viral or due to other microorganisms. They tend to prevent re-infection, but if formed early enough in the primary infection they could block the attachment of the microorganism to susceptible cells or cell surfaces (see Table 2, pp. 20–21) and thus interfere with the spread of infection. Their actual function in recovery, however, is doubtful. As was pointed out earlier, virus infections that are limited to epithelial surfaces and do not have a time-consuming spread of infection through the body, have incubation periods of no more than a few days. There is little opportunity for the slowly evolving immune response to play an important role in recovery, and virus replication is often inhibited before there has been a detectable IgA response. On the other hand, it must be remembered that antibodies (IgG or IgA) can be produced locally within a few days after experimental respiratory tract infections, for instance, and they would not be detected routinely when bound to viral antigens at this stage. But interferon is produced by the first infected cell, and is likely to have an important local antiviral action. If the process of infection takes longer, then secretory IgA antibodies have more opportunity to aid recovery. When the intestinal protozoan *Giardia lamblia* cause symptoms, these are not seen until 6–15 days after infection. A role for secretory IgA antibodies is indicated because patients with a shortage of these antibodies show troublesome and persistent giardial infection.

Quite clearly, as discussed in Ch. 4, the antibody response to streptococci, staphylococci and various encapsulated bacteria such as the pneumococcus is of particular importance. These are the common pyogenic (pus-forming) infections. For its antibacterial function antibody needs to operate together with phagocytic cells and complement and, if either of these are missing, resistance to pyogenic infections is impaired. Children with agammaglobulinaemia suffer repeated infections with pyogenic bacteria.* The spleen is an important site of antibody formation, and when the spleen has been removed surgically, or rendered incompetent in children with sickle cell disease (see p. 275) there is increased susceptibility to such infections. On the other hand, many bacterial infections (tuberculosis, syphilis, typhoid, gonorrhoea) can persist or can re-infect in spite of the presence of large amounts of antibody. This is discussed more fully in Ch. 7, and it is a reminder of the frequent inability of antibodies to ensure recovery.

---

* Infants with congenital (inherited) forms of agammaglobulinaemia remain well until about 9 months of age because the gift of maternal IgG via the placenta gives passive protection during this period.

Antibodies are vital in recovery from diseases caused by toxins, such as diphtheria and tetanus. As soon as antibodies have been formed to neutralize the powerful toxins and prevent further tissue damage, recovery is possible; without antibody the other antibacterial forces may operate in vain. In diphtheria the patient often recovers and is immune to the toxin without having controlled the infection itself, and he remains a carrier.

Circulating antibodies are probably important in the recovery from infection with certain protozoa such as malaria. Here, in particular, antibody must be directed against the relevant stage of the microorganism (especially the merozoite) and also against the relevant antigen on the microorganism. Merozoites are the forms that specifically absorb to red blood cells and parasitize them, and protective antibodies coat the merozoite surface and inhibit this absorption, at the same time promoting phagocytosis by the reticuloendothelial system.

Host defences against fungi are less clearly defined but there are indications that CMI is more important than antibody. Disseminated infection with certain fungi (*Coccidioides, Histoplasma*) occurs even in the presence of high antibody titres, and in such cases there is usually no CMI demonstrable by skin tests (Table 15, p. 142), suggesting that CMI matters most. Local infections with fungi elicit good CMI responses but poor antibody responses, and the patient recovers. Severe mucocutaneous candidiasis is seen in those with defective CMI, in spite of normal antibody production.

Small microorganisms such as viruses may have no more than one or two different antigens on their surface. The surface of influenza virus, for instance, consists of repeating subunits of the haemagglutinin antigen, interlaced with smaller numbers of subunits of the neuraminidase antigen. Antibodies to either antigen protect against infection, the antihaemagglutinin probably preventing virus attachment to the susceptible cell. Antibody to the neuraminidase does not prevent infection of the cell, but holds up virus release from the infected cells,* thus hindering the spread of infection. The mechanism of antibody protection can be worked out in a relatively simple microorganism of this sort.† Larger microorganisms, however, gen-

---

* The enzyme neuraminidase was once thought to physically dissolve away mucus and help the virus reach the susceptible cell in the respiratory tract. This crude picture is misleading, but the neuraminidase can release the haemagglutinin attached to (trapped by!) neuraminic acid residues in mucus, so that it can bind to receptors on the susceptible cell. It may also function by digesting the cell's haemagglutinin receptors, to which the newly formed virus is bound, thus enabling virus to escape from the infected cell.

† The haemagglutinin of influenza virus as the first viral protein for which a three-dimensional model was obtained after sequencing of the protein and analysis with monoclonal antibodies. Antibodies binding to any of three domains on the molecule neutralize infectivity, and these are the domains that are the sites of antigenic variation (p. 173).

erally have many different antigens on their surface. Some of these will be concerned with vital steps in the process of infection, and antibodies to such antigens will be protective. Antibodies to other surface antigens will not be protective, and when they are attached to the microbial surface may even physically interfere with (block) the action of protective antibodies. In addition, a large assortment of antibodies are produced to irrelevant internal components of the microorganism. Antibodies themselves differ in the firmness of the combination they make with antigens and may be of high or low affinity or avidity (see Glossary). Thus the quality of the antibody also matters. Protection by antibody is therefore a complicated matter, and if there is no protection in spite of the presence of large amounts of antibody, one has to ask first what components of the microbe these antibodies are combining with, and whether they are important components. Second, one needs to ask whether the antibody itself is of good quality.

Cell-mediated immunity

There is good evidence that cell-mediated immunity (CMI) is of supreme importance in recovery from a variety of microbial infections. These tend to be infections in which the microorganism replicates intracellularly (see Table 28). Tissue responses in the host bear the hallmarks of CMI involvement, the infiltrating cells consisting primarily of lymphocytes and macrophages. Macrophages are often infected. Delayed hypersensitivity is usually demonstrable by skin testing (Table 15, p. 142). Infections of this nature include tuberculosis, brucellosis, tularaemia, syphilis, tuberculoid leprosy (see p. 238) and leishmaniasis. Recovery is associated with the development of a vigorous CMI response, which also makes an important contribution to the pathology of the disease. As pointed out earlier, CMI develops in many other infections but is not very clearly associated with recovery. On infection with *Streptococcus pyogenes*, for instance, delayed hypersensitivity to the streptococcal products streptokinase and streptodornase develops, but it is less important than antibody in recovery from infection. An interesting distinction can be made between different types of infectious agent and the immune strategy most likely to be effective (Table 27).

The clearest picture about CMI in recovery comes from certain virus infections, particularly herpes viruses, pox viruses and measles virus, and it is first necessary to refer to important features of these infections which make the CMI response important. Antibodies neutralize free virus particles liberated from cells, but often fail to influence events in infected cells. Action on the infected cell seems necessary for recovery from the above virus infections. The destruction of cells infected with viruses takes place in

Table 27. Immune defences appropriate to different types of infection

Type of infectious agent	Primary immune defence	Immune mechanism	Further possible immune defences	Examples
1. Multiplies inside tissue cells	Prevent entry into cells by coating microbial surface with specific antibody	Antibody production (IgG, IgA, IgM)	Kill infected cell[a]	Many viruses Rickettsias, malarial merozoites
2. Multiplies inside phagocytes	Activate phagocytes and thus render them resistant to infection	T cells generate lymphokines	Kill infected[a] phagocyte	Certain viruses *Mycobacterium tuberculosis* *Leishmania*, trypanosomes (see Table 7, p. 87)
3. Multiplies outside cells	Kill microbe extracellularly or intracellularly	Complement-mediated lysis[b] Opsonized phagocytosis and killing	Neutralize microbial toxins	Most bacteria Trypanosomes
4. Multiplies outside cells, but attachment to body surface necessary for invasion	Prevent attachment by coating microbial surface with specific antibody	Antibody production (mainly secretory IgA)	As under 3	Streptococci *Neisseriae* *E. coli* etc. (see Table 2, pp. 20–1)

[a] Mechanisms are antibody + complement, antibody + K cell, cytotoxic T cell, or natural killer cell (see Ch. 6).
[b] NK cells (e.g. in *Toxoplasma gondii* infection) or T cells, K cells, may have a role.

Table 28. Antibody and CMI in resistance to systemic infections[a]

Type of resistance	Antibody	CMI

Recovery from primary infection	Yellow fever
	Polioviruses
	Coxsackie viruses
		Poxviruses
		  e.g. ectromelia (mice)
		    vaccinia (man)
		Herpes-type viruses
		  Herpes simplex
		  Varicella-zoster
		  Cytomegalovirus

	Streptococci Staphylococci *Neisseria meningitidis* *Haemophilus influenzae* Malaria? *Candida* spp. *Giardia lamblia*	LCM virus (mice) Measles Tuberculosis Leprosy Typhoid Systemic fungal infections Chronic mucocutaneous candidiasis?
Resistance to re-infection	Nearly all viruses including measles Most bacteria	Tuberculosis Leprosy
Resistance to reactivation of latent infection	Herpes simplex?	Varicella-zoster Cytomegalovirus Tuberculosis *Pneumocystis carinii*

[a] Either antibody or CMI is known to be the major factor in the examples given. But in many other infections there is no information, and sometimes both types of immunity are important.

various ways, but depends on the mechanism of virus maturation in the cell. Many viruses, such as poliovirus or papilloma viruses, replicate and produce fully infectious particles inside the cytoplasm. These particles are nucleocapsids, consisting of the basic nucleic acid core with its protein coat (capsid), and they are liberated from the cell and exposed to antibody when it dies and disintegrates (Fig. 33). Other viruses do not have to wait for cell disruption, but are liberated by a process of budding through the cell membrane. The basic viral nucleocapsid in the cytoplasm becomes closely associated with the cell membrane, causing viral antigens to be incorporated into it (Fig. 33). The virus particle finally matures by budding through the altered cell membrane, acquiring an envelope as it does so. Such viruses are referred to as "enveloped" and include herpes viruses, myxo and paramyxo viruses etc. (pp. 300–1). It is as if the virus is excreted or egested from the living cell.

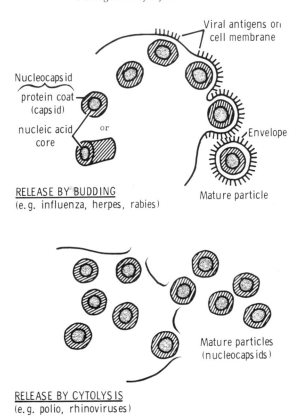

Viral antigens on cell membrane

Nucleocapsid
protein coat (capsid)
nucleic acid core
or

Envelope

Mature particle

RELEASE BY BUDDING
(e.g. influenza, herpes, rabies)

Mature particles
(nucleocapsids)

RELEASE BY CYTOLYSIS
(e.g. polio, rhinoviruses)

Fig. 33. Diagram to illustrate mechanisms of virus release from infected cell. Nucleocapsids may be spherical (herpes viruses) or tubular (influenza). Budding may also take place from nuclear membrane (herpes viruses) or from the membrane lining cytoplasmic vacuoles (coronaviruses, flaviviruses).

There are two important consequences of this mechanism of virus maturation. First, virus can be released even though the cell remains alive and intact. Second, the foreign viral antigens appearing on the cell surface are recognized by the host and an immune response is generated with the infected cell as the target. The significance of this is that the infected cell can be destroyed before virus has been liberated,* and can also be destroyed in oncogenic and other virus infections in which virus is liberated from the cell over long periods.

* Viral antigens often appear on the cell surface very early in the replication process, many hours before progeny virus particles have been formed. These antigens can be identified by fluorescent antibody staining, or by the susceptibility of the infected cell to lysis after treatment with antiviral antibody plus complement. As many as five distinct viral antigens (glycoproteins) appear on the envelope in the case of a large virus such as herpes simplex.

Viral antigens are also formed on the cell surface during the replication of certain nonenveloped viruses such as adenoviruses. The surface antigens are not incorporated into the virus particle, but the infected cell bearing the antigens can be recognized and destroyed by immune mechanisms. Also, although destruction of infected host cells has long been considered a feature of viral rather than other infections, there is growing evidence that it is a possibility in certain other infections. Host cells infected *in vitro* with protozoa (*Plasmodia* and *Theileria*), with rickettsia (*Coxiella burneti*) and probably with certain bacteria (*Listeria*) express microbial antigens on their surface and thus should be vulnerable to immune lysis.

The immune mechanisms for the destruction of cells bearing foreign antigens on their surface are as follows:

(1) Specifically sensitized T cells make intimate contacts with foreign antigen in association with MHC Class 1 antigens on the target cell surface. The target cell membrane is damaged at the site of contact, leaving a gaping hole 40 nm in diameter that cannot be repaired, so that when the T cell moves away 30–60 s later there is a leakage of cell components, an influx of water, and the target cell swells up and dies.* The T cell can kill again.

(2) Macrophages, polymorphs, and also certain mononuclear cells (K cells, see Ch. 6) which are not macrophages or typical T lymphocytes have the ability to destroy target cells with the assistance of specific antibody. Antibody combines with antigen on the infected cell surface, and K cells attach to the antibody-coated cells via the Fc receptor. The final killing mechanism is not clear but the K cell releases oxygen radicals (see pp. 68–9) which produce "burns" (Professor Peter Lachmann) involving lipid oxidation on the target cell. The Fc receptors on eosinophils enable them to function in the same way and kill multicellular parasites such as schistosomes (see p. 65) after adhering in large numbers to the antibody-coated surface of these parasites.

(3) Antibodies combine with antigen on the target cell surface, complement is activated locally, making "holes" in the cell membrane and leading to cell disruption (see p. 147). CMI is not involved. This type of cell destruction generally needs much more antibody and in that sense is less efficient than the antibody-dependent destruction by mononuclear cells described under 2.

*The exact mechanism is not clear, and *lymphocytotoxin*, a soluble cytotoxic factor produced by T cells may play a role. *Tumour necrosis factor*, a product of activated macrophages and lymphocytes (now cloned and with a similar sequence to lymphocytotoxin) also kills cells, and has an ill-defined role in macrophage-mediated cytotoxicity. Tumour necrosis factor also inhibits viral replication in cells, like interferon (see pp. 243–5). But it acts on its own rather than by inducing interferon production, and as little as 1ng ml^{-1} is effective. Its role *in vivo* is not yet clear.

In herpes-type virus infections (herpes simplex, varicella, CMV etc.), virus antigens appear on the surface of infected cells 12–24 hours before virus multiplication is completed, so that cells can be destroyed early in infection by CMI or by the other mechanisms listed above. Herpes viruses tend to spread directly from cell to cell without entering extracellular fluids, and antibodies cannot enter cells to neutralize virus. By acting directly on infected cells, immune cytolysis helps prevent this type of spread. Immune cytolysis has a similar action on cells infected with poxviruses and measles virus.

The sequence of events with herpes virus, poxvirus and measles virus infections appears to be as follows. At sites of virus multiplication T lymphocytes, in the course of their normal movements through the body (see p. 138) encounter virus antigens that have become bound to the surface of a macrophage or other antigen-presenting cell (see pp. 123–4). When a T cell encounters the antigen to which it is specifically sensitized, the CMI response is initiated as described in Ch. 6. The T cell differentiates and divides to give fresh supplies of specifically sensitized T cells. Lymphokines are liberated to attract macrophages and other leucocytes and focus them onto the site of infection. Infected cells are destroyed by cytotoxic T lymphocytes and other cells, and virus material and cell debris is phagocytosed and disposed of by activated macrophages. Similar events occur in lymph nodes to which virus or virus antigens have been brought by lymphatics.

In experimental infections, CMI can be removed without affecting antibody or interferon responses, and changes in the disease are then studied. For instance, the selective removal of CMI* in mice infected with ectromelia (mouse pox) virus has profound effects on the disease. The virus normally causes focal liver necrosis, and in CMI-depleted mice inflammatory responses in foci of liver infection are inhibited so that virus continues to grow and destroy hepatic cells, proving fatal in spite of the presence of antibodies. If immune T cells are transferred to such an animal, there is a prompt cellular infiltration into foci of infection and inhibition of virus growth. Immune T cells react with viral antigens in tissues and focus macrophages onto the site of infection, inhibiting virus growth by the mechanisms described above and in Ch. 6.

The best way of discovering the function of a bodily mechanism or organ is to see what happens when it is removed (see also agammaglobulinaemia, p. 228). Thus, convincing evidence for the importance of CMI in the control

*This was done in adult mice by treatment with antilymphocyte serum. Nowadays a better defined depletion can be achieved by using monoclonal antibodies reactive with different types of T cell.

of infections comes from studies on patients with defective CMI. Very rarely infants are born with an absent or poorly developed thymus gland (thymic aplasia or hypoplasia). Their T lymphocytes fail to differentiate and develop, giving rise to severe CMI deficiency, but there is a normal antibody response to most antigens. Congenital immunodeficiencies are often mixed in nature with defects in CMI, antibody response or phagocytic cells; thymic aplasia, although so rare,* is a "pure" deficit and gives some insight into the importance of CMI in infectious diseases. Affected infants show normal ability to control most bacterial infections, but a greatly increased suscepti- bility to infections with various viruses and certain other intracellular microorganisms. After measles infection, for instance, there is no rash but an uncontrolled and progressive growth of virus in the respiratory tract, leading to fatal giant cell pneumonia. Evidently the CMI response controls the infectious process and at the same time plays a vital role in the development of skin lesions. If affected children are vaccinated against smallpox with vaccinia virus, the virus grows as usual in epidermal cells at the inoculation site to give an increasing zone of skin destruction. In normal infants there is an inflammatory response at the edges of the lesion after 6–8 days and this leads to inhibition of virus growth, then scabbing and healing of the lesion. The infant with thymic aplasia, however, does not show this response and the destructive skin lesion continues to enlarge, occupying an ever increasing area of the arm and shoulder. The infection can be controlled by local injection of immune lymphocytes from a closely related donor, but not by antibody. Infants with this type of immune deficiency also tend to suffer severe generalized infections with herpes simplex virus. In addition they show increased susceptibility to other intracellular microorganisms. When they are vaccinated against tuberculosis with live BCG vaccine, the attenuated bacteria, instead of undergoing limited growth with induction of a good CMI response, multiply in an uncontrolled fashion and may eventu- ally kill the patient. The CMI response is therefore necessary for the control of infection with intracellular bacteria of this type.

---

*Mixed antibody and CMI deficiencies are commoner. The infants suffer from superficial *Candida albicans* infections, and commonly die with *Pneumocystis carinii* (see Glossary) pneumonia or generalized infections with vaccinia, varicella or measles. Immune deficiencies (mostly CMI) are seen in adults with Hodgkin's disease, or after immunosuppression for organ transplants. In these patients, who have encountered the common infections in early life, there is reactivation of persistent infections such as varicella-zoster, tuberculosis, herpes simplex, cytomegalovirus, warts, *Pneumocystis carinii* infection. Gram-negative bacterial pneumonia may also occur. In many immunodeficiencies the primary defect is unknown. Patients lacking adenosine deaminase, an enzyme in the purine salvage pathway, develop a severe combined immunodeficiency. Their lymphocytes fail to mature, macrophage activation is defective, and they die early as a result of infection.

There are two more clinical examples of the importance of CMI in recovery from nonviral intracellular infections. Leprosy, caused by *Mycobacterium leprae*, exists in a spectrum of clinical forms. At one end of the spectrum is tuberculoid leprosy. Here, the infection is kept under some degree of control, with infiltrations of lymphocytes and macrophages into infected areas such as the nasal mucous membranes. In the lesions there are very few bacteria and all the signs of a strong CMI response. Injection of lepromin (leprosy antigens) into the skin of the infected patient gives a rather slowly evolving but strong delayed hypersensitivity reaction. This type of leprosy is called tuberculoid leprosy because the host response is similar to that in tuberculosis. At the other end of the leprosy spectrum* (lepromatous leprosy) there are very few lymphocytes or macrophages in the lesions and large numbers of extracellular bacteria. Associated with these appearances indicating less effective control of the infection, there is a weak or absent skin response to lepromin. Lepromin is a crude bacterial extract and the exact antigens to which the lepromatous patient fails to respond are not known.† Antibodies are formed in larger amounts than in tuberculoid patients and indeed may give rise to immune complex phenomena in lepromatous patients (see Ch. 8), but these antibodies fail to control the infection. The second clinical example of the importance of CMI in recovery concerns the disease chronic mucocutaneous candidiasis. Children with immunodeficiency diseases sometimes develop severe and generalized skin lesions caused by the normally harmless fungus *Candida albicans*. Antibody to candida is formed but the CMI response is often inadequate and these patients can be cured by supplying the missing CMI response. This can be given in the form of repeated injections of transfer factor (see Glossary).

The CMI response may have additional antimicrobial effects in chronic infections with certain intracellular organisms. When the microorganism persists as a source of antigenic stimulation and the CMI-induced influx of mononuclear cells continues, a granuloma may be formed (see below). The focus of infection tends to be walled off, and this is often associated with the inhibition of microbial growth. Granulomas are a feature of respiratory tuberculosis, contributing to pulmonary fibrosis. Granulomas, however, can result from chronic accumulation of immune complexes as well as from chronic local CMI reactions (see Ch. 8).

---

*To some extent there is also a clinical spectrum in tuberculosis, according to the type of immune response, some (more susceptible) patients showing strong antibody responses and weak cell-mediated immune responses.

†Lymphocytes from patients show normal transformation responses to other mycobacteria such as BCG and *Mycobacterium lepraemurium* (see Ch. 7).

Phagocytosis

Phagocytes play a central role in resistance to and recovery from infectious diseases (see pp. 89–90). In the old days physicians saw the formation of pus (see p. 71) as a valiant attempt to control infection, and referred to it as "laudable pus", especially when it was thick and creamy. An account of the antimicrobial functions of phagocytes and the consequences of phagocyte defects is given in Ch. 4.

Inflammation

Inflammation, whether induced by immunological reactions, tissue damage or microbial products plays a vital role in recovery from infection (see also Chs 3 and 6). Inflammation is necessary for the proper functioning of the immune defences because it focuses all circulating antimicrobial factors onto the site of infection. The circulating antimicrobial forces that arrive in tissues include polymorphs, macrophages, lymphocytes, antibodies, activated complement components, and materials like fibrin that play a part in certain infections.* The increased blood supply and temperature in inflamed tissues favour maximal metabolic activity on the part of leucocytes, and the slight lowering of pH tends to inhibit the multiplication of many extracellular microorganisms.

The prompt increase in circulating polymorphs during pyogenic infections is caused in the first place by the release of cells held in reserve in the bone marrow, but there is also an increase in the rate of production. Monocyte release and production is controlled independently. At least four colony stimulating factors, all glycoproteins, control the mitosis of polymorph and macrophage precursors, and their final differentiation and activity. One of them is Interleukin-3 (Il-3), which acts mainly on polymorph precursors. They are present in increased amounts in serum during infection, and in animals the serum levels are dramatically raised by the injection of endotoxin.

---

*There have been numerous reports of antimicrobial factors present in normal serum. Doubtless some of these involved alternative pathway activation of complement, as in the case of pathogenic *Neisseria* (see below). Trypanocidal factors in normal human serum may be related to natural resistance to trypanosomiasis. It has been known since 1902 that *Trypanosoma brucei*, which is not infectious for man, is lysed by something present in normal human serum, whereas *Trypanosoma rhodesiensi* and *Trypanosoma gambiensi* which infect man and cause sleeping sickness, are relatively resistant. The trypanocidal factor has been shown to be a high density lipoprotein.

Circulating polymorphs show increased functional activity during pyogenic infections and readily take up and reduce a certain yellow dye (nitroblue-tetrazolium), forming dark blue deposits in the cytoplasm. An increase in the proportion of polymorphs showing this reaction reflects their increased activity, but the test is of no value in the diagnosis of pyogenic infections because of false positive and false negative results. In any case, increased reduction of the dye is not necessarily associated with increased bactericidal activity.

When inflammation becomes severe or widespread there is a general body response with the appearance of acute-phase proteins in the blood (see p. 59). As a result two classical changes can be detected in the blood. The first is an increase in the erythrocyte sedimentation rate (ESR), and this is a clinically useful indication that inflammation or tissue destruction is occurring somewhere in the body. The exact mechanism of the increase is not understood. The second change is the appearance in the blood of increased quantities of a β globulin synthesized in the liver and detected by its precipitation after the addition of the C carbohydrate of the pneumococcus. It is therefore called C-reactive protein. Very small amounts are present in the blood of normal individuals, but there is a 1000-fold increase within 24 h of the onset of inflammation. After binding to substances derived from microorganisms and from damaged host cells, it activates the complement system, acts as an opsonin, and possibly serves a useful function. Both the ESR and C-reactive protein changes are nonspecific sequelae to inflammation of any sort, whether infectious or noninfectious.

When the infection is persistent, inflammation may become chronic, lasting weeks or months. Infections do not generally last for long periods if they induce acute polymorphonuclear inflammation; the battle between host and microbe is decided at an early stage.* Chronic inflammation depends on a constant leakage of microbial products and antigens from the site of infection. The type of infection that persists and causes chronic inflammation is generally an intracellular bacterial or fungal or chlamydial infection. In these infections there is a chronic CMI response, with proliferation of lymphocytes and fibroblasts in infected areas, a steady influx of macrophages and the formation of giant and epithelioid † cells. Episodes of tissue necrosis alternate with repair and the formation of granulation tissue, then fibrous tissue. It is a ding-dong battle between microorganisms and host

---

* Occasionally this is not so, and there is continued polymorph infiltration, as for instance in chronic osteomyelitis or a pilonidal sinus.

† Epithelioid cells are poorly phagocytic, highly secretory, and about 20 μm in diameter, whereas giant cells, formed by the fusion of macrophages, are up to 300 μm in diameter, containing up to 30 nuclei.

antimicrobial forces. The resulting granuloma (see also above) can be regarded as an attempt to wall off the infected area. Chronic infections with chronic inflammation and granuloma formation include tuberculosis, syphilis, actinomycosis, leprosy, lymphogranuloma inguinale and coccidiodomycosis. Chronic viral infections are not associated with chronic inflammatory responses, probably because virus growth is often defective and no more than minute amounts of antigen are liberated.

Complement

Complement has been discussed and invoked on many occasions in Chs 6, 7, 8 and in this chapter. It should be remembered that some of the complement components are quite large molecules, and do not readily leave the circulation except where there is local inflammation. Complement can carry out antimicrobial activities in the following ways.

1. Complement lysis. Complement reacts with antibody that has attached to the surface of infected cells or to the surface of certain microorganisms, and destroys the cell or microorganism after making holes in the surface membrane. Gram-negative bacteria are killed in this way, and also enveloped viruses such as rubella and parainfluenza. Because of the amplification occurring in the complement system (see Ch. 6), especially when the alternative pathway is also activated, antibody attached to the surface of a microorganism is more likely to induce complement lysis than it is to neutralize it. Complement lysis is therefore perhaps more important when antibody molecules are in short supply, early in the immune response. Bacteria with surface polysaccharide components can activate complement without the need for antibody (see 5 below), as can host cells infected with viruses such as measles. In the latter case alternative pathway activation by itself does not do enough damage to kill the cell, presumably because less severe membrane lesions can be repaired; antibody must also be present for lysis.

2. Complement opsonization. Complement reacts with antibody attached to the surface of microorganisms, providing additional receptor sites for phagocytosis by polymorphs or macrophages. Phagocytosis is also promoted by each molecule of antibody attached to the microorganism because of the Fc receptors on phagocytes, but when complement is activated there are many more molecules of C3b present as a result of the amplification phenomenon. Therefore complement often has a more pronounced opsonizing effect than antibody alone and for some bacteria, such as the pneumococ-

cus, opsonization actually depends on complement. Complement opsonization is important when the antibody is IgM, because human phagocytes do
not have receptors for the Fc region of IgM. Complement can also act as an
opsonin though not always so effectively, in the absence of antibody (see 5,
below).

3. Complement-mediated inflammation. Specific antibodies react with
microbial antigens that are either free or on the surface of microorganisms.
Following this antigen–antibody reaction, complement is activated, with
generation of inflammatory and chemotactic factors. These substances focus
antimicrobial serum factors and leucocytes onto the site of infection.

4. Complement-assisted neutralization of viruses. In the case of viruses
coated with antibody, complement adds to the mass of molecules on the
virus surface and further hinders attachment of virus to susceptible cells.
This action is more likely to be important when antibodies are in short supply
early in the immune response.

5. Complement-assisted K cell lysis. C3b deposition on infected host cells
not only opsonizes (see above) but also augments K cell-mediated cytotoxicity (ADCC, see p. 135).

6. Complement opsonization via alternative pathway. Complement reacting
with endotoxin on the surface of Gram-negative bacilli, with capsular
polysaccharide of pneumococci etc., or with *Candida*, is activated via the
alternative pathway (see p. 147) and C3b mediated opsonization takes place.
It seems likely that this is important in natural resistance to infection.

Unfortunately, there is little direct evidence that the above antimicrobial
activities of complement are in fact important in the body. The rare patients
with C3-deficiency develop repeated pyogenic infections, and C3-deficient
mice show increased susceptibility to plague and to staphylococcal infections. Mice with C5 deficiency (controlled by a single gene) are more
susceptible to *Candida* infection, probably because of inadequate opsonization. Patients with C5–C8 deficiency, however, are often particularly susceptible to disseminated or recurrent neisserial infection. In this case the
bactericidal rather than the opsonizing action of complement seem important. But observations on complement deficiencies are probably too limited
to draw firm conclusions and there have been few clearly defined deficiencies. The system is a highly complex one, with alternative pathways, positive
feedback amplification and multiple inhibitors. A similar complement system occurs in a wide range of vertebrates and it must be assumed that such a

complex, powerful system confers some biological advantage, presumably by giving resistance to microbial infections.

Interferons

The interferons are a family of cell-regulatory proteins produced in all vertebrates. Most of the human interferon genes have been cloned and the different interferon molecules sequenced. There are three types of interferon, which are chemically and antigenically distinct. Alpha and beta interferons are made by nearly all cells in the body, including epithelial cells, neurons, muscle cells etc. in response to viral and other infections. Gamma interferons are produced by lymphocytes following antigen-specific stimulation, and are lymphokines (see pp. 139–140), with immunoregulatory functions as well as the antimicrobial action described below.

Viruses are the most important inducers of α and β interferon, the stimulus to the cell being in most cases the foreign double-stranded RNA formed during virus replication (Fig. 34). Interferons act on uninfected cells, binding to a receptor on the surface and inducing the synthesis of a series of enzymes. These enzymes prevent the replication of all viruses by causing other enzymes to destroy viral messenger RNA by inactivating the peptide chain initiation factor, and possibly other effects.* Interferons are exceedingly potent *in vitro*, being active at about 10^{-15} M. Interferons have no direct action on virus itself and do not interfere with viral entry into the susceptible cell. The interferons produced by different species of animals are to a large extent species specific in their action. Mouse interferon, for instance, has no action on chick or human cells, and monkey interferon has only slight action on human cells.

Interferon liberated from infected cells can reach other cells in the vicinity by diffusion and protect them from infection.† The cell that has been acted on by interferon is then protected from infection with all viruses for a period of up to 24 h. It would seem inevitable that interferon is important in recovery from virus infections, whether on epithelial surfaces or in solid tissues. Interferon, moreover, has an independent effect on host resistance because it activates NK cells (see p. 139). It has proved difficult to show

---

* In addition to their antiviral effects, interferons appear to protect against infection with certain streptococci and shigella, but the mechanism is not known. There is also a wide range of additional effects, including inhibition of cell division and changes in the plasma membrane, and interferons have therefore been called hormones.

† Interferon is also induced by non-viral agents such as rickettsiae and certain bacteria, and will protect cells from various nonviral intracellular microorganisms.

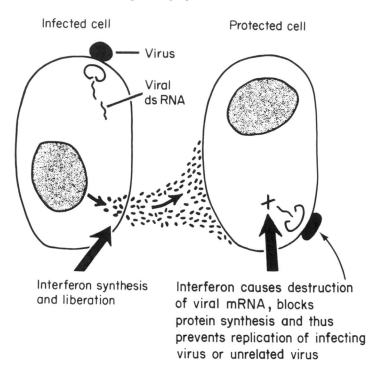

Infected cell   Protected cell

Interferon synthesis
and liberation

Interferon causes destruction
of viral mRNA, blocks
protein synthesis and thus
prevents replication of infecting
virus or unrelated virus

Fig. 34. Mechanism of induction and action of α and β interferon. Interferon attaches to receptor on uninfected cell on right and protects it against virus infection. Interferon from T cells acts in the same way. Interferons also increase NK cell activity.

conclusively that interferon is a vitally important part of the body's defence against viruses. If there were naturally occurring deficiencies in interferon production, or naturally occurring insensitivity to interferon it would be possible to decide what interferon does, but deficiencies are not known to occur, partly because in men there are about 12 genes for α interferon, although only one each for β and for γ interferon.* However, interferon can be selectively inhibited in mice by treatment with antibody to interferon. When this is done, enhanced susceptibility to certain virus infections is observed. Interferon has also been given passively to experimental animals and can be effectively induced by the administration of a synthetic ds RNA preparation (poly I:poly C). Antiviral results are demonstrable in experi-

*A recent study of 30 children who suffered from recurrent respiratory tract infections identified four with impaired interferon production. When these particular children were infected with common cold viruses, α interferon could not be detected in nasal washings. Their peripheral blood leucocytes also failed to produce α interferon on repeated testing *in vitro*, although γ interferon production was normal.

mental infections, and are most clearly seen in infections of epithelial surfaces such as the conjunctiva or respiratory tract, and when treatment is begun before rather than after infection.

Interferon would seem to be the ideal antiviral chemotherapeutic agent for use in man, being produced naturally by human cells, nonallergenic and active against a broad spectrum of viruses. So far, results in human patients have not been dramatic. For instance, volunteers infected intranasally with influenza B and other respiratory viruses have been given either poly I : poly C or repeated very large doses of purified human interferon by the same route, but with disappointingly slight protection. Perhaps not enough of the administered or induced interferon reaches the cells that need protecting early enough in the infection. The "toxic" effects of large doses of pure interferon were referred to on p. 185. At present, 30 years after its discovery, it is still of no practical importance in infectious diseases. However, very large quantities of pure human α and β interferon are now available, and further trials in virus infections are in progress.

Temperature

In man the mean daily body temperature is 36.8°C with a daily variation of only 1.3°C, the maximum being at about 18.00 h, the minimum at about 03.00 h. This almost constant body temperature, like the almost constant level of blood sugar, illustrates Claude Bernard's dictum that "*La fixité du milieu intérieur est la condition de la vie libre*". If the individual is to function steadily in spite of changes in the external environment, the internal environment must remain constant. The brain is one of the most sensitive parts of the body to departures from normality. At temperatures below 27.7–30.0°C people become unconscious, at 40.5°C or above they become disoriented and may be maniacal; above 43.3°C they are comatose. A rise in body temperature is one of the most frequent and familiar responses to infection, whether the infection is largely restricted to body surfaces (common cold, influenza) or is obviously generalized (measles, typhoid, malaria). During fever the appetite is often lost and headache may result from dilation of meningeal blood vessels. The temperature rise is largely due to an increase in heat production, and the raised metabolic rate, together with reduced food intake, results in a high excretion of nitrogen in the urine. There is rapid wasting of body fat and muscles if the fever is prolonged.

In infectious diseases there is a common mediator of the febrile response known as endogenous pyrogen (interleukin-1). It is present in inflammatory exudates and in the plasma during fever, and acts on the temperature-regulating centre in the anterior hypothalamus, resetting the body thermostat.

Endogenous pyrogen is produced by macrophages and certain other cells, and as little as 30–50 ng causes fever in rabbits. It can be induced by immunological mechanisms. Fever is a common accompaniment of generalized antigen–antibody reactions. For instance, rabbits immunized with bovine serum albumin develop fever when injected with this antigen. Systemic virus infections such as the exanthems (see Glossary) are characterized by an asymptomatic incubation period during which virus replicates and spreads through the body, followed by a sudden onset of illness with fever. The febrile reaction is mainly due to the immune response to the virus; hence its relatively sudden onset a week or two after infection. The CMI response (see below) as well as the antibody response is involved. Antigen–antibody reactions, in addition to causing fever, can also give rashes, joint swelling and pain, even glomerulonephritis (see Ch. 8). The first signs of illness in hepatitis B, before jaundice, are often "allergic" in nature and mediated by antigen–antibody interactions, with fever, joint pains and fleeting rashes.

The generalized CMI response in the infected host is also a cause of fever. This certainly contributes to the fever in tuberculosis, brucellosis and perhaps staphylococcal and cryptococcal infections. When tuberculin is added to alveolar macrophages from an immunized animal endogenous pyrogen (interleukin-1) is generated, and patients with chronic brucellosis develop fever when injected with 10 μg of purified brucella.

Certain bacterial products are pyrogenic. The peptidoglycan in the cell wall of staphylococci causes monocytes to liberate endogenous pyrogen. More importantly, endotoxins from Gram-negative bacteria also have this effect, as little as 2 ng of Salmonella endotoxin per kg causing fever in man. Endotoxin is present in the circulation during systemic infection with Gram-negative bacteria, but tolerance to endotoxin-induced fever develops quite rapidly, and endotoxin itself probably makes no more than a partial contribution to the febrile response, even in infections such as typhoid and dysentery. There is no good evidence that other microbial products or toxins cause fever other than by immunological mechanisms. In the old days before penicillin, pneumococcal pneumonia used to give one of the highest fevers known in man with dramatic and severe onset, the temperature often rising to 40°C within 12 h. These bacteria, however, have no endotoxin or other pyrogens and the mechanisms were presumably immunological.

Since fever is such a constant sequel of infection, it is natural to suppose that it has some antimicrobial function: Thomas Sydenham in the seventeenth century wrote that "Fever is a mighty engine which nature brings into the world for the conquest of her enemies". Bodily functions are profoundly disturbed by fever. Metabolic activity is increased in phagocytic cells, and studies *in vitro* show that there are big increases in T cell proliferation and in antibody production at febrile temperatures. The evidence, however, is disappointing. Temperature-sensitive mutants of certain viruses are often less virulent, and experimental virus infections can sometimes be made more severe by preventing fever with antipyretic drugs. When fever is induced in infected animals by raising the environmental temperature there are also other complex physiological changes, making it difficult to interpret such experiments. In two bacterial infections, gonorrhoea and syphilis, the microbes themselves are actually killed by febrile temperatures, but in the natural disease these temperatures are rarely reached. Before the introduction of antibiotics, patients with these two diseases were infected with malaria in order to induce body temperatures high enough to eradicate the infection (following which the malaria was treated with quinine).

Is fever, then, a purely accidental consequence of the immune response to an infectious agent and of little value to the host? Perhaps it would be wisest to reserve judgement. Fever is costly in energy and is an ancient bodily response, having evolved with the vertebrates over hundreds of millions of years. Perhaps one day some more convincing evidence will emerge to give substance to Sydenham's eloquent convictions.

Tissue Repair

Once the multiplication of the infecting microorganism has been controlled, and the microorganism itself perhaps eliminated from the body, the next step in the process of recovery is to tidy up the debris and repair the damaged tissues. Four examples will be given, in the skin, respiratory tract, liver and the foetus.

In the skin

During recovery from a boil or smallpox vaccination, the sequence of events is as follows. Superficial tissue debris, including necrotic epidermis, inflammatory cells and plasma exudate, dries off as a scab. This gives mechanical protection, acts as a barrier to further infection, and can be shed to the exterior after repair is completed. Below the scab, phagocytic cells clear up the debris and fibroblasts move in, multiply, and lay down a mucopolysaccharide matrix over the underlying intact tissues. New blood vessels are formed, and later on lymphatics, by sprouting of the endothelial cells of neighbouring vessels into the fibroblast matrix. The newly formed capillaries advance into the damaged zone at 0.1–0.6 mm a day. They are fragile and leaky, and there is a continuous extravasation of polymorphs, macrophages and fibroblasts into the matrix. As seen from the surface, each collection of capillary loops in the fibroblast matrix looks like a small red granule and this soft vascular material is therefore called granulation tissue. It bleeds easily and with its rich blood supply and abundant phagocytic cells is well protected against infection. Meanwhile, epidermal cells at the edges of the gap have been multiplying. The newly formed layer of cells creeps over the granulation tissue, and the epidermis is thus reconstituted. Fibroblasts in the granulation tissue lay down reticulum fibres, and later collagen. If the area of epidermal cell destruction is large, and when underlying sebaceous glands, hair follicles etc. are destroyed, a great deal of collagenous fibrous tissue is formed to repair the gap. The newly formed collagen in fibrous tissue contracts and tends to bring the skin edges together. Contracting collagen can strangle an organ like the liver but in the skin it merely forms a scar. A scar is a characteristic sequel to vaccination against smallpox, vaccination with BCG, or to a bacterial infection involving sebaceous glands, as seen in severe acne.

In the respiratory tract

After infection with a rhinovirus or influenza virus, there are large areas where the epithelial cells are destroyed, mucociliary transport is defective (see Ch. 2) and the underlying cells vulnerable to secondary bacterial infection. Phagocytic cells must now ingest and dispose of tissue debris, and the epithelial surface must be reconstituted by a burst of mitotic activity in adjacent epithelial cells. To some extent pre-existing cells can slide across the gap, but repair depends on mitosis in cells at the edges. The process of repair takes several days, and the mechanism is the same whether the damage is caused by viruses, bacteria or chemicals. Epithelial regeneration is particularly rapid in respiratory epithelium, and also in conjunctiva, oropharynx and mucocutaneous junctions, but it is delayed if the infection continues. After chronic bacterial or chemical damage there is an increase in mucus-producing goblet cells in the respiratory epithelium, and sometimes impairment of mucociliary mechanisms, resulting in the condition called chronic bronchitis. As a rule, however, recovery is complete.

In the liver

During recovery from focal hepatitis, polymorphs and macrophages are active in areas of tissue damage, phagocytosing dead and damaged hepatic cells, Kupffer cells, biliary epithelial cells, inflammatory cells and microorganisms. As this proceeds neighbouring hepatic cells and bile duct epithelial cells divide to replace missing cells. This, together with cell movement and rearrangement, leads to remodelling of the lobules and the restoration of normal appearances. If supporting tissues have been significantly damaged, and particularly if there are repeated episodes of necrosis, healing involves scar formation. When this is widespread it is referred to as cirrhosis, the bands of fibrous tissue dividing up the organ into irregular islands. The regenerating islands enlarge to form nodules, the fibrous tissue thickens and contracts and there is obvious distortion of structure, with circulatory impairment, biliary obstruction and liver dysfunction.

In most tissues, repair with restoration of structural integrity can be achieved by fibrous tissue formation. Recovery of function depends more on the ability of differentiated cells in damaged tissues to increase their numbers again and thus restore functional integrity. Liver cells or epithelial cells have a great capacity for mitosis, and the intestinal epithelium, respiratory epithelium or liver can be restored to normal without great difficulty. In the case of cardiac muscle, striated muscle or brain, the differentiated cells show little if any mitotic capacity and destruction in these tissues results in a permanent deficit in the number of cells. This may be of no consequence in a muscle as long as firm scar tissue repairs the damage, but it may be important in the central nervous system. Anterior horn cells destroyed by poliovirus cannot be replaced, and if enough are destroyed there will be a permanent paralysis, although some restoration of function takes place by learning to use muscles more effectively and by the recovery of damaged anterior horn cells.

In the foetus

Tissue repair in the foetus is in some ways easier and in others more difficult. In general there is a very great capacity for repair and reconstitution of damaged tissues. Primitive mitotic cells abound, organs are in a state of plasticity, and in the developmental process itself tissue destruction and repair accompanies mitosis and construction. On the other hand, at critical times in foetal life, there is a programmed cell division and differentiation in the course of constructing certain major organs. If one of these organs is damaged at this critical time, the developmental process is upset and the organ is malformed. This is what happens when rubella virus infects the human foetus during the first three months of pregnancy. Depending on the exact organ system being formed at the time of foetal infection, there may be damage to the heart, eyes, ears or brain, resulting in congenital heart disease, cataract, deafness or mental retardation in the infant. Other infectious agents (see Table 10, p. 117) affect particularly the central nervous system of the foetus (toxoplasmosis, cytomegalovirus, syphilis) and sometimes bones and teeth (syphilis).

If the foetal infection is severe, as is the rule with vaccinia virus or with most bacteria, foetal death and abortion is the inevitable consequence. There are only a small number of microorganisms that infect the foetus and interfere with development without proving fatal. This type of nicely balanced pathogenicity is needed if the infected foetus is to survive and be born with a malformation. Even the infections that cause malformations (teratogenic infections) are sometimes severe enough to kill the foetus. In most congenital infections the microorganism remains present and is detectable in the newborn infant (cytomegalovirus, rubella, syphilis etc.), often persisting for many years. It is a striking feature of most teratogenic foetal infections (rubella, cytomegalovirus, toxoplasmosis) that the mother suffers a very mild or completely inapparent infection.

Certain microorganisms infect the foetus and damage developing organs, but are then eliminated from the body. The damaged organs are formed as best as possible, and at birth there are no signs that the malformation was caused by a microorganism. Tissues are sterile, and no inflammatory responses are visible histologically. Thus when a pregnant hamster is infected with K virus, there is infection of the dividing cells that are to form the molecular layers constituting the bulk of the cerebellum. These cells are destroyed, the cerebellum therefore fails to develop normally, and the newborn hamster shows severe signs of cerebellar dysfunction, although it is perfectly well in every other way. The affected cerebellum is small and greatly depleted of cells, but there is no evidence of past microbial infection.

Resistance to Re-infection

Resistance to re-infection depends on the immune response generated during primary infection. Passive immunization with antibody is known to protect humans against measles, hepatitis A, hepatitis B, rabies etc., and the passively acquired (maternal) immunity of the newborn child or calf to a great variety of infections is another example of the resistance conferred by specific antibody. Most resistance to re-infection is antibody-mediated (Table 28, p. 233). IgG antibodies generally continue to be formed in the body for many years following the initial infection; IgA antibodies are less persistent than IgG antibodies. Even if antibody levels have sunk to undetectable levels, memory cells from the initial infection are often present in large enough numbers to give an accelerated (anamnestic) response within a few days of re-infection. This is especially important in infectious diseases with incubation periods measured in weeks because there is time enough for the anamnestic response to operate and terminate the infection during the incubation period, before production of clinical disease. Sometimes resistance to re-infection is maintained by repeated subclinical infections, each of which boosts the immune response. For instance, children catching rubella at school can re-infect their immune parents subclinically, and this is detected by a rise in antibody levels. Resistance to rubella, diphtheria and perhaps other infectious diseases is maintained in this way.

Antibodies protect against infection in a number of ways (see pp. 134–6). For instance they attach to the microbial surface and promote its uptake by phagocytic cells, acting as opsonins. Other antibodies protect against re-infection by combining with the microbial surface and blocking attachment to susceptible cells or body surfaces. Microorganisms that need to make specific attachments are listed in Table 2, pp. 20–1. Circulating IgG or IgM antibodies coat polioviruses, coxsackie viruses or adenoviruses and thus block their attachment to susceptible cells. Secretory IgA antibodies are particularly important because they can act on the microorganism before its attachment to a body surface. They do not act as opsonins; they do not lyse microorganisms because there is no complement on body surfaces, and in any case they fix complement poorly. But by preventing the attachment of microorganisms such as *Vibrio cholerae* to intestinal epithelium, the gonococcus to urethral epithelium, or chlamydia to the conjunctiva, IgA antibodies can ensure that these microorganisms are carried away in fluid secretions rather than initiate infection. Acquired resistance to infection of the surface of the body is often of short duration. For instance resistance to gonorrhoea or parainfluenza viruses following natural infection seems to last only for a month or so, and in childhood repeated infections with respiratory syncytial virus and *Mycoplasma pneumoniae* are common. Presumably the IgA antibodies that mediate resistance are short lived and IgA memory cells do not generate a good enough or rapid enough secondary response.

Resistance to re-infection, since it is immunological in nature, refers especially to the antigenic nature of the original infecting microorganism. Resistance to measles or mumps means resistance to measles or mumps wherever or whenever they occur, because these viruses are of only one type (monotypic) immunologically. Resistance to the disease influenza or poliomyelitis, however, depends on the separate acquisition of resistance to a number of distinct antigenic types of influenza or polio virus. Resistance to streptococci depends on the acquisition of antibodies to the M protein in the bacterial cell wall, and since there are at least 10 M types that circulate quite commonly in communities (40–50 M types altogether), repeated infections with *Streptococcus pyogenes* occur as antibodies are gradually developed against the various types. Often, however, different serological types of a given microorganism show some overlap so that antibodies to one type can confer partial resistance to another.

When resistance to a disease appears not to develop, the possibility of multiple antigenic types must be considered. There are multiple antigenically distinct types of gonococcus, for instance, as discussed on p. 172, a fact that helps account for successive attacks of gonorrhoea. Numerous attacks of nonspecific urethritis are to be expected because of the variety of microorganisms that cause this condition. In one study 40% of attacks were due to chlamydia, but there are twelve known antigenic types.

Resistance to re-infection can also be mediated by CMI. The CMI response generated on primary infection last weeks or perhaps months rather than years, and there is an accelerated CMI response on re-infection, although less vigorous than in the case of antibodies. Nearly always a persistent infection is needed to give continued CMI resistance and infections showing this are usually intracellular in nature. For instance, resistance to re-infection with tuberculosis, syphilis and possibly malaria, depends on the active presence of the microorganism in the body, with continuous stimulation of the antibody and CMI responses. In most of these instances, resistance to re-infection is CMI-mediated. There are a few examples, however, such as measles, in which recovery from primary infection is largely due to CMI, but resistance to re-infection is attributable to antibody.

References

Dinarello, C. A. (1984). Interleukin-1 in the pathogenesis of the acute phase response. *New Engl. J. Med.* **311**, 1413–1418.

Friedman, R. M. (1977). Antiviral effect of interferon. *Bact. Rev.* **41**, 543.

Isaacs, D. *et al*. (1981). Deficient production of leukocyte interferon (interferon γ) *in vitro* and *in vivo* in children with recurrent respiratory tract infections. *Lancet* **ii**, 950.

Lee, T. J. *et al*. (1978). Familial deficiency of the seventh component of complement associated with recurrent bacteremic infections due to Neisseriae. *J. Inf. Dis.* **138**, 359–368.

Grieco, M. H. (Ed.) (1980). "Infections in the Abnormal Host". Yorke Medical, USA.

Hahn, H. and Kaufmann, S. H. E. (1981). The role of cell-mediated immunity in bacterial infections. *Rev. Inf. Dis.* **3**, 1221.

Kirchner, H. (1986). The interferon system as an integral part of the defense system against infections. *Antiviral Res.* **6**, 1–17.

Mauel, J. and Behin, R. (1974). Cell-mediated and humoral immunity to protozoal infections. *Transplant. Rev.* **19**, 121–146.

Pepys, M. B. (1981). C-reactive protein fifty years on. *Lancet* **i**, 653–656.

Rifkin, M. R. (1978). Identification of the trypanocidal factor in normal human serum: High density lipoprotein. *Proc. Natn. Acad. Sci. U.S.A.* **75**, 3450–3454.

Roberts, N. J. (1979). Temperature and host defence. *Microbiol. Rev.* **43**, 241–259.
Rogers, T. J. and Balish, E. (1980). Immunity to *Candida albicans*. *Microbiol. Rev.* **44**, 660–682.
Wiley, D. C., Wilson, I. A. and Skehel, J. J. (1981). Structural identification of the antibody binding sites of Hong Kong influenza haemagglutinin and their involvement in antigenic variation. *Nature* **289**, 373.
Wyatt, H. V. (1973). Poliomyelitis in hypogammaglobulinaemics. *J. Inf. Dis.* **128**, 802.

10

Failure to Eliminate Microbe

There are many infections in which the microorganism is not eliminated from the body, but persists in the host for months, years or a life time. Examples of persistent infections are given in Table 29. One way of looking at persistent infections is to regard them as failures of the host defence mechanisms which are designed to eliminate invading microorganisms from tissues. There are various ways in which the host defence mechanisms can fail and various methods by which the microbes can overcome them. Microbial adaptations to the encounter with the phagocytic cell are described in Ch. 4 and the ways in which the immune responses are by-passed are described in Ch. 7. Persistent infections are not significant causes of acute illness, but they are particularly important for four reasons.

(1) They enable the infectious agent to persist in the community (see below).
(2) They can be activated in immunosuppressed patients.
(3) They are sometimes associated with immunopathological disease (see pp. 211–4).
(4) They are sometimes associated with neoplasms (see Table 19, pp. 182–3).

Persistent infections cannot by definition be acutely lethal; in fact they tend to cause only mild tissue damage or disease in the host. The mild diseases caused by persistent infections with adenoviruses, herpes viruses, typhoid or malaria can be contrasted with the serious diseases caused by the nonpersistent microorganisms of plague, cholera, smallpox or paralytic poliomyelitis.

In certain acute infections the patient appears to recover, but there is later a relapse. Following typhoid, for instance, 8–10% of patients suffer relapses, although usually mild. In such instances the infection is not strictly persistent, but it seems as if the host's immune forces need repeated stimulation before there is complete elimination of the infectious agent.

Latency

Persistent infections have a greatly enhanced ability to remain present in the host population as well as in the infected individual. Measles, for instance, is not normally a persistent infection, and after an individual has been infected and suffered the characteristic illness and rash, the immune response controls the infection and eliminates the virus from the body. Immunity to re-infection is life long, and a continued supply of fresh susceptible hosts must be found if the virus is to persist in the community. The virus does not survive for long outside the body, and therefore cannot persist in a community unless there is, at all times, someone actually infected with measles. Before the general use of measles vaccine, measles used to come to towns and cities every few years, infecting the susceptible children who had appeared since the last epidemic, and then disappearing again. The virus had to be reintroduced into the community at intervals because there were not enough susceptible children appearing to keep the infection going all the time. From studies of island communities it has been shown that the minimum sized population to maintain measles without introduction from the outside is about 500 000. Chickenpox, in contrast to measles, causes a persistent infection (see below). During childhood infection with chickenpox the virus ascends to the dorsal root ganglia of sensory nerves supplying the affected skin areas, and stays there in a noninfectious state after recovery and elimination of virus from the rest of the body (Fig. 35). The disease, chickenpox, disappears temporarily from the community. Virus in the dorsal root ganglia is kept under control by CMI, but the strength of the CMI response weakens as individuals age, and there is an increasing likelihood in older people that the noninfectious virus in one of the ganglia will activate. If this happens, the infection then spreads down the peripheral nerve to the skin and causes a crop of vesicles restricted to the distribution of that particular nerve. This disease is called zoster (shingles) and the vesicles are rich in virus and capable of causing chickenpox in any susceptible children who have appeared in the community. Studies of island communities have shown that chickenpox can maintain itself indefinitely in a community of less

Table 29. Examples of persistent infections (mainly human)

	Microorganism	Site of persistence	Infectiousness of persistent microorganism	Consequence	Shedding of microorganism to exterior
Viruses	Herpes simplex	Dorsal root ganglia	−	Activation, cold sore	+
		Salivary glands	+	None known	+
	Varicella zoster	Dorsal root ganglia	−	Activation, zoster	+
	Cytomegalovirus	Lymphoid tissue	−	Activation ± disease	+
	EB virus	Lymphoid tissue	−	Lymphoid tumour	−
		Epithelium		Nasopharyngeal carcinoma	−
		Salivary glands	+	None known	+
	Hepatitis B	Liver (virus shed into blood)	+	Chronic hepatitis; liver cancer	+
	Adenoviruses	Lymphoid tissue	−	None known	+
	Polyomavirus (mice)	Kidney tubules	+	None known	+
	Polyomaviruses BK and JC (man)	Kidney	−	Activation (pregnancy, immunosuppression)	+
	Leukaemia viruses (mice, man)	Lymphoid and other tissues	±	Late leukaemia	−
	Measles	Brain	±	Subacute sclerosing panencephalitis	−
	HIV	Lymphocytes, macrophages	+	Chronic disease	+

Chlamydia	Trachoma	Conjunctiva	+	Chronic disease and blindness	?
	Psittacosis	Lung (rarely in man)	?	None known	–
		Spleen (of bird)	±	Activation	+
Rickettsia	*Rickettsia prowazeki*	Lymph node	?	Activation	+
	Rickettsia burneti (sheep)	Spleen?	–	Activation; source of human Q fever	+
Bacteria	*Salmonella typhi*	Gall bladder	+	Intermittent shedding in urine, faeces	+
		Urinary tract	+		+
	Mycobacterium tuberculosis	Lung or lymph node (macrophages?)	?	Activation, tuberculosis in middle aged	+
	Treponema pallidum	Disseminated	±	Chronic disease	–
Protozoa	*Plasmodium vivax*	Liver	?	Activation, clinical malaria	+
	Toxoplasma gondii	Lymphoid tissue, muscle, brain	±	Activation, neurological disease	–
	Trypanosoma cruzi	Blood, macrophages	±	Chronic disease	–

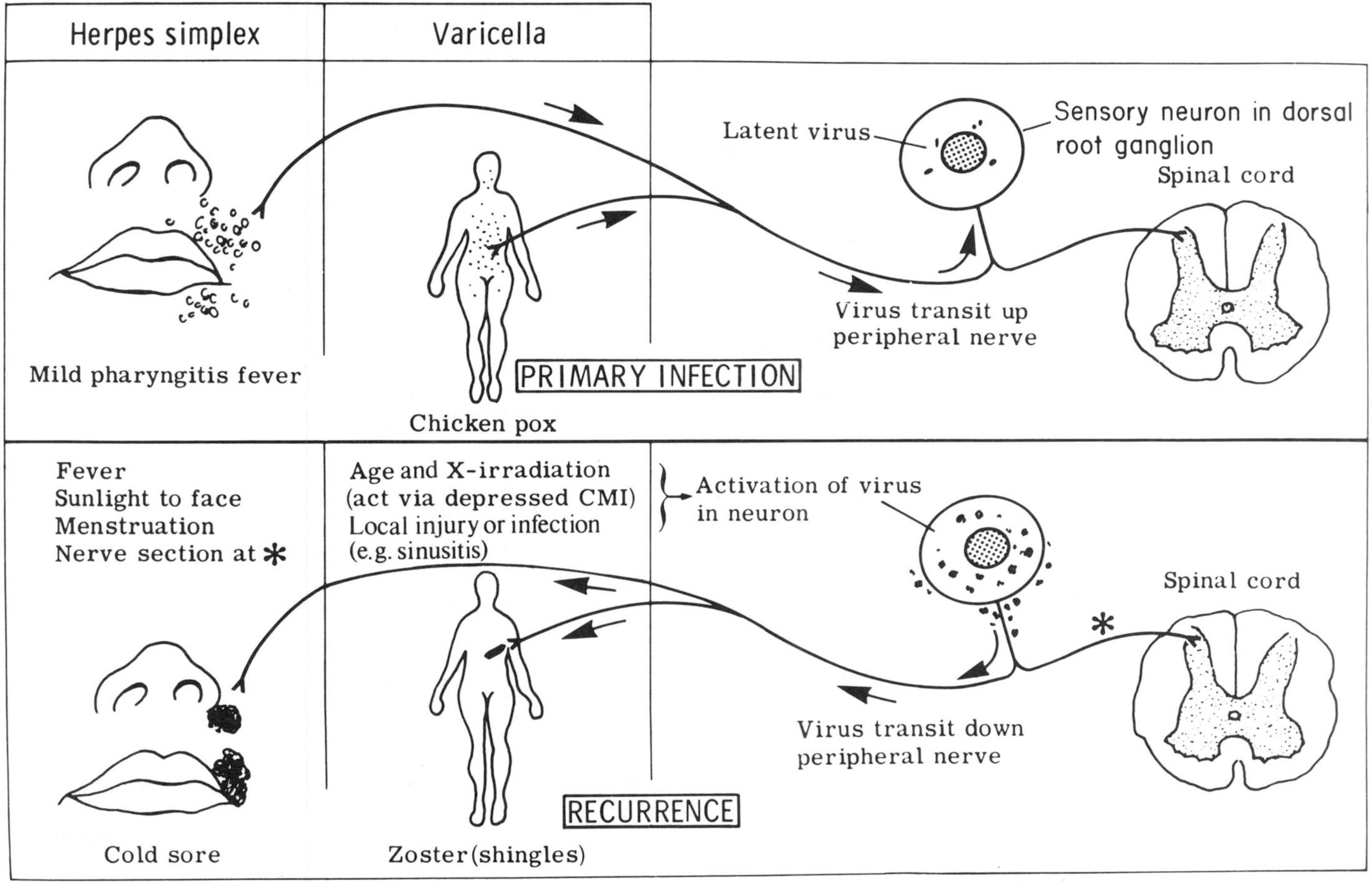

Fig. 35. Mechanism of latent herpes simplex and varicella-zoster virus infection in man

than 1000 individuals.* Chickenpox is a persistent infection characterized by latency, meaning that there is apparent recovery from the original infection but disease reappears later in life and the microorganism is once again shed to the exterior.

Herpes simplex virus gives rise to an exactly comparable latent infection. Infection normally occurs during infancy or early childhood, and causes a mild illness with stomatitis and slight fever. The virus travels up the axons of sensory nerves to the trigeminal ganglion supplying the mouth and related areas, and after apparent recovery from the initial infection, virus remains in a noninfectious state (latent) in neurons in the ganglion (Fig. 35). At intervals later in life virus can be activated in the ganglion, travel down the nerve and cause a vesicular eruption, usually round the lips or nostrils. This is called a cold sore, and virus from the cold sore can infect a susceptible individual. Cold sores occur particularly in certain individuals and the factors that activate virus in the ganglion include colds and other fevers, sunlight, menstruation and psychological factors. Their mode of action is not understood. The eruption is restricted to the area supplied by the particular sensory ganglion that was involved during the original childhood infection. Herpes simplex may infect other areas of the body. A small child falls and hurts its knee, the knee is kissed better by an aunt with a cold sore, and the knee is now the primary site of infection. Recurrent "cold sores" in this individual involve the knee. Likewise venereally transmitted herpes simplex, causing primary infection of the penis or cervix, will give recurrent lesions in these areas if reactivated later in life.

We still know little about the mechanism of latency and reactivation of herpes simplex or varicella-zoster. During the latent stage, herpes simplex virus DNA is present in neurons in dorsal root ganglia, but there is a block in transcription and few if any viral proteins are formed. The latent state seems to be delicately balanced, because the virus is activated merely by exposing without touching the trigeminal ganglion at operation. At the cellular and molecular level, however, reactivation events are shrouded in mystery. It has been suggested from experimental work with mice that activation is quite common in ganglion cells, but immune responses generally suppress virus replication before the full pathogenic sequence can be enacted. The virus must first travel down the nerve (apparently in the axon

---

*The viruses that maintain themselves in small, completely isolated Indian communities in the Amazon basin are therefore persistent viruses (see Table 29) rather than nonpersistent viruses such as polioviruses, influenza or measles. This was shown from antibody surveys carried out shortly after first contact of these communities with the outside world. Other infections which can be maintained in small populations are those in which there is persistent shedding of the microorganism (typhoid, tuberculosis, see below) or in which there is a reservoir of infection in some other host species (yellow fever, plague).

and at about 9 mm h^{-1}), then infect dermal cells and finally epidermal cells, before a lesion is produced. Looked at this way, each clinical lesion represents a failure to control the growth and spread of reactivating virus. After virus has reactivated in sensory neurons sensations such as itching are generated in the areas supplied by affected neurons, perhaps before virus actually reaches the skin. When pseudorabies, a similar virus, multiplies in sensory neurons in pigs, these phenomena are prominent enough to give the condition the name "mad itch". With reactivation of varicella-zoster virus in man the skin lesions may be small (or even absent) in comparison with the area affected by pain or paraesthesia. Herpes simplex reactivations can occur without visible skin or mucosal lesions. At times, therefore, immune forces seem to control the infection before skin lesions can be produced. Whatever the stage of reactivation that is under immune control, it is clear that CMI is involved. For unknown reasons the CMI response to varicella-zoster is selectively depressed in the elderly and in patients with lymphomas (see below), whereas responses to other persistent infections such as herpes simplex and cytomegalovirus are unaffected. Thus varicella-zoster is the persistent infection that commonly reactivates to cause disease in these individuals.

Brill's disease is a rickettsial example of latency. Following complete clinical recovery from typhus, the rickettsias sometimes persist in lymph nodes or the reticuloendothelial system. After 10 or more years, unknown influences cause the latent infection to be activated and the individual suffers a mild illness, less severe than the original typhus but with the rickettsias once again present in the blood. If the human body louse is present it can acquire the infection following a blood feed and transmit it as typhus to susceptible individuals. Sheep become latently infected with *Rickettsia burneti*. The infection may reactivate in late pregnancy, and very large numbers of organisms are then shed in urine, faeces, amniotic fluid and placenta. A stable infectious aerosol is formed which can cause Q fever in susceptible farmers or veterinary surgeons.

Malaria provides a classic example of protozoal latency. After clinical recovery, particularly from vivax malaria, the parasite persists in the liver without infecting red blood cells and thus without causing disease. Subsequently, often after many years, the parasite in the liver re-infects red blood cells to give a fresh clinical attack of malaria. Malarial latency is particularly striking in those from temperate climates who become infected in the tropics, return home, and suffer an attack of malaria many years later.

Tuberculosis sometimes gives a type of latent infection. The bacteria remain dormant in the body after the initial infection and recovery and can later be reactivated to give clinical disease. In the old days before BCG vaccination many town and city dwellers were infected in early life, but in most cases the infection in the lung or lymph node was controlled and remained subclinical giving rise to a healed primary focus. After the age of about 40, perhaps with the general age-related decrease in the strength of CMI, there is an increasing likelihood that the bacteria in a primary focus will become active again and cause clinical disease. Respiratory tuberculosis in the middle-aged patient generally arises in this way.

Persistent Infection with Shedding

There are other microorganisms that persist in the individual and are also shed more or less continuously, often for many years, without causing further disease. After recovery from typhoid, for instance, bacteria sometimes persist for long periods in the gall bladder. Scarred, avascular areas of the gall bladder are colonized, where the bacteria enjoy a certain freedom from the blood-borne antimicrobial forces of the host. Typhoid bacilli are discharged intermittently into the bile and thus the faeces. Two to five per cent of typhoid cases become faecal excretors and nearly all of them are women, because gall bladder damage and scarring is commoner in women. Such carriers of typhoid are important apparently healthy sources of infection. "Typhoid Mary" was a carrier who was employed as a cook in the USA, and moved from one place to another, cooking for eight different families and causing more than 200 cases of typhoid before she was finally caught and pensioned off. Typhoid can also persist in the urinary tract, especially in the presence of schistosomiasis, giving urinary spread of disease from the carrier. One serious outbreak of typhoid in Croydon, London, in 1937 was traced to a carrier who had been employed during work on water pipes supplying the affected area, and had urinated on nearby ground and contaminated the water supply. There were 310 cases, with 43 deaths.

A carrier state is also seen in certain bacterial infections of the body surfaces. After recovery from diphtheria, scarlet fever or whooping cough, the bacteria often persist in the nasopharynx for many months, serving as a source of infection for susceptible individuals. The mechanisms of persistence are not understood, but it must be remembered that the normal resident bacteria of the nasopharynx by definition are also persistent, and often include potentially pathogenic bacteria such as the meningococcus, the pneumococcus and pathogenic strains of group A streptococcus or *Staphylococcus aureus*. It is uncommon for these bacteria to give trouble; for every person suffering from meningococcal disease there are about 1000 unaffected carriers. The fact that bacteria capable of causing diphtheria, scarlet fever or whooping cough can also persist in this site is perhaps not surprising.

Entamoeba histolytica often causes a persistent infection, and cysts can be shed in the faeces for many years after recovery from amoebic dysentery or after subclinical infection. The cysts are highly resistant and infectious.

Persistent virus infections include EB virus and herpes simplex virus infections, and these are shed in saliva, often for long periods after the initial infection. EB virus continues to be detectable in throat washings for at least a month or so. Herpes simplex virus reappears in the mouth later in life if there are cold sores, and repeated tests on given individuals have shown that the virus is also intermittently present in oral secretions at other times. Hepatitis B virus sometimes persists in the blood for long periods, and perhaps for life. About 0.1% of apparently normal individuals in northern Europe and North America are carriers, and the incidence is much higher in India and SE Asia (3–5%) and Oceanic Islands (10–15%). The blood of a carrier is infectious and can be transmitted to susceptible individuals via blood transfusions, the contaminated syringes of drug addicts and the tattoist's, acupuncturist's, or ear-piercer's needle.* Other viruses are shed in urine. Polyoma virus, for instance, causes a natural infection of mice and establishes foci of infection in kidney tubules, whence it is discharged into the urine. Mice remain perfectly well, but infection is persistent and urine is the major vehicle for the spread of infection between individuals.† Cytomegalovirus is present in the urine of about 10% of children under the age of five in London, but it is unlikely that this is important in the spread of infection. Certain viruses, such as mammary tumour virus of mice and cytomegalovirus in man are shed persistently in milk, and among the bacteria both *Brucella* and tubercle bacilli are present in the milk of persistently infected cows.

There are several human infections in which the microorganism often persists in tissues for long periods and at the same time causes chronic disease. These include tuberculosis, leprosy, syphilis, brucellosis and trachoma. In these infections the disease is the result of a long drawn out battle between the microorganism and the immune and tissue defences of the host, sometimes one and sometimes the other gaining the upper hand. In the cases of leprosy and tuberculosis, bacteria continue to be shed to the exterior and infect others. Each of these infections is a tribute to the ability

---

* Hepatitis B infection also often occurs in individuals who have not been transfused with blood or injected with contaminated needles. Evidently there are other important mechanisms for the transmission of this infection. It is common in male homosexuals, and in some carriers the virus is detectable in saliva and semen.

† The human polyomaviruses (JC and BK), in contrast, show latency rather than persistence with shedding. They persist as noninfectious virus DNA in the kidneys of many adults, and are reactivated and shed in urine during normal pregnancy, and also in the immunosuppressed kidney transplant patient.

of the microorganism to survive and multiply in the face of host defence responses, and the progressive tissue damage is partly a direct result of bacterial activity, but largely attributable to the host responses (see Ch. 8). The protozoa of malaria and trypanosomiasis also give rise to chronic infections, and the ways in which these microorganisms evade host immune responses are discussed in Ch. 7.

A rare group of infectious agents persist in the body after infection, and give rise to progressive and fatal neurological disease after prolonged incubation periods. These are scrapie, transmissible mink encephalopathy, kuru and Creutzfeld-Jacob disease. Scrapie is a naturally occurring disease of sheep that has been present in Europe and the UK for hundreds of years. The brain is involved, and the disease is so called because affected sheep itch, and scrape themselves against posts and fences to relieve this symptom. In the laboratory scrapie is transmissible to mice and other animals, and the feeding of infected sheeps' heads to mink on mink farms in the USA has given rise to the disease called transmissible mink encephalopathy. Kuru is a rare and fast disappearing neurological disease of man in New Guinea, spread by cannibalism. Those dying with kuru were eaten by relatives as a mark of respect. The women and children ate the brain and acquired the disease, whereas the men preferred extraneural tissues and consequently were not affected. At one time up to half the women in affected villages were suffering from kuru. Cannibalism in New Guinea is now dying out and so, therefore, is the disease. Creutzfeld-Jacob disease is another rare neurological disease of man, occurring sporadically all over the world, caused by microorganisms similar to those of scrapie and kuru, but with an unknown mode of transmission.* In all these diseases, the incubation period represents a large fraction of the life span of the host — six months with mouse scrapie, two years with sheep scrapie, 12–15 years with kuru in man. During this time the microorganism steadily replicates, first in lymphoid tissues and then in the brain. The process of infection and production of pathological changes is slow but proceeds inexorably. One prominent pathological feature is a fine vacuolation in the brain and this group of diseases was therefore called the "spongiform encephalopathies". Scrapie has now been transmitted experimentally to primates, and Creutzfeld-Jacob disease to the domestic cat and to mice. As the host susceptibility of these infectious agents widens they seem less and less distinct, and this raises interesting possibilities

---

*Transmission from patient to patient has been recorded following the use of neurosurgical instruments contaminated with this resistant agent, and also after corneal transplantation from a donor who turned out to be infected. Presumably there are less artificial routes of transmission than these! It may turn out that infection is quite common but is usually extraneural and asymptomatic. Unfortunately we cannot test for this possibility because antibodies are not formed and serological surveys cannot be carried out.

of cross-infection. Almost nothing is known about the mechanism of disease production or about the natural routes of transmission (see also p. 175). They are not typical viruses, their mode of replication is a mystery and indeed, so far, they have not been shown to contain either DNA or RNA.

Epidemiological Significance of Persistent Infection with Shedding

There are obvious advantages to a microorganism if it persists in the host and is shed from the body for long periods after the initial infection. Maintenance of the infection in a host community is made easier, and herpes simplex, varicella-zoster, tuberculosis, typhoid and other conditions have already been discussed from this point of view.

The epidemiological advantages of prolonged shedding of micro-organisms to the exterior are well illustrated in the cases of myxomatosis and cholera. They are not truly persistent infections, but show the results of an increased period of shedding during the acute disease and convalescence. Each provides an excellent example of the natural evolution of an infectious disease. Myxomatosis is a virus disease of rabbits, spread mechanically by biting arthropods. When introduced into Australia in 1950, it caused nearly 100% mortality in the rabbit population. But rabbits were never eliminated from Australia because within the next 5 years or so a new and more stable host–microbe balance evolved. There was a change in both the virus and in the host species. First, rabbits with a genetically based susceptibility to myxomatosis were weeded out, leaving a rabbit population that was by nature more resistant, only 25% of them dying after infection with virulent virus. Second, the virus changed. Infected rabbits develop virus-rich swellings on the ears and face, and these skin lesions serve as sources of infection for the mosquitoes that carry virus to other rabbits. In the early stages of the Australian epidemic, when the infection was very severe, rabbits died a few days after developing these swellings. Later, however, a strain of virus emerged which was much less lethal and allowed the rabbit with the virus-rich swellings to live for a week or two, even to survive, and this gave greatly increased opportunities for virus spread by mosquitoes. The less lethal strain of virus therefore replaced the original virulent strain in the rabbit population.

Cholera is an intestinal infection transmitted by faecal contamination of water supplies, and it is always spread with great rapidity and efficiency in crowded human communities in the absence of satisfactory sanitary arrangements. This was so in the nineteenth century in London, and nowadays in India or the Middle East. Classically there is very short illness, characterized by vomiting, diarrhoea, dehydration and shock, which is often lethal within

24 h. The bacteria persist in water for a week or so and convalescent patients may continue to excrete bacteria in faeces for a few weeks. Classical cholera, however, is gradually being replaced in many regions with a less virulent type of cholera. This is the El Tor strain.* It is less virulent, but more infectious, and gives a much larger number of symptomless carriers, who continue to excrete bacteria for longer periods than in classical cholera. It is also less readily inactivated, and can thus spread from person to person by contact, feeding utensils etc, as well as by faecal contamination of drinking water. The El Tor strain is replacing classical strains of cholera, mainly because it is shed from the patient for a longer period and does not depend for its transmission on the contaminated water supply.

Persistent Infection without Shedding

A large proportion of the microorganisms that persist in the body are rarely it ever shed to the exterior. Their importance is for the individual rather than for the community. Most of them give rise to no ill effects, but one or two may cause trouble if the immune responses are weakened, and one or two can ultimately cause cancer. Most of them are viruses, and viruses have a unique ability to persist and multiply in cells, often in a defective (noninfectious) form (see Ch. 7). Many adenoviruses, for instance, persist in lymphoid tissues after initial infection, causing no disease, but still recoverable from normal adenoids or tonsils. There is little or no infectious virus in these tissues because of effective control by immune or other mechanisms, but when the tissue is removed and placed in culture where the controls are no longer present, the infectious virus appears. Adenoviruses are recoverable from one-third of all adenoids and tonsils removed during the first decade of life, and they must be regarded as part of the normal microbial flora of man. Certain herpes viruses including EB virus, cytomegalovirus and Marek's disease virus in chickens, also show persistent infection of lymphoid tissue.

In the case of EB virus, circulating leucocytes contain noninfectious virus, and the viral nucleic acid can be demonstrated by nucleic acid hybridization; cytomegalovirus is present in leucocytes of about 5% of normal people (e.g. healthy blood donors) so that infection occurs after blood transfusions.

In the early days of tissue culture, when normal monkey and human kidney cells were used for the propagation of polio and other viruses, a number of viruses were isolated from the kidneys of normal individuals.

---

* El Tor was a quarantine camp in Sinai, where in 1905 strains of *V. cholerae* were isolated from dead pilgrims from Mecca who had shown no signs of cholera-type disease. Of those infected with the El Tor strain as few as 1 in 50 develop clinical disease, compared with about 1 in 6 with classical cholera.

These included reoviruses, measles virus, cytomegaloviruses, and a papovavirus (SV40) in monkey kidneys (see p. 316). The form in which they existed in the normal kidney is not known, but this provides another illustration of the principle that many viruses persist after infection in the normal individual.

There is a final group of persistent viral infections that are nearly all the time completely harmless to the host, but sometimes, often a very long period after initial infection, they cause malignant change. These are the retroviruses that cause mammary tumours in mice, and leukaemias (sometimes other types of tumour) in mice, humans and other mammals. Retroviruses are RNA viruses that contain a reverse transcriptase enzyme, which transcribes viral RNA into cDNA as a necessary part of the replication cycle. When this DNA becomes integrated into the genome of the infected cell it behaves as a genetic character. Thus if the egg is infected (or the sperm in the case of mouse mammary tumour virus) the viral genome is present in all embryonic cells and is transferred from one generation to the next, via the offspring. This is an example of vertical transmission (see p. 3), and these viruses are endogenous retroviruses. Some of them never produce infectious progeny, remaining as DNA in the host genome, protected, replicated, and handed down the generations as if they were the host's own genes. This surely represents the ultimate, the final logical step in parasitism!* It becomes difficult to determine which is host and which is parasite, and the word infection loses much of its meaning. Indeed if the host benefited from the presence of the viral genome, the association could be classed as symbiotic. Other retroviruses more regularly undergo a full cycle of replication in cells throughout the body, and are shed in saliva, milk, blood etc., to infect other individuals. These can be transmitted horizontally and are called exogenous retroviruses. Cats infected with cat leukaemia virus for instance excrete in their saliva up to 10^6 infectious doses ml^{-1}.

These particular retroviruses are generally completely harmless, with no detectable effect on the health or function of the cell, even when full replication takes place. Thus, the various mouse leukaemia viruses are present from birth in all individuals of all known strains of mice, but leukaemia is a relatively uncommon and late consequence of infection. From the virus point of view, leukaemia is an irrelevant result because it does not help viral persistence in the individual nor transmission to fresh individuals.† The incidence

---

* Tests for endogenous viral nucleic acid sequences show that they are very common in the host genome of vertebrates. In mice for instance, they account for 0.04% of the entire host genome, and some of the viruses are present in defined genetic loci.

† Virus innocence was confirmed when it became clear that the cancer-producing part of the viral genome, the *onc* gene, originated in evolution from oncogenes present in host cells, where they play a role in the control of normal cell growth and differentiation (see p. 219 footnote).

and type of leukaemia depends on the virus and on the genetic constitution of the mouse, but the mechanism of leukaemia induction is not completely understood. In man, HTLV1 (see p. 183) infects T cells, increasing the density of Il-2 receptors (see pp. 140, 327) on these cells and thus ensuring their continued and eventually malignant growth.

The lentiviruses ("slow" viruses) are another group of retroviruses, which includes visna of sheep and goats, equine infectious anaemia of horses, and HIV (see pp. 161–2) of humans. All are persistent infections, causing chronic disease and showing antigenic variation in the infected host (see pp. 170–4). As is so often the case in persistent virus infections, many of which are listed in Table 16 (p. 161), macrophages and lymphocytes are infected.

For an infection transmitted exclusively vertically, via the egg or sperm, there is of course no need for the virus ever to mature into an infectious particle. Its continued presence in the descendant host generations is ensured. Some transmission between individuals sometimes occurs, however, after birth, as with the mammary tumour virus of mice transmitted via milk to the offspring or leukaemia virus of cats transmitted horizontally between individuals, and in these circumstances infectious virus must be produced.

The phenomenon of integration of viral genome into host cell genome is not unfamiliar to microbiologists. It is a feature of the so called temperate (nonlysogenic) infection of bacteria with bacteriophages. The infection is harmless, but the bacteriophage genome may show some activity, causing the formation of certain proteins in the host bacterium (e.g. the toxins of the diphtheria bacillus). Following treatment with certain inducing agents or occasionally spontaneously, the infection reverts to a lytic one in which infectious phage is produced and the host bacterium is destroyed. Integration also occurs experimentally when certain papovaviruses such as SV40 in monkeys or polyoma virus in mice enter the right kind of host cell. The cell is transformed, developing new viral surface antigens and malignant properties. These papovaviruses, however, are not known to cause malignant tumours under natural conditions.

Significance for the Individual of Persistent Infections

Persistent infections that are normally held in check by immune defences can be activated when immune defences are weakened. This occurs when patients for kidney transplantation are given immunosuppressive drugs, and the persistent but normally harmless cytomegalovirus for instance is activated in most patients within a month or two, often giving rise to fever, pneumonitis or hepatitis. Even warts are activated and appear sometimes in large numbers. The CMI response is depressed in patients with certain tumours of lymphoid tissues, such as Hodgkin's disease, and these patients may suffer from activation of persistent tuberculosis, varicella-zoster, or cytomegalovirus infections. Not all persistent infections are activated, and there is no evidence for an increased incidence of herpes simplex cold sores because CMI impairment is specific for varicella-zoster rather than herpes simplex.

Persistent infections induce persistent immune responses, and these, although failing to eliminate the microorganism, are sometimes causes of pathological changes. The continued immune response to infections such as tuberculosis, syphilis etc, leads to chronic disease, as mentioned above. In many cases the granuloma is the characteristic lesion formed round persistent foci of infection, making a major contribution to the disease itself. Persistent infections are often associated with persistence of microorganisms or microbial antigens in the blood. Circulating immune complexes are formed under these circumstances (see Ch. 8), and can give rise to a number of pathological changes, including glomerulonephritis. If the lesions at the sites of microbial persistence are trivial, immune complex formation is sometimes the major disease process. This seems to be the case in some types of chronic glomerulonephritis in man.

One consequence of persistent infection of major significance for the individual is that persistent microorganisms may eventually induce tumour formation. The viral leukaemias, sarcomas, mammary carcinomas and leukoses of mice, cats, chickens and other animals are caused by persistent RNA tumour viruses, when present in individuals of suitable age and genetic constitution. In man (see Table 19, p. 183) certain types of leukaemia are caused by human T cell leukaemia viruses 1 and 2 (HTLV1 and 2). The human wart is a benign tumour caused by a persistent virus, and cancer of the cervix is now very closely associated with two of the sexually transmitted papilloma (wart) viruses. Burkett's lymphoma and nasopharyngeal carcinoma appear to be due to EB virus, and liver cancer to hepatitis B virus. By no means everyone infected with these viruses develops a malignant tumour, and various cofactors are probably necessary, but have not yet been identified.

Conclusions

Microbial persistence, in summary, is a common sequel to viral, chlamydial and intracellular bacterial infections. Many of the severe infections causing illness and death in communities (smallpox, poliomyelitis, plague, yellow fever, cholera) are not persistent, and the microorganisms are eliminated from the body after recovery. Persistent infections are often important from the microbe's point of view, enabling it to be maintained in small or isolated host communities. Persistent infections also generally present problems in the development of vaccines (see Vaccine addendum). They are becoming relatively more important, both for the individual and for the community, as the nonpersistent infections are eliminated by public health measures and by vaccination. Not only may they reactivate and cause troublesome infections in immunocompromised or immunosuppressed patients, but some of them can cause malignant tumours.

References

Bishop, J. M. (1985). Viral oncogenes. *Cell* **42**, 23–28.

Gibbs, C. J. and Gajdusek, D. C. (1978). Atypical viruses as the cause of the sporadic, epidemic and familial chronic diseases in man: slow viruses and human diseases. *Perspect. Virol.* **10**, 161–194. (Kuru, Creutzfeld-Jakob Disease etc.).

Heritage, J., Chesters, P. M. and McCance, D. J. (1981). The persistence of papovavirus BK DNA sequences in normal human renal tissue. *J. Med. Virol.* **8**, 143–150.

Horn, T. M., Huebner, K., Croce, C. and Callaban, R. (1986). Chromosomal locations of members of a family of novel endogenous human retroviral genomes. *J. Virology* **58**, 955–959.

Howard, C. R. (1986). The biology of hepadnaviruses. *J. Gen. Virology* **67**, 1215–1235.

Kimberlin, R. H. (1986). Scrapie: how much do we really understand? *Neuropath. Applied Neurobiol.* **12**, 131–147.

Klein, R. J. (1982). The pathogenesis of acute, latent and recurrent herpes simplex infections. *Arch. Virol.* **72**, 143.

Miller, A. E. (1980). Selective decline in cellular immune response to varicella-zoster in the elderly. *Neurology* **30**, 582–587.

Mims, C. A. and White, D. O. (1984). "Viral Pathogenesis and Immunology", Chapter 6. Blackwell Scientific Publications, Oxford.

Mims, C. A. (1981). Vertical transmission of viruses. *Microbiol. Rev.* **45**, 267–286.

Weiss, R. A. (1982). "The Persistence of Retroviruses" (B. W. J. Mahy, A. C. Minson and G. K. Darby, eds), pp. 267–288. 33rd Soc. Gen. Microbiol. Symposium. Cambridge University Press.

11

Host and Microbial Factors Influencing Susceptibility

A host may be susceptible to infection by a given microorganism but rarely suffer harmful effects. In the old days everyone was susceptible to infection with polioviruses or tubercle bacilli, but relatively few became paralysed or developed pulmonary tuberculosis. Not only this, but host susceptibility to infection often varies independently of susceptibility to disease. From the microorganism's point of view, infectiousness or transmissibility is not the same as pathogenicity. Transmissibility in fact depends on the extent of shedding of microorganisms from the infected individual, on the stability of microorganisms outside the host, and on the ease with which infection is established in new hosts. Each of these factors shows great variation. Variations in the ease with which infection is established are illustrated in Table 30. It can be seen that the dose required to produce infection, disease or death, depends on the microorganism, the route of infection, the host, and on other factors.

The word virulence is sometimes used to refer to the infectiousness or transmissibility of a microorganism, but the word as used here will refer instead to its pathogenicity, or ability to cause damage and disease in the host. An infection can be totally harmless and asymptomatic or lead to a lethal disease, depending on the results of the encounter between microorganism and host. The characteristics of both the microbe ("seed") and the host ("soil") contribute to the outcome of an infection, and either can exercise a determining influence. To put it as a platitude, it takes two (microbe and host) to make an infection or a disease. Some of the host and microbial factors influencing susceptibility to disease are discussed in this chapter.

Table 30. Examples of variations in the dose of microorganisms required to produce infection, disease or death in the host

Microorganism	Host	Routes of infection	Minimal infections (ID) disease producing (DD) or lethal dose (LD)
Rhinovirus	Man	Nasal cavity	1 TCID 50[a] (DD)
		Conjunctiva	16 TCID 50 (DD)
		Posterior pharyngeal wall	200 TCID 50 (DD)
Salmonella typhi	Man	Oral	$\leqslant 10^5$ bacteria (DD)
Shigella dysenteriae	Man	Oral	10 bacteria (DD)
Vibrio cholerae	Man	Oral	10^8 bacteria (DD)
		Oral (together with bicarbonate, see Ch. 2)	10^4 bacteria (DD)
Giardia lamblia	Man	Oral	10 cysts (ID)
Mycobacterium tuberculosis	Man	Inhalation	1–10 bacteria (ID)
Ectromelia (mousepox) virus; virulent strain	Mouse (C57 B1 or WEHI strain)	Footpad	1–2 virus particles[b] (ID)
	Mouse (WEHI strain)	Footpad	25 virus particles (LD)
	Mouse (C57 B1 strain)	Footpad	10^7 virus particles (LD)

Examples from man, together with one example from an experimental animal (mouse) to show host genetic effects (mouse strain differences).

[a] Tissue culture infectious doses.

[b] By electron microscopy.

Genetic Factors in the Microorganism

The microorganism's ability to infect a given host is genetically determined and many microorganisms infect only one particular host species. For instance, measles, trachoma, typhoid (*Salmonella typhi*) and warts are exclusively human infections. Others are less specific, rabies and anthrax seeming capable of infecting all mammals. Pathogenicity or virulence is also a function of the microbial genome. Virulence often depends on numerous factors, such as adherence, antiphagocytic activity, production of toxins etc., and it is not surprising that it often depends on more than one gene. Changes in pathogenicity or virulence take place very easily, often involving only trivial changes in the genome. Minor changes in the M protein that coats group A streptococci can lead to major changes in bacterial virulence. The differences between variola minor and variola major used to be a matter of life and death when human beings were infected, but are only detectable with difficulty in the laboratory. A fresh pandemic strain of influenza A virus is able to spread readily in the community because one of the surface proteins of the virus shows a major difference from pre-existing strains and therefore no one has immunity to infection (see Ch. 7). The change in surface protein must be associated with a high level of transmissibility but may or may not be associated with an increase in virulence. The Hong Kong strain (1968), for instance, was avirulent in comparison with the devastating strain of 1918. Artificial influenza viruses can be made in the laboratory; the surface components of new strains and the avirulence characters of other strains are welded together by a process of genetic recombination to give hybrid viruses that are useful as vaccines.

The pathogenicity for a given host is often dramatically altered following the repeated growth of a microorganism under unfamiliar circustances outside the body. The laboratory passage of pathogenic viruses in cultured cells often leads to great reductions in pathogenicity (attenuation) in the original host, and this has been a standard procedure for the production of live virus vaccines (see Addendum). The attenuated strain breeds true and is a genetic variant. A similar phenomenon is seen with bacteria. For instance, BCG (Bacille Calmette Guerin) vaccine consists of a strain of bovine tubercle bacillus, highly attenuated after passage for more than 10 years in glycerin–bile–potato culture medium. Also, gonococci cultivated in artificial media after isolation from the human urethra show rapid change to an almost nonpathogenic form. Until recently little was known of the genetics of animal viruses because it was not easy to find good genetic markers and use classical approaches such as recombination. The reoviruses, however, have a genome consisting of 10 discrete segments (genes) of dsRNA, and when cells are infected with more than one type of reovirus the different genes undergo reassortment in the progeny virus. Painstaking studies of the properties of strains of virus produced in this way have enabled scientists to identify genes and gene products that control the virulence of reoviruses in mice. For instance, there is a viral surface (capsid) polypeptide that binds the virus to neurons which is obviously important in the produc-tion of encephalitis, and a surface polypeptide that confers resistance to intestinal proteases gives the virus the capacity to infect via the alimentary canal. When the genes for both these polypeptides are present in a virus strain, it can infect by mouth and cause encephalitis. The genetic analysis of virus virulence is now changing as a result of powerful new research methods such as the cloning of DNA sequences, and their application to viruses (and also to bacteria) is transforming microbial genetics. For instance, by introducing genome segments from virulent microbial strains into avirulent strains the virulence genes can be identified. Viruses have a smaller, simpler genome than other microorganisms, and for many viruses the nucleic acid sequence of the entire genome has been established, and functions are slowly being assigned to specific sequences. But it may not be possible to account for virulence in terms of a single specific gene product because virulence is often multifactorial. Also, even when a gene product is closely associated with virulence, it is likely to be a perplexing further step to say how it operates *in vivo*. Nevertheless, genetic engineering techniques will greatly accelerate progress, and we look forward to exciting advances in our understanding of virulence.

All viruses undergo mutation, and the selection of mutant viruses is the mechanism for the changes that take place during attenuation. Changes in the pathogenicity of myxoma virus during the evolution of the virus in wild rabbit populations have been referred to in Ch. 10, but nothing is known of the mechanisms or genetic basis of these changes. Sometimes the mechanism of the change in pathogenicity of a virus variant has been elucidated. Mousepox is an infectious disease of mice, comparable to smallpox in man, caused by ectromelia virus. There is a virulent strain that kills all infected mice following extensive growth of virus in the liver. After repeated growth of this strain in an unnatural laboratory host, the chick embryo, a variant virus strain emerged that is well adapted for growth in the chick embryo but has a greatly reduced pathogenicity and is nonlethal for mice. It has been shown that the virulent strain of virus grows readily in liver macrophages (Kupffer cells) and subsequently infects hepatic cells to cause extensive liver necrosis, whereas the avirulent variant infects liver macrophages with difficulty and therefore infects no more than the occasional hepatic cell. In this instance decreased virulence is due to decreased ability to infect macrophages (pp. 105–9).

For bacteria one of the important types of change in genetic constitution is mutation. The progeny of a single bacterial cell are not genetically homogeneous; a small proportion of them are mutants. The mutation rate for a given genetic change varies between 1 in 10^7 and 1 in 10^{10}, and the spontaneous mutants only replace the original type if they are favoured (selected) by the environment. There are about 6000 genes in a bacterium such as *E. coli*, and mutations may involve changes in structure, biochemical activity, antigenic properties, ability to produce toxins etc. any of which could lead to changes in pathogenicity. Much of bacteriology consists of a study of mutants, especially those that acquire new antigens or toxins. Smooth–rough variation is an important type of mutation affecting pathogenicity. Certain bacteria owe their pathogenicity to a surface component or capsule that interferes with phagocytosis by polymorphs and macrophages (see Ch. 4). This surface material often gives the bacterial colonies formed on artificial media a "smooth" appearance. The surface material is lost during long periods of growth of bacteria in the laboratory, and in the host this leads to more efficient phagocytosis and decreased pathogenicity. The colonies now have a "rough" appearance. Smooth to rough variations are common in salmonellas, shigellas and pneumococci, and represent bacterial mutations. Genetic changes in bacteria are frequently due to extrachromosomal genetic elements called plasmids (see p. 194). Plasmids also often carry determinants for toxin production (e.g. *E. coli* enterotoxin, *S. aureus* exfoliative toxin), or for colonization (pili of enteropathogenic *E. coli*) or invasiveness (*Shigella flexneri*). Plasmids are transferred between bacteria and are important in the transfer of antibiotic resistance between intestinal bacteria.

We understand much less about the genetic control of pathogenicity in protozoa. An individual with trypanosomiasis is persistently infected because the parasite undergoes periodic changes in surface coat proteins. These are programmed from the trypanosome genome (see p. 171), and enable it to evade host immune defences. Twenty two different types of *Entamoeba histolytica* can be distinguished by isoenzyme electrophoresis, and 12 appear to be nonpathogenic, failing to invade tissues and cause disease (see p. 222). But the basis for amoebic pathogenicity is not understood, and it is not clear whether these types are genetically stable.

Genetic Factors in the Host

Susceptibility to infectious disease is always influenced and is sometimes determined by the genetic constitution of the host. An impressive example of individual differences in susceptibility that are assumed to be to a large extent genetic in origin was provided in Lubeck in 1926. Living virulent tubercle bacilli instead of vaccine was inadvertently given to 249 babies. There were 76 deaths, but the rest developed minor lesions, survived, and were alive and well 12 years later. The infecting material and the dose was in each case identical. Overstating the point, one could say that for a given microorganism there are almost as many different diseases as there are susceptible individuals.*

* Another unfortunate example occurred in 1942 when more than 45 000 US military personnel were vaccinated against yellow fever but were inadvertently injected at the same time with hepatitis B virus which was present as a containment in the human serum used to stabilize the vaccine. There were 914 clinical cases, of which 580 were mild, 301 moderate and 33 severe. Even with a given vaccine lot, the incubation period varied from 10 to 20 weeks. Serological tests were not then available, so the number of subclinical infections is not known. In this case, physiological as well as genetic differences in susceptibility presumably played a part.

Sometimes the mechanism of genetic susceptibility can be defined with some precision. People with the sickle cell trait show a markedly decreased susceptibility to malaria. Malarial merozoites parasitize red blood cells and metabolize haemoglobin, freeing heme and utilizing globin as a source of amino acids. A single gene present in these individuals causes a substitution of the amino acid valine for glutamic acid at one point in the β polypeptide chain of the haemoglobin molecule. The new haemoglobin (haemoglobin S) become insoluble when reduced, and precipitates inside the red cell envelope, distorting the cell into the shape of a sickle. In the homozygote there are two of these genes and the individual suffers from the disease sickle cell anaemia, but in heterozygous form (sickle cell trait) the gene is less harmful, and provides a resistance to severe forms of falciparum malaria that ensures its selection in endemic malarial regions. Parasitized red cells readily sickle following utilization of oxygen* by the developing parasite. Perhaps the haemoglobin S crystals kill the parasite, and in any case such cells are removed from the circulation at an early stage by the reticuloendothelial system. This probably accounts for the resistance to malaria of those with the sickle cell trait. The gene would be eliminated from populations in 10–20 generations unless it conferred some advantage, and restriction endonuclease analysis of the gene in peoples in India and West Africa show that it has arisen independently in these malarious countries. It is not often that genetic susceptibility to infectious disease of man has been defined in this way, both genetically and at the biochemical level in the infected individual. A similar protection against malaria is conferred on those with another type of abnormal haemoglobin called haemoglobin C, also produced by a single amino acid change in the polypeptide chain. Both are hereditary conditions and are found in malarious countries. The Duffy antigen provides another example of powerful genetic selection by an important pathogen. Red blood cells from most West Africans, in contrast to those from Europeans, lack the Duffy antigen which acts as an attachment site for *Plasmodium vivax*. This type of malaria is accordingly almost unknown in West Africa.

Human susceptibility to diseases such as tuberculosis and rheumatic fever is influenced by the genetic constitution of the host, as indicated in familial studies (rheumatic fever) and differences in racial susceptibility (tuberculosis). During the great ravages of pulmonary tuberculosis in European countries in the seventeenth, eighteenth and nineteenth centuries, genetically susceptible individuals were weeded out. As recently as 1850, mortality

---

* People with the sickle cell trait (heterozygotes) do not suffer clinically, but the homozygotes often die during childhood. They not only develop anaemia (their red blood cells are more fragile because they sickle and unsickle under normal circumstances while circulating), but also show increased susceptibility to infection. Pneumococci in particular cause trouble, probably a sequel to spleen dysfunction (see p. 229) which in turn is a result of the repeated infarcts that occur in the spleen, as well as in other organs.

rates in Boston, New York, London, Paris and Berlin were higher than 500 per 100 000. With improvements in living conditions these fell to 180 per 100 000 by 1900, and they have fallen greatly since then, but it appears that the present populations have a certain amount of genetic resistance to the disease (see also Ch. 1). Previously unexposed inhabitants of Africa, the Pacific Islands and elsewhere show greater susceptibility. Extensive lung involvement is still common in infected Africans,* and in the Plains Indians living in the Qu'Appelle Valley reservation in Saskatchewan, Canada in 1886, the disease spread through the body affecting glands, bones, joints, meninges, to give a death rate of 9000 per 100 000. Yellow fever, on the other hand, appears to have originated in Africa, and African people show greater resistance to the disease than Europeans. Yellow fever was transported to the Americas (together with the transmitting mosquito *Aedes aegypti*) on the slave ships, and the first American cases were recorded in Yucatan in 1640. The disease was more lethal in the previously unexposed and genetically more susceptible people of Central and South America. Genetic influences in man are often difficult to dissociate from nutrition and other socio-economic factors, but the genetic effect is clearly shown to be distinct from environmental effects in studies of the occurrence of diseases such as tuberculosis in identical twins who have lived apart. In one classical study with tuberculosis, it was shown that 87% of identical twins also had the disease, whereas only 26% of nonidentical twins were affected. The identical twins, moreover, showed a similar type of clinical disease. Naturally occurring changes in the genetic resistance of rabbits to myxoma virus are referred to on p. 264.

The picture is much clearer in certain experimental infections in animals. For instance the susceptibility of mice to certain viruses and to enteric bacteria such as *Salmonella* is under genetic control, and susceptible and resistant strains have been developed by breeding. Susceptibility of mice to *Salmonella* infections is under the control of many genes. In one instance, that of susceptibility to the lethal effect of intracerebrally injected yellow fever virus, resistance is inherited as a single dominant genetic factor. The basis of resistance in the brain is not understood, but it presumably involves the susceptibility of neurons to infection with yellow fever virus. Resistance to mouse hepatitis virus is also under simple genetic control and this seems to operate by restricting virus growth in liver macrophages, and thus preventing infection of liver cells (see also mousepox, above). Genetic factors presumably control the behaviour and characteristics of macro-

---

* Altogether 10–15 million people in the World are actively infected, mostly in developing countries. But even in England and Wales this ancient and preventable disease continues at a scandalous level. About 8000 fresh cases are notified each year–if it were typhoid or leprosy this would be regarded as intolerable.

phages, and macrophages play a central role as determinants of pathogenicity in many viral, bacterial and other infections.

Species differences in susceptibility to infection, of course, are also genetically determined, and in some instances the mechanisms have been identified. Guinea-pigs are resistant to South American strains of *Yersinia pestis*, and this is because asparagine, a bacterial growth requirement, is missing from guinea-pig serum, which contains the enzyme asparaginase. Bacterial growth is accordingly slower, giving time for the immune response to control the infection. Susceptibility of the bovine placenta to *Brucella abortus* is associated with the presence of a bacterial growth stimulant, erythritol. This is not present in the human placenta which is therefore resistant to infection. Accordingly cows but not people abort when infected with *Brucella abortus*.

Genetic susceptibility of the host to infectious disease may operate at the level of the immune response and there is increasing evidence that this is an important phenomenon. The development of immune responsiveness in general is under genetic control, as illustrated by the failure of development in congenital agammaglobulinaemia and thymic aplasia (see Ch. 9), but genetic control also operates at a more specific level because immune responses to antigens are under the control of specific immune response (Ir) genes. There are hundreds of these genes in mice or men, most of them situated very near to the genes that determine the major tissue (histocompatibility) antigens. Many of them code for Class 2 antigens (HLA-DR, DQ, DP on chromosome 6 in man; H2 I-A on chromosome 17 in mice) which control immune responses by interacting with and presenting foreign antigens to the immune system (see pp. 123–4). Individuals with a gene conferring a poor immune response* to a given microbial antigen, especially a surface antigen, are likely to have difficulty controlling infection with that particular microorganism. On the other hand, those with a poor response are less likely to suffer any immunopathological consequences of the infection. Tissue typing for the various histocompatibility or transplantation antigens is now a sophisticated and commonly used test, performed on a person's blood lymphocytes. HLA type correlates with susceptibility to certain types of infectious diseases presumably because genes controlling susceptibility are located near to (linked to) the HLA genes. For instance, patients with the familial form of tuberculoid leprosy show an excess of HLA-DR2. The HLA association is clearest when there is a strong autoimmune component in susceptibility, and the most striking example is ankylos-

---

* In the case of antibody a poor immune response may mean production of antibody too slowly, in small amounts, of the wrong class, of low avidity, or against less relevant microbial antigens (see pp. 165–7).

ing spondylitis, where 92% of patients are HLA-B27, compared with 9% in the general population. The mechanism is not clear, but it has been suggested that when HLA-B27 individuals make an immune response to antigens of *Klebsiella** or possibly other gut bacteria it cross-reacts with antigens on their own lymphocytes and in joint tissues. This leads to a crippling "autoimmune" disease. Also, in rheumatoid arthritis, a disease not known to be of infectious origin (see p. 181) 70% of patients are HLA-DR4 compared with 28% of normal people. There is a genetic component in susceptibility to rheumatic fever (see p. 206), which perhaps operates via the immune response genes controlling the production of the streptococcal antibodies that cross-react with heart muscle.

There is a good example in mice of the independent control of immune responses to different microbial antigens. Adult mice of most strains infected with LCM virus generally show severe pathological changes as a result of the cell-mediated immune response to the virus (see Ch.8). Virus multiplies in exactly the same way in mice of the C57 B1 strain but they do not develop disease because they have a weak CMI response to the LCM virus antigens. However, mice of the C57 B1 strain generate a vigorous immune response to ectromelia (mousepox) virus. This virus grows in the liver and is often lethal in many strains of mice, but the vigorous immune response of C57 B1 mice ensures the early inhibition of virus multiplication in the liver, and allows them to survive. In both these examples C57 B1 mice show greater resistance to disease; resistance to LCM virus disease because of a weaker immune response, and resistance to the disease mousepox because of a stronger immune response.

There are obviously other ways in which genetic factors in the host influence susceptibility,† but little is known. For instance, the production of α interferon (see pp. 243–5) in man is regulated by twelve different genes, and in mice interferon responses to a given virus infection appears to be under genetic control, and this may influence susceptibility. Susceptibility to many virus infections depends on the presence of specific virus receptors on the surface of host cells. Virus receptors are genetically determined, and a poliovirus receptor gene is known to be located on chromosome 19 in man.

---

* A monoclonal antibody to HLA B27 reacted also with defined antigens on a certain strain of *Klebsiella pneumoniae*, providing an example of molecular mimicry (see pp. 156–8). But there are indications that the bacterial antigens can interact with the B27 molecule and make it immunogenic, and in any case other factors must be involved because not all spondylitics have the B27 antigen.

† *Tinea imbricata* is a fungal infection of the skin that is very common in parts of New Guinea. Susceptibility is inherited as an autosomal recessive trait, and there is evidence that it is determined by the composition of sweat. Sweat from affected individuals (collected in rubber "sleeves" worn during village football matches) shows defective inhibition of fungal growth.

Genetically determined receptors also control susceptibility to certain bacterial infections (see pp. 20–1). For instance, pigs susceptible to *E. coli* K88 diarrhoea have receptors for the K88 surface component on their intestinal epithelial cells. Receptors are controlled by an autosomal dominant gene.

A fascinating type of parasitism that is at the borderland between infection and heredity should be mentioned here. The vertically transmitted RNA tumour viruses studied in mice and chickens (leukaemia and leukosis viruses) have become integrated as DNA into the genome of the host animal and are transmitted vertically (see Ch. 7). There are interactions between viral and host genomes, and viral functions show all degrees of expression from zero to the production of fully infectious viral progeny in cells. This type of infection can itself properly be regarded as a genetic feature of the host.

Age of host

There are hardly any infectious agents that cause exactly the same disease * in infancy, adult life and old age. Susceptibility is generally greater in the very young and the very old, as for example in Q fever, bacillary dysentery, or bacterial pneumonia, and this is for a number of different reasons. In the first place immune responses are weaker in immature and in ageing individuals. Men over the age of 40 years show a gradual decline in the magnitude of antibody and cell-mediated immune responses to standard antigens, and there is a similar effect in mice. All types of infections therefore tend to be controlled less successfully at these ages, but at the same time there is less immunopathology. Infections in infants sometimes spread rapidly and prove fatal without the evolution of the characteristic clinical and pathological changes seen in adults. The infant's greater freedom from immunopathology is illustrated in LCM virus infection of mice. Adult mice die when virus is injected into the brain, as a result of the CMI response to infection, but infant mice remain well because their response is much weaker. Certain latent infections are kept under control by CMI forces, and in older people with failing CMI these infections are more likely to undergo activation. Thus, older people show an increased incidence of activation of healed pulmonary tuberculosis and of activation of varicella virus in dorsal root ganglia to cause zoster (see Ch. 10).

---

* This is distinct from age-related differences in the *incidence* of infection. It is not surprising that most infections are commonest in children, especially after first contact with other children at school. Exposure can be an important factor. Sexually transmitted diseases are largely restricted to adolescents and adults, but the occasional case of gonococcal vulvovaginitis in girls before puberty shows that the incidence of such diseases is restricted by exposure rather than by susceptibility.

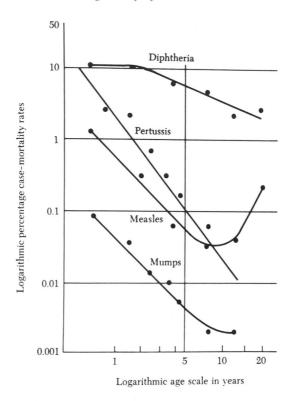

Fig. 36. The effects of age on the case-mortality rates of some bacterial and viral infections of man, plotted on logarithmic scales. (From Burnet, F. M. (1952). The pattern of disease in childhood. *Australas Ann. Med.* **1**, 93.)

Immunological immaturity makes newborn animals highly susceptible to viral, bacterial and other infections. Some of the human infections that are more severe in early infancy are illustrated in Fig. 36. They become progressively less severe as the child grows up. The commonest infantile infections are those that cause respiratory illness and those that give diarrhoea and vomiting. Infections that are prevalent in the community, however, will at some time have infected the mother, and the transfer of maternal antibodies to the infant via placenta or milk confers protection during this vulnerable period of life. In the rare human infant who is born without maternal antibodies, viruses such as herpes simplex or varicella can cause lethal diseases. Newborn mice also, in the absence of maternal antibodies, are notoriously highly susceptible to a great variety of virus infections. In man, IgM antibodies are not transferred from mother to infant, and in so far as these antibodies are important in resistance to

Gram-negative bacterial sepsis, infants are particularly susceptible to coliform sepsis. Maternal antibody, whether to herpes simplex, malaria or streptococci is transferred mainly via the placenta in man, but in other animals transfer through the milk is more important. A newborn foal, for instance, takes a feed of antibody-rich milk (colostrum) within minutes of birth and thereby acquires a protective umbrella against a great number of infectious agents.

Age-related differences in susceptibility are at times attributable to physical or physiological differences. The increased susceptibility of old people to respiratory infection is partly due to things like the loss of elastic tissue round alveoli, weaker respiratory muscles and a poorer cough reflex. Both old people and infants sometimes fail to show the usual signs of infection, such as fever. The lungs of infants are particularly susceptible to whooping cough and other bacterial pneumonias, partly because the airways are narrow and more readily blocked by secretion and exudate. Infants are also the first to suffer the effects of fluid and electrolyte loss, so that infections characterized by fever, vomiting or diarrhoea tend to be more serious at this time of life. Often the reasons for increased susceptibility in infancy are not clear. Respiratory syncytial virus, for instance, often causes serious illness in infancy and early childhood with croup, bronchiolitis or bronchopneumonia. In adults the virus causes a minor upper respiratory infection, but in early life there is invasion and growth of virus in the lower respiratory tract. It is not known whether this is because respiratory epithelium and alveolar macrophages are more vulnerable to infection than in older individuals, or because host defences are less effective. As an example of age-related susceptibility based on a local physiological difference, the skin of children becomes less susceptible to fungus infections ("ringworm") at puberty, and this is connected with the marked increase in sebaceous secretions at puberty. However, the same increase in sebaceous secretion at puberty leads to greater susceptibility to the skin disease acne, induced by bacteria whose headquarters are sebaceous glands. It is thought that lipases from *Proprionibacterium acnes* hydrolyse triglycerides in sebum to form fatty acids that are responsible for the inflammation in the lesions (and scars in mind and skin).

Certain virus infections are usually milder in childhood, and more likely to be severe in adults. These include varicella, mumps, poliomyelitis and EB virus infections. Varicella often causes pneumonia in adults, and mumps involves the testicle after puberty, giving a troublesome orchitis. Infections with polioviruses are nearly always asymptomatic in early childhood. When polioviruses first came and caused a "virgin-soil" epidemic in certain isolated Eskimo communities in the 1940s and in the island of St. Helena in 1947, there was a strikingly high incidence of paralysis in adults, but mostly inapparent infections in childhood and old age. Therefore it might be expected that in developing countries in Africa, Central America etc. where infection during childhood is the rule, paralytic disease would be uncommon.* In developed countries, on the other hand (North America, northern Europe etc.), where there has been a certain amount of interruption of the faecal–oral spread of infection (see Ch. 2), poliovirus infection is often delayed until adolescence or adult life, and as a result paralytic disease had been quite common (until the development of vaccines). EB virus is excreted in saliva, and in developing countries most individuals are infected as young children, undergoing an inapparent infection. In developed countries where childhood infection is less common, first infections often occur in adolescence or early adult life, following the extensive salivary exchanges that take place during kissing. In this age group, and in these countries, therefore, EB virus causes the more serious disease, glandular fever. It is not known why these infections are more severe in adults, but a more powerful immunological contribution to pathology and disease might be suspected.

Sex of host

There is a slight excess of males over females at birth, but males have a higher mortality, and by old age there is an excess of females. The higher mortality in males is distinct from that due to accidents and wars, and perhaps a slightly increased susceptibility to infectious diseases plays a part. This is also suggested by the observation that in mice the difference in mortality between the sexes disappears in the germfree state.

There are a few examples of sex-related susceptibility to infectious disease but the differences are usually small and almost nothing is known about mechanisms. For instance, women show greater mortality from tuberculosis than do men, but later in life the situation is reversed. Mortality and morbidity in whooping cough and infectious hepatitis is also slightly higher in women. A difference in susceptibility, of course, must be distinguished from a difference in exposure. Women have a lower incidence of leptospirosis and jungle yellow fever because they are less often exposed to infection.

It seems likely that hormonal influences are important in sex-related susceptibility, and this is partly because of effects on the immune system. Females generally have higher IgG and IgM levels, develop stronger CMI

---

* Although this might be expected, surveys from rural Ghana show that paralytic poliomyelitis is quite common in children. There have been suggestions that this is associated with injections of antibiotics, vaccines etc. into affected limbs (see p. 292).

responses, and are more susceptible to autoimmune diseases. Mechanisms are not clear, but sex hormones (especially oestrogens) influence the differentiation, maturation and migration of lymphocytes, NK cell activity, and phagocytosis by macrophages. Pregnancy certainly affects the severity of many infectious diseases. Smallpox is particularly severe in pregnant women, often invading the foetus and causing abortion; malaria is more severe, both hepatitis A and hepatitis B are more likely to be lethal, and paralytic poliomyelitis is more common. Hormonal changes during pregnancy are complex. Various new hormones appear, together with substances with known effects on the immune response such as α-foetoprotein, and there are changes in levels of oestrogens, progesterone and corticosteroids. Increases in corticosteroids would tend to decrease the control of the infectious process (see below) and at the same time inhibit inflammatory responses in the tissues. One should not overemphasize these effects. Pregnancy inevitably brings its own risks, and perhaps some interference with immune responsiveness is unavoidable, but Nature would surely not have tolerated a severe or generalized immunosuppressive handicap. Malnutrition may play a part in the increased susceptibility of pregnant women, especially in developing countries.* In pregnant women bacterial infections of the bladder are much more likely to ascend to the kidney and cause pyelonephritis. This is partly because in pregnancy the ureter peristalsis that normally "milks" urine down to the bladder is reduced, making it easier for infection to ascend to the kidney. CMI responses to cytomegalovirus infection weaken during pregnancy and this virus then reactivates and is shed from the genitourinary tract. Papovaviruses also, are reactivated and shed in urine during normal pregnancy (see. p. 262).

The increased susceptibility to infectious disease of pregnant women shoud be distinguished from the susceptibility of the foetus. The pregnant woman can be regarded as the site of development of a novel set of tissues, including the foetus, placenta, lactating mammary gland etc., each providing a new and possibly susceptible target for infectious agents. The foetus is exquisitely susceptible to nearly all microorganisms, but access is normally restricted by the placenta. Microorganisms that can infect the placenta, such as syphilis, toxoplasmosis, cytomegalovirus, rubella and smallpox, are then at liberty to infect the foetus (see Table 10, p. 117).

---

*As well as effects on the pregnant mother, malnutrition leads to lower birth weight and reduced survival of offspring. Babies born weighing 4–5 lb are much more likely to die than those of normal weight. In the Gambia, where the average woman has 10–12 children, a superbiscuit containing peanuts, dried milk and wheat-soy flour given twice daily has greatly reduced the number of underweight babies, and contributed to a dramatic reduction in child mortality.

Malnutrition of the host

Malnutrition can interfere with any of the mechanisms that act as barriers to the multiplication or progress of microorganisms through the body. It has been repeatedly demonstrated that severe nutritional deficiencies will interfere with the generation of antibody and CMI responses, with the activity of phagocytes, and with the integrity of skin and mucous membranes. Often, however, nutritional deficiencies are complex, and the identification of the important food factor is difficult. This is reflected in the use of inclusive terms such as "protein-calorie malnutrition". Also at times it is impossible to disentangle the nutritional effects from socio-economic factors such as poor housing, crowding, inadequate hygiene and microbial contamination of the environment. In developing countries, where communicable diseases still stand as the main public health problem, the five most lethal infections in terms of the total numbers killed each year are respiratory tuberculosis, respiratory infections (general), dysentery (all forms), whooping cough and measles. This is because certain specific infections and the variety of infections included under "respiratory infections" or "dysentery", occur in individuals with malnutrition, poor hygiene and accompanying protozoal and parasitic infection. The period just after weaning is often the most vulnerable, when the nutritional state is poor and there are many common microorganisms still to be encountered. A study of children in Guatemalan villages provides a good illustration of the synergism between malnutrition and infection. A group of children were studied individually from birth, and their colonization by various microorganisms and parasites was recorded. There was a loss in body weight after the sixth month, at the time of weaning from breast milk to a deficient diet. Further interruptions in weight gain, and sometimes temporary weight loss, were correlated with measles, various respiratory infections and infection with *Shigella* and *Entamoeba histolytica*. Body weights at two years of age were sometimes little more than a half of those of American children, and there was often almost no gain in weight during the second and third year of life.

Nutrition is affected when there is a bacterial overgrowth in the upper small intestine (see also p. 18). This is common in developing countries and is associated with heavy bacterial contamination of water supplies. The increased numbers of bacteria degrade bile salts to cause maladsorption of fat (steatorrhoea), they impair absorption of carbohydrate, they bind vitamin B12 whose shortage leads to anaemia, and they further interfere with absorption of nutrients when they produce enterotoxins. Children in Jakarta with malnutrition had more than 10^5 bacteria ml^{-1} in the upper jejunum (and as many as 10^7–10^8 ml^{-1}) whereas normal children had less than 10^4 bacteria ml^{-1}.

It seems clear that protein deficiency tends to depress in particular the CMI response, which, together with reduced C3 levels, lowered production of secretory IgA, and reduced killing of bacteria by polymorphs, causes an increased susceptibility to many infectious diseases. Children with protein deficiency, the extreme form being represented by the clinical condition called kwashiorkor, are uniquely susceptible to measles. This is a result of their weaker CMI response to the infection, the lowered resistance of mucosal surfaces of the body, and perhaps to the higher contamination of the environment with the microorganisms that cause secondary infections. All the epithelial manifestations of measles are more severe. Life-threatening secondary bacterial infection of the lower respiratory tract is common, as well as otitis media, sinusitis etc. Conjunctivitis occurs, especially if there is associated vitamin A deficiency, and at times progresses to severe eye damage and blindness. The tiny ulcers in the mouth that constitute Koplik's spots in normally nourished children can enlarge to form massive ulcers or necrosis of the mouth (cancrum oris). Instead of an occasional small focus of infection in the intestine, there is extensive intestinal involvement with severe diarrhoea which exacerbates the nutritional deficiency.* Even the skin rash is worse, with numerous haemorrhages that give the condition referred to as "black measles". The scarcity of good medical care and antibiotic therapy adds to the serious outcome of the illness, and measles is about 300 times as lethal in developing countries as it is in the countries of northern Europe and North America. The case fatality approaches 10%, and in severe famines reaches the tragic figure of 50%. The severe form of measles is seen in children in tropical Africa, in aboriginal children in certain parts of Australia, and it was also seen in children in European cities in the nineteenth century. The virus ("seed") has not altered, but changes in the "soil" (host) dramatically enhance the severity of the disease. Increased susceptibility to herpes simplex and *P. carinii* (see Glossary) infection and to Gram-negative septicaemia, is also seen in protein deficiency. Because of the effect on CMI, there is greater susceptibility to tuberculosis. Tuberculosis has often been noted to increase in frequency in times of famine, and this has also been observed in the inmates of concentration camps.

On the other hand, it looks as if certain infections are less severe in malnourished individuals. Typhus, for instance, is said to cause a higher mortality in well-fed than in malnourished individuals, and clinical malaria was suppressed in Somali nomads during the 1970s famines, only to be

---

* $\frac{1}{2}$–2 year old W. African children suffering from acute measles enteritis were found to lose 1.7 g albumin a day in faeces, the ideal daily intake of protein being 9–10 g a day. Thus measles exacerbates malnutrition as well as vice versa, and not only because of diarrhoea, but also because during systemic febrile infections like measles there is always a greatly increased breakdown and excretion of body nitrogen.

reactivated 5 days after refeeding. A four-year study of 100 000 prisoners in the UK in the 1830s showed that those given the most food (costing three shillings per week) had a 23% mortality, presumably largely due to infection, whereas those given least food (costing 10 pence per week) had a 3% mortality. It is not known why malnourished individuals are sometimes less susceptible to infection. A decrease in the vigour of host inflammatory and hypersensitivity responses would be expected, and perhaps there are adverse effects on the nutrition of the infectious agent itself, with depressed replication in the malnourished host.

Vitamin A, B and C deficiencies are known to lead to impaired integrity of mucosal surfaces, which in turn causes increased susceptibility to infection, and adds to the complexity of the picture.

Hormonal Factors and Stress

Hormones have an important role in maintaining homoeostasis and in regulating many physiological functions in the body. The hormones with a pronounced effect on infectious diseases are the corticosteroids. This is largely because corticosteroids are vital for the bodily response to stress (see Glossary) and infection, like injury or starvation, is a stress (see Fig. 37). It has long been known that the adrenal glands are needed for resistance to infection and trauma. Corticosteroids of various types have a complex and wide range of actions; the most important for infectious diseases are the glucocorticosteroids, which inhibit inflammation and depress immune responses. These corticosteroids also stabilize cell membranes and lysosomes, giving cells some protection against damage or destruction. There is, moreover, a great deal of interaction between the neuroendocrine and the immune system which is not included in Fig. 37. Not only are immune cells influenced by corticosteroids (see below) and by other mediators generated via the hypothalamic–adrenal axis, but the immune cells themselves produce endorphins, ACTH and other hormones.

Inflammation makes an important contribution to tissue damage and pathology in infectious disease (see Ch. 8) and injected corticosteroids (or ACTH) have a pronounced anti-inflammatory effect, their therapeutic use in infectious diseases depending on a reduction in the inflammatory pathological components at sites of infection. At the same time they tend to inhibit immune responses. This last action is not completely understood. There is an ill-defined effect on lymphocytes, some of which have receptors for corticosteroids, and inhibition of production and action of immune

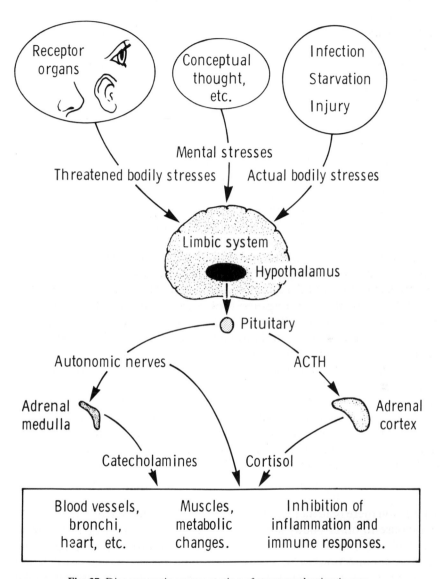

Fig. 37. Diagrammatic representation of stress mechanism in man.

mediators such as Il-1 and Il-2. Corticosteroids also prevent the inflammatory expression of the immune response in tissues by blocking the movement of plasma and leucocytes from blood vessels, and this is partly due to inhibition of prostaglandin production.

The inflammatory and immune responses, although on the one hand they contribute to pathological changes and disease, are also powerful antimicrobial forces (see Ch. 9). This dual role is reflected in the results of giving corticosteroids in infectious disease. Herpes simplex keratoconjunctivitis or encephalitis, for instance, is temporarily improved by corticosteroids because of the reduction in inflammation, but the simultaneous weakening of antimicrobial forces means that the infection progresses more readily. The net effect is to make the disease worse. For the same reasons a large number of different experimental infections in animals are made more severe by corticosteroid administration.

All the above remarks apply to corticosteroids administered artificially, often in large doses. It is perhaps more relevant to ask what effect the individual's own corticosteroids have on the course of an infectious disease. It is first necessary to say something about the function of the corticosteroid response to stress. Small areas of tissue injury give rise to quite severe but nevertheless locally useful inflammation, mediated by various inflammatory factors. If exactly the same response took place in multiple sites of infection in the body or in response to more extensive tissue injury, the immediate overall result in terms of vasodilation and loss of fluid into tissues would be harmful. An individual who is infected or wounded may need to retain bodily functions for running or fighting, and the effect of multiple unmodified local inflammatory responses might well be incapacitating. When inflammation occurs on a large scale, therefore, it is an advantage to make an overall reduction in its severity, so that the general impact on the host is lessened. This is a teleological way of looking at the function of corticosteroid hormones, which also makes sense of their metabolic function in mobilizing energy sources. The response to stress of the autonomic nervous system, involving adrenalin-mediated changes in preparation for bodily action (fight or flight) is more obviously interpreted in these terms. During an infection there is an increase in the rate of corticosteroid secretion, just as in response to other bodily stresses such as hunger, injury or exposure to cold. Rises in urinary 17-ketosteroids are seen, for instance, in Q fever and sandfly fever injections in man. There is also an increased rate of utilization of corticosteroids by tissues. Inflammatory and immune responses thus take place against the dampening and modifying background of increased corticosteroid levels, which ensure that continued bodily function and balance (homoeostasis) is maintained. When the corticosteroid response is depressed, as in Addison's disease (see Glossary) the consequences of infection or tissue injury are very severe, and affected patients therefore have to be given increased doses of corticosteroids during infections.* Bilaterally adrenalectomized animals usually show greatly increased susceptibility to tissue damage and death in experimental infectious diseases.

It can be concluded therefore that increased circulating levels of corticosteroid hormones are necessary for a successful host response to infectious disease. Administering additional amounts of corticosteroids is not necessarily of value unless the host's own corticosteroid response is known to be subnormal, or if it is for the moment more important to reduce inflammation than to control infection. Otherwise, additional corticosteroids tend to promote the infection by decreasing the effectiveness of antimicrobial forces, as discussed above.

When corticosteroids are given they not only make any infection that happens to occur at the time more severe, but also favour the lighting up of persistent infections that are normally held in check by immune forces. Tuberculosis in man is often activated or made worse by corticosteroid administration. Stress tends to act in the same way, probably because of increased secretion of corticosteroids. One classical example in animals is psittacosis, a chlamydial infection of parrots and budgerigars. These birds normally carry the microorganism as a persistent and harmless infection, localized in the spleen. Following the stress of transport in cages, exposure to strange surroundings or inadequate diet, the infection is activated in the bird, and the microorganism begins to be excreted in the faeces. Human infection can then take place by inhalation of dried droppings from the cage, causing the troublesome disease psittacosis, with pneumonia as a common feature.

In human beings, mental stress in the form of anxiety calls into action the same physiological changes which were designed to deal with physical stresses (see Fig. 37). For instance, in a university boat race the crew had increases in corticosteroid production that enabled them to sustain the physical stress of the race, but the coxswain was found to have an increase of equal magnitude. It is possible but not proven that sustained mental stress, by causing persistent rises in circulating corticosteroids, lowers resistance to persistent infections and other infections that occur during the period of stress (see illness clustering below).

---

*It may be noted that in Cushing's syndrome there is also a greatly increased susceptibility to infection because of excessive production of corticosteroids from the adrenal cortex. Abnormally high corticosteroid levels promote infection for reasons referred to above, and bacterial infections have been leading causes of death in these patients.

Infections are sometimes more severe when the host animal lives under crowded conditions. Increased transmission as well as stress responses, can play a part. Intestinal coccidiosis in domestic animals is generally asymptomatic, but clinical disease is seen when a heavy parasite load is carried. This is favoured under crowded conditions because of increased transmission. It is distinct from the increased rate of meningococcal and streptococcal disease when people are crowded together, because this is associated with an increased rate of infection.

The adrenal cortex itself is not often involved in infectious diseases, but if it is the infection in the cortex tends to be extensive. Examples include tuberculosis and histoplasmosis in man and various viral, bacterial, fungal and protozoal infections in experimental animals. Infectious agents localizing in the adrenal cortex encounter a high concentration of corticosteroid hormones originating from cortical cells. Antimicrobial forces are therefore weakened locally, and the infection is exacerbated. Active adrenal foci of infection are often seen at a time when foci elsewhere in the body are healing.

There is usually a change in susceptibility to infection during pregnancy, as discussed earlier in this chapter, and this is due to hormonal changes. The relative importance of oestrogens, progesterone and corticosteroids is not clear. Oestrogens are necessary for maintaining the resistance of the adult vagina to most bacterial infections, as described on p. 29. The male sex hormones responsible for the changes in the testicle at puberty can be regarded as causing this organ's susceptibility to mumps virus infection. Insulin is also worth mentioning because the metabolic changes in poorly controlled diabetes in some way increase susceptibility to staphylococcal, fungal and tubercular infections (see p. 34). Clearly there are hormones that control the health and wellbeing of cells and tissues in all parts of the body and, in this sense, serious hormonal disturbances could always affect the course of infectious diseases. It would be surprising for instance if untreated cretins showed a completely normal response to infections. Such effects would scarcely be worth mentioning were it not for the existence of this category called "hormonal factors".

Other Factors

A host of miscellaneous factors influence the course of infectious diseases, and some of them merit particular mention. Certain lung conditions resulting from the inhalation of particles have an important effect on respiratory infection. Silicosis is a disease due to the continued inhalation of fine particles of free silica. It occurs in coal miners and in various industries where sandstone and similar materials are used. There is a great increase in susceptibility to tuberculosis, which is more likely to cause serious or fatal disease. This is because lung macrophages, which play a central role in resistance to respiratory tuberculosis, become damaged or destroyed following the phagocytosis of the free silica particle. When intact macrophages containing nonlethal amounts of silica phagocytose tubercle bacilli, the bacteria grow faster, the cell dies, and the progeny bacteria are released sooner.

The air is polluted in many towns and cities, especially with substances derived from the combustion of commercial, domestic and automobile fuels. Although these form a small proportion of the total mass of particles suspended in air, they are important because they occur in small ($<2\,\mu$m diameter) particles, which are stable, penetrate deep into the lungs and may contain toxic elements such as lead. The commonly measured pollutants are SO_2 and particulates (smoke). For both, the upper limit (24 h mean) recommended by the WHO is 100–150 μm m^{-3}, but these values are commonly exceeded. Can atmospheric pollution increase the severity of respiratory infections? It has been reported that people with chronic bronchitis produce larger volumes of morning sputum and note a worsening of symptoms when SO_2 values in air reach 250 μg m^{-3}, and there is an increase in respiratory mortality when levels exceed 750 μg m^{-3}. In the great London smog of 1952, before the Clean Air Bill greatly improved the quality of London air, SO_2 levels reached 8000 μg m^{-3}, and there were 4000 excess respiratory deaths. The morbidity and mortality, however, is seen in the respiratory cripples (chronic bronchitis etc.), in the very old and in other susceptible individuals.* One feels that atmospheric pollution must also be having a long-term harmful effect on the lungs of normal people, but so far the evidence has been unsatisfactory. Nor is there any convincing evidence that normal people exposed to atmospheric pollution experience an increase in the severity of acute respiratory infections. A careful study of 20 000 children and adults in four geographical areas of the USA has shown that high levels of SO_2 and suspended sulphates are significantly associated with excess acute respiratory disease, much of which can be assumed to be infectious. The effect was most marked after more than three years exposure, and it was independent of cigarette smoking and socio-economic status, two of the factors that had always been difficult to dissociate from atmospheric pollution in previous studies. Cigarette smoking can be regarded as a self-induced atmospheric pollution, and many interesting observations have been made. For instance, cigarette smoke inhibits ciliary

---

*The same vulnerable groups also experience increased mortality in influenza epidemics.

activity, the debris-laden alveolar macrophages of smokers show less bactericidal activity, and lung pathogens such as pneumococci and *Haemophilus influenzae* attach more readily to pharyngeal cells from smokers. Cigarette smoking is certainly associated with chronic bronchitis, but the evidence linking cigarette smoking with susceptibility to acute respiratory disease in otherwise healthy individuals is conflicting. For instance, one study of 1800 students at a military college in the USA during the Hong Kong 'flu epidemic showed that those who smoked 21 cigarettes a day had a 21% higher incidence of clinical influenza, but other studies have failed to show an effect.

It is a widespread popular belief that people are less resistant to infectious diseases when they are in a poor mental state, and there is in fact some evidence that psychological factors influence susceptibility. This is seen in the phenomenon of illness clustering. In two studies in the USA, the illnesses and significant life events of several thousand people were recorded over a period of about 20 years. It was found that in a given individual illnesses of all kinds, not only psychosomatic conditions such as peptic ulcers but also bacterial infections and tumours, tended to occur in clusters. There was a significant association of these illness clusters with stressful life situations such as the death or serious illness of a close relative, personal injury, career crises etc. Little is known of the mechanism by which such events influence infectious diseases. Presumably it involves the stress response and the known effects of the nervous system on immune responses (see above).

Simple fatigue generally has little effect on susceptibility to infection, but violent exercise in the early stages of poliomyelitis is known to predispose to paralysis in the exercised muscles. The exercise must be done during the preparalytic stages of infection, when virus is spreading from the alimentary canal to the central nervous system. It is associated with dilation of capillary blood vessels supplying the spinal cord neurons that innervate the exercised muscles. Perhaps circulating virus is more likely to invade such regions of the spinal cord. Paralytic poliomyelitis also tends to involve muscles that receive injections during the preparalytic stages of the infection, especially with materials such as pertussis vaccine. In this case too, the injection causes capillary dilation in the appropriate region of the spinal cord.

Exposure to changes in temperature and sitting in draughts are traditionally regarded as influencing infectious disease. Careful studies with common cold viruses have not provided any evidence for this. Volunteers infected intranasally with a standard dose of virus were exposed to cold, but failed to show detectable changes in the incidence or severity of infection, even after standing naked in draughty corridors. The effect of changes in relative humidity has been less carefully studied. Experimentally, ciliary activity in segments of respiratory epithelium is impaired by reductions in the relative humidity of the overlying air. Increases in air temperature in heated buildings lead to substantial reductions in relative humidity unless the air is humidified. The lower respiratory tract would tend to be protected because of humidification of inhaled air by the turbinate mucosa, but the nasal mucosa would be exposed to the dry air and an effect on ciliary activity and thus on respiratory infection might be expected.

The local concentrations of key elements sometimes determine microbial growth in tissues. For instance, nearly all bacteria require iron, but the body fluids of the host contain iron-binding proteins such as lactoferrin and transferrin, which limit the amount of free ion available. Hence certain bacteria show greatly increased virulence after administration of iron to the host, and patients with excess iron in the blood may show increased susceptibility to infection. The lethality for mice of *Pseudomonas aeruginosa* is increased 1000-fold by the injection of iron compounds to saturate the iron-binding capacity of serum transferrin. The ability of bacteria to compete with the host for iron can be an important factor, and virulent bacteria such as pathogenic *Neisseria* and enteric bacilli that produce their own iron-binding compounds (collectively called siderochromes), are able to circumvent the host restriction on the availability of iron.* Oxygen is a key element for other bacteria. It is essential for many, such as the tubercle bacillus, but *Clostridium perfringens*, for instance, is strictly anaerobic and multiplies best in tissues that are anoxic as a result of interruption to their blood supply. Bacterial multiplication is actually inhibited in the presence of oxygen, and patients with gas gangrene are treated by exposure to oxygen in a pressure chamber. *Clostridium tetani* also requires local anoxic conditions in tissues, whether produced by severe wounds or by trivial injuries due to splinters, thorns or rusty nails. It may be noted that some of the most successful invaders of the respiratory tract show optimal growth in the presence of up to 5–10% CO_2 (e.g. tubercle bacilli,† pneumococci). The gases bathing the lower respiratory tract normally contain about 5% CO_2.

Foreign bodies in tissues often act as determinants of local microbial virulence. The term foreign bodies includes foreign particles that are too large to be phagocytosed. Foreign bodies presumably act by interfering with the blood supply and also by serving as a continuous source of multiplying microorganisms, giving them physical protection in nooks and crannies from phagocytes and other antimicrobial forces. Foreign bodies potentiate various clostridial infections (see above) and particularly staphylococcal infec-

---

*Malaria parasites induce the formation of transferrin receptors on the surface of infected red blood cells.

†Tubercle bacilli commonly cause lesions in the apical regions of the lung, perhaps because oxygen and CO_2 tensions in these regions favour bacterial growth or depress host defences.

tions. Necrotic bone fragments in chronic osteomyelitis act as foreign bodies, hindering treatment and giving a source of bacteria for flare-up of infection many years later. The ability of staphylococci to cause a local lesion after introduction into the skin is increased about 10 000-fold if the bacteria are implanted on a silk thread. Skin is generally more susceptible to infection when wet, as well as following injury. Wet pastures and minor foot injuries predispose to various types of "footrot" in cattle, sheep and pigs, due to infection with *Fusiformis* spp. or other bacteria.

Certain drugs influence resistance to infectious disease, and of the self-administered drugs alcohol is the commonest. In various studies, intoxicated animals have been found to have impaired ciliary activity, impaired removal of inhaled bacteria, defects in phagocytosis or poor closure of the glottis. Most of these phenomena have not been satisfactorily demonstrated in man, and polymorph function, for instance, appears normal, although there is impaired migration of polymorphs from blood vessels. The position is clearer for chronic alcoholics, many of whom have alcoholic liver disease. These individuals have reduced polymorph counts in the blood and are more likely to develop bacterial (especially pneumococcal) pneumonia. Alcoholics also show increased susceptibility to pulmonary tuberculosis, but it is not clear how much is due to impaired host defences and how much to the alcoholic life style. Lung infections can also be acquired by inhaling anaerobic bacteria from the mouth while in a drunken stupor.*

Those who inject themselves with narcotics are particularly susceptible to infection. To a large extent this is due to the insanitary techniques used, and it results in skin sepsis or more serious systemic infections such as endocarditis. In heroin addicts, staphylococcal infections are not so common as might be expected, apparently because street heroin contains quinine which has antistaphylococcal action. Shared syringes may transmit hepatitis B virus infection or HIV (the causative agent of AIDS), and as with alcohol susceptibility to pulmonary infection is increased during drug-induced stupor. One disadvantage of regular marihuana smoking is that it lowers stomach acid and thus increases susceptibility to bacterial infection of the intestine (see p. 19).

The influence of immunosuppressive drugs on infection is an important feature of hospital medicine at the present time, and is referred to in Ch. 9.

---

*During sleep normal individuals often aspirate material from the nasopharynx. This can be demonstrated by introducing 1.0 ml of a [111]Indium-Cl solution into the nose every half hour during sleep; a gamma scan carried out after waking reveals the presence of the labelled material in the lungs. In other words, the lungs are regularly contaminated during sleep with microorganisms from nose and throat, but this does not lead to trouble as long as host defences (see pp. 12–17) are intact.

References

Ahmed, S. A., Penhale, W. J. and Talal, N. (1985). Sex hormones, immune responses and autoimmune diseases: mechanisms of sex hormone action. *Am. J. Pathol.* **121**, 531.

Chandra, R. K. (1983). Nutrition, immunity and infection: present knowledge and future directions. *Lancet*, March 26, 688.

Cockburn, W. C. and Assaad, F. (1974). Some observations on the communicable diseases as public health problems. *Bull. W.H.O.* **49**, 1–12.

Fields, B. N. and Byers, K. (1983). The genetic basis of viral virulence. *Phil. Trans. R. Soc. Lond. B* **303**, 209 (survey of reovirus studies).

French, J. G. *et al.* (1973). The effect of sulfur dioxide and suspended sulfates on acute respiratory disease. *Archs Environ. Health* **27**, 129–133.

Gardner, I. D. (1980). The effect of ageing on susceptibility to infection. *Rev. Inf. Dis.* **2**, 801–810.

Gracey, M. S. (1981). Nutrition, bacteria and the gut. *Br. Med. Bull.* **37**, 71–75.

Huxley, E. J. *et al.* (1978). Pharyngeal aspiration in normal adults and in patients with depressed consciousness. *Am. J. Med.* **64**, 564–568.

Kan, Y. W. and Dozy, A. M. (1980). Evolution of the hemoglobin S and C genes in world populations. *Science, N.Y.* **209**, 388.

Keusch, G. T. and Scrimshaw, H. S. (1986). Selective primary health care: strategies for control of disease in the developing world. XXIII. Control of infection to reduce the prevalence of infantile and childhood malnutrition. *Rev. Inf. Dis.* **8**, 273.

Loag, D. G. (1981). Air pollution: the "classical" pollutants. *Br. Med. J.* **282**, 723–725.

Luzatto, L. (1979). Genetics of red cells and susceptibility to malaria. *Blood* **54**, 961–976.

Mata, L. J. (1975). Malnutrition—infection interactions in the tropics. *Am. J. Trop. Med. Hyg.* **24**, 564–574.

Murray, J. and Murray, A. (1977). Suppression of infection by famine and its activation by refeeding—a paradox? *Perspect. Biol. Med.* **20**, 471–484.

O-Amaan, S. *et al.* (1977). Is poliomyelitis a serious problem in developing countries?—lameness in Ghanaian schools. *Br. Med. J.*, April 16, 1012.

Ogasawara, M., Kono, D. H. and Yu, D. T. Y. (1986). Mimicry of human histocompatibility HLA-B27 antigens by *Klebsiella pneumoniae*. *Infect Immunity* **51**, 901.

Phair, J. P. (1979). Ageing and infection; a review. *J. Chronic Dis.* **32**, 535.

Report of Study Group (1979). Acne. *J. Investig. Dermatology* **73**, 434–442.

Weinberg, E. D. (1978). Iron and infection. *Microbiol. Rev.* **42**, 45–66.

Zinkernagel, R. M. (1979). Association between major histocompatibility antigens and susceptibility to disease. *Ann. Rev. Microbiol.* **33**, 201–213.

Appendix

Table 31. Bacteria of human importance

Organism	Diseases	Other features
Gram-positive cocci		
Staphylococcus aureus	Boils, septicaemia, food poisoning	Common skin commensal. Phage typing identifies virulent strains. Enterotoxin causes food poisoning.
Streptococcus pyogenes	Tonsilitis, scarlet fever, erysipelas, septicaemia	Also causes glomerulonephritis, and rheumatic fever, with immunopathological basis.
Streptococcus viridans group (*Streptococcus sanguis* etc.)	Infective endocarditis	Oral commensals settle on abnormal heart valves during bacteraemia.
Streptococcus mutans	Dental caries	Regular inhabitant of mouth; initiates plaque on tooth surface.
Streptococcus pneumoniae	Pneumonia, otitis meningitis	Normal upper respiratory tract commensal, can spread to infected or damaged lungs.
Gram-negative cocci		
Neisseria gonorrhoeae	Gonorrhoea	Obligate human parasite.
Neisseria meningitidis	Meningitis	Obligate human parasite; increased upper respiratory carriage in epidemics.
Gram-positive bacilli		
Corynebacterium diphtheriae	Diphtheria	Natural host man. Noninvasive disease due to toxin.
Bacillus anthracis	Anthrax	Pathogen of herbivorous animals, who ingest spores. Occasional human infection.
Clostridium spp.	Tetanus, gas-gangrene botulism	Widely distributed in soil and intestines.
Gram-negative bacilli		
E. coli	Urinary tract infections, infantile gastro-enteritis	Normal inhabitant intestine (man and animals). Many antigenic types.
Salmonella spp.	Enteric fever; food poisoning	*Salmonella typhi*—natural host man; invasive. Other *Salmonella*—1000 species, mainly animal pathogens.
Shigella spp.	Bacillary dysentery	Obligate parasites man. Local invasion only.

Table 31. (*Cont.*)

Organism	Diseases	Other features
Proteus spp.	Urinary tract and wound infection	Common in soil, faeces. Occasionally pathogenic.
Klebsiella spp.	Urinary tract and wound infection, otitis, meningitis, pneumonia	Present in vegetation, soil, sometimes faeces. Pathogenic when host resistance lowered.
Pseudomonas aeruginosa	Urinary tract and wound infection	Common human intestinal bacteria. Resists many antibiotics.
Haemophilus influenzae	Pneumonia, meningitis	Human commensal. Invades damaged lung
Bordetella pertussis	Whooping cough	Specialized human respiratory parasite.
Yersinia pestis	Plague	Flea-borne pathogen of rodents. Transfer to man as greatest infection in human history.
Brucella spp.	Undulant fever	Pathogens of goats, cattle and pigs with secondary human infection.
Acid-fast bacilli		
Mycobacterium tuberculosis	Tuberculosis	Chronic respiratory infection in man; 10–15 million active cases in the world. Enteric infection with bovine type via milk.
Mycobacterium leprae	Leprosy	Obligate parasite of man. Attacks skin, nasal mucosa and nerves. 15 million lepers in the world.
Miscellaneous		
Vibrio cholerae	Cholera	Obligate parasite of man. Non-invasive intestinal infection.
Treponema pallidum	Syphilis	Oligate human parasite. Sexual transmission. Related nonvenereal human bacteria.
Actinomyces israeli	Actinomycosis	Normal inhabitat human mouth.
Leptospira spp.	Leptospirosis (Weil's disease etc.)	Mostly pathogens of animals. Human infection from urine of rats, etc.
Legionella pneumophila	Legionnaire's disease	Respiratory pathogen of man, often acquired from contaminated air-conditioning units.

Table 32. Comparison of bacteria with smaller microorganisms

	Bacteria	Mycoplasmas	Rickettsias	Chlamydias	Viruses
DNA and RNA	+	+	+	+	–
Cell wall muramic acid	+	–	+	+	–
Binary fission	+	+	+	+	–
Growth nonliving media	+	+	–	–	–
Examples of microbe	Staphylococci *Mycobacterium tuberculosis* *Treponema pallidum*	*Mycoplasma pneumoniae*	*Rickettsia prowazeki* *Rickettsia burnetii*	*Chlamydia psittaci* *Chlamydia trachomatis*	Herpes simplex Rhinovirus
Human diseases produced	Abscesses Tuberculosis Syphilis	Atypical pneumonia	Typhus Q fever	Psittacosis Trachoma	Cold sore Common cold

Table 33. Fungi and protozoa of human importance

Organism	Disease	Features
Fungi		
Candida albicans	Thrust dermatitis etc.	Normally present on body surfaces; occasionally pathogenic
Dermatophytes (*Trichophyton* spp. *Epidermophyton* spp. *Microsporum* spp.)	Ringworm	Infection of skin, hair, nails (e.g. *Tinea pedis* – athlete's foot) Some species acquired from animals.
Cryptococcus neoformans	Meningitis	Occurs in soil; occasionally gives also skin, lung or systemic disease in man
Blastomyces spp.	Blastomycosis	Soil fungi in the Americas; systemic infection in man
Histoplasma capsulatum	Histoplasmosis	Soil fungus in the Americas; can give lung lesions and systemic illness in man
Protozoa		
Plasmodia (4 species)	Malaria	Mosquito transmitted; persistent infection in man
Toxoplasma gondii	Toxoplasmosis	Widely distributed in animals and birds; transplacental infection in man
Trichomonas vaginalis (flagellate)	Trichomoniasis (urethritis, vulvo-vaginitis)	Genito-urinary infection in both sexes, often asymptomatic
Giardia lamblia (flagellate)	Low-grade intestinal disease	Water-borne outbreaks occur
Trypanosoma spp. (flagellate)	Trypanosomiasis	Transmission by biting insects (animal reservoir); three species pathogenic for man
Leishmania spp. (flagellate)	Leishmaniasis (kala-azar, oriental sore etc.)	Transmission from animal host to man via sandflies
Entamoeba histolytica	Amoebic dysentery	Invasion of intestinal mucosa; may spread to liver
Balantidium coli (ciliate)	Dysentery	Infection of man from pigs

Table 34. Viruses of human importance

Nucleic acid	Virus group	Example	Envelope from infected cell	Miscellaneous properties
ss DNA	Parvovirus	Human parvovirus	–	Infects blood-forming cells in bone marrow
ds DNA	Poxvirus	Smallpox (variola) Vaccinia Myxoma, moll. contagiosum	–[a]	Large complex viruses
	Herpesvirus (herpes = creeping)	Herpes simplex Varicella-zoster EB virus, cytomegalovirus	+	Latency and oncogenicity
	Adenovirus (adeno = gland)	Adenovirus (types 1–33 in man)	–[a]	May give latent infections of lymphoid tissue
	Papovavirus (PAPilloma POlyoma Vacuolating virus)	Wart virus, polyoma (JC and BK) viruses, SV40	–[a]	Oncogenic in experimental animals, persistent infection common
	Hepadnavirus	Hepatitis B virus	+	Not readily grown *in vitro*
ss RNA	Picornavirus (pico = small + RNA)	(a) Enteroviruses 3 Polioviruses 33 Echoviruses 30 Coxsackie viruses Hepatitis A virus (b) Rhinoviruses (100 types)	–	Acid stable (pH 3) Coxsackie viruses pathogenic for baby mice Common cold viruses, acid labile (pH 3)
	Togavirus (toga = cloak)	Alphaviruses—Semliki forest, Sindbis etc. viruses	+	Multiply in arthropods, 200 different togaviruses

Type	Family	Viruses		Notes
		Flaviviruses—Yellow fever, dengue	+	
		Pestivirus	+	Bovine viral diarrhoea; hog cholera
		Rubivirus	+	Rubella in man
	Orthomyxovirus (myxo = mucin)	Influenza types A, B and C	+	Respiratory infections (intestinal in birds)
	Paramyxovirus	Parainfluenza types 1–4 Respiratory syncytial virus Mumps, measles viruses	+	Respiratory ± generalized infection
	Coronavirus (corona = crown)	Common cold agents	+	Group includes mouse hepatitis virus
	Retrovirus	Leukaemia viruses (man, mouse, cat etc.) mammary tumour viruses	+	Includes human immuno-deficiency virus (HIV), causative agent of AIDS
	Rhabdovirus (rhabdo = bullet)	Rabies, vesicular stomatitis of horses	+	
	Arenavirus (arena = sand)	Lymphocytic choriomeningitis, S. American haemorrhagic fevers, Lassa fever	+	Normally infect rodents; may give serious disease in man
ds RNA	Reovirus (Respiratory Enteric Orphan)	Reoviruses types 1–3	−	Harmless in man
		Rotaviruses (rota = wheel)	−	Infantile gastroenteritis
Unknown	Not typical viruses	Kuru, scrapie, Creutzfeld-Jacob	?	SLOW agents distinct from conventional viruses

a Do not have a conventional envelope, but viral antigens appear on surface of infected cells which are then susceptible to immune lysis.

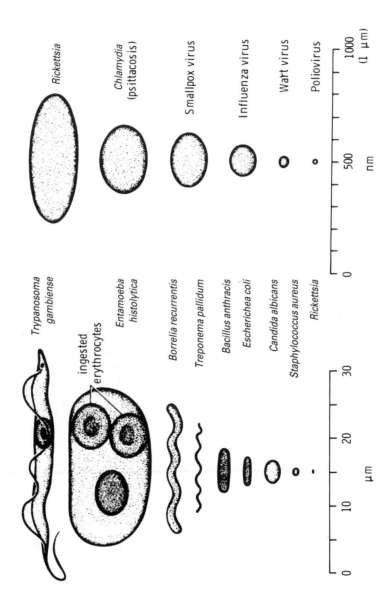

Fig. 38. Relative size of microorganisms.

Vaccines—An Addendum

Introduction

Probably the greatest achievement in medicine in the twentieth century has been the great reduction in the incidence of infectious disease. Smallpox has been eliminated, and most of the old scourges such as tuberculosis, cholera, diphtheria and typhoid have been brought under control, at least in the developed countries of northern America, northern Europe, Australia etc. giving us the opportunity to die of other things later in life. This revolution in infectious diseases was in the first place the result of dramatic improvements in sanitation and public health, which provided clean water supplies, adequate disposal of sewage and better housing. The downward trends in many infectious diseases were in progress early in the twentieth century, well before antibiotics and vaccines had been invented.

Improvements in water supplies and sewage disposal obviously have a great impact on enteric diseases such as cholera and typhoid. Better housing and nutrition have had an important influence on other diseases. Tuberculosis, referred to as the Great White Plague in the cities of nineteenth century Europe, and notoriously promoted by crowding and poverty, has been steadily declining as a cause of death as standards of housing and nutrition have improved. Infectious diseases like typhus and plague have receded as people and their dwellings have become free from the lice, fleas and rats that were necessary for the spread of these diseases. But all these infections are still present in the world and the people of developed countries are protected from them only so long as they continue to be protected from lice, fleas, rats, poverty, crowding and contaminated food and water. A general breakdown in the organization and structure of modern society would lead to food shortages and allow the lice, fleas, rats and contaminated water to return, together with many of the old diseases. This is what happens on a limited scale during wars and in natural disasters such as earthquakes. War, famine and pestilence traditionally ride together. Once an infectious agent has been totally eradicated on a global scale it cannot of course return. This is difficult to achieve with infections such as malaria, plague and yellow fever, because they have vectors and animal reservoirs (see Glossary), but

303

infections restricted to man and involving no other host can be totally eradicated if all human infection is prevented. Smallpox comes into this last category, and it has now been totally eradicated from the world by a relentless vaccination programme carried out by the WHO. Smallpox eradication was also made easier because the virus does not persist in the body and therefore cannot reactivate (see pp. 255–261). Other infections restricted to man and which do not cause persistent infection and reactivation include whooping cough, bacillary dysentery, and measles. The US authorities have almost eliminated measles from the country by a vigorous programme of vaccination. Reintroduction into the USA from outside is controlled by public health measures as in the days of smallpox.

Although many infectious diseases were already declining following general improvements in public health, the decline was greatly accelerated by the development of vaccines to prevent diseases and antibiotics to treat diseases. Vaccines, used on a large scale, have been a major antimicrobial force in the community. As each microbial agent has been isolated and identified, its cultivation under artificial conditions has generally led within a short time to the development of a vaccine. Many infections, especially virus infections such as smallpox and poliomyelitis, have receded wherever effective vaccines have been used. Some vaccines are better than others. Yellow fever has proved to be one of the best vaccines, while vaccines against typhoid and cholera have so far remained comparatively unsatisfactory. There has been complete failure to develop effective vaccines for many important human diseases such as trachoma, malaria, syphilis and gonorrhoea.

Infectious diseases remain the greatest health problem for most people and for most animals in the world. More and more, the practitioners of medicine or veterinary science will be concerned with the prevention rather than with the cure of diseases. Current advances in immunology and microbiology are leading to the development of many new vaccines, and many better vaccines, and it is the purpose of this addendum to survey some of the principles governing the development and use of vaccines.

What is a vaccine?

A vaccine* is a material originating from a microorganism or other parasite that induces an immunologically mediated resistance to disease.† Material

---

*The word vaccine (vacca, Latin = cow) derives from the vaccinia (cowpox) virus inoculated to protect against smallpox.

†Vaccines are distinct from specific antibodies which are given to confer passive immunity. Immunoglobulin pooled from normal adults generally contains enough antibody to hepatitis A virus to confer protection for a few months. But for other viruses (hepatitis B, rabies, mumps, varicella-zoster) immunoglobulin from known immune donors is necessary.

with similar structure and activity can also be produced artificially rather than obtained from the actual microorganism or parasite.

What do we ask of an ideal vaccine?

(1) That it promotes effective resistance to the disease, but not necessarily to the infection.
(2) That resistance lasts as long as possible.
(3) That vaccination is safe, with minimal and acceptable side effects. Standards have changed for human vaccines, and today we are more fussy than we used to be. The present smallpox vaccine, which has remained more or less unchanged for more than a hundred years, would never have been licensed if introduced a few years ago. Rather lower safety standards are acceptable for most veterinary vaccines. A vaccine, even if not completely safe, should be safer than exposure to the disease, assuming that the risk of exposure is significant. Attitudes to a given vaccine's safety depend on whether the safety of the individual or the protection of the community is under consideration. When a vaccine gives protection to the community, the community owes a debt to any individual damaged by the vaccine.
(4) That the vaccine is stable, and will remain potent during storage and shipping. The fact that yellow fever virus can be freeze-dried and transported unrefrigerated in the tropics has been a great asset favouring the success of this vaccine.
(5) That the vaccine is reasonably cheap, if it is for large scale use, or for use in developing countries.

General Principles

Effective resistance to infection or disease depends on the vaccine having certain properties, and there are often different requirements for different types of infection. Some important general principles are listed below.

1. The vaccine should induce the right type of immune resistance

The relative importance of antibody and CMI in resistance to disease has been discussed in Chs 6 and 9. Vaccines should induce the type of immunity that is relevant for the particular microorganism. Resistance to tuberculosis or typhoid seems to require effective cell-mediated immunity, whereas resistance to yellow fever or poliomyelitis requires a good antibody response. If the wrong type of response is induced protection is inadequate, and once or twice the disease when it occurred has even been made more serious. Early killed measles vaccines, for instance, induced circulating antibody rather than CMI. It was also directed against the wrong viral antigen (see below); and this did not prevent re-infection. Subsequent infection with either natural ("wild") measles or live measles vaccine virus resulted in immunopathological events in the skin and lungs with an unusual type of disease.

2. The vaccine should induce an immune response in the right place

For resistance to infections of epithelial surfaces it is more appropriate to induce secretory IgA antibodies than circulating IgG or IgM antibodies. Thus, secretory IgA antibodies might give valuable protection against influenza or cholera, but not against rabies or yellow fever which by-pass epithelial surfaces and enter the body through bite wounds (see Ch. 2). Even the secretory antibody response must be in the right place; antibodies in the intestine will not protect the nose or throat. Unfortunately, in spite of attention to these principles, live polio vaccine (Sabin) remains almost the only one that induces a good IgA-mediated immunity.

3. The vaccine should induce an immune response to the right antigens

A given microorganism contains many different antigens, as discussed in Ch. 6 and as illustrated by number of genes (Table 12, p. 135). There are many hundreds or thousands of antigens in the case of protozoa, fungi* and bacteria, and in virus infections from as little as three (polyoma virus) to more than 100 (herpes and poxviruses) are produced. Immune responses to many of these antigens develop during infection. Resistance to infection, however, depends principally on immune responses to the smaller number of antigens on the surface of the microorganism. The relevant surface antigens have been isolated and characterized for certain viruses, but much less is known of the surface antigens that induce resistance to chlamydia, bacteria, fungi and protozoa. Vaccines consisting of killed whole bacteria, for instance, inevitably induce a very large number of irrelevant immune responses.

* *Candida albicans,* for instance, contains at least 78 water-extractable antigens, and from *E. coli* 1100 proteins have been resolved by two-dimensional gel electrophoresis.

4. Resistance to some infectious diseases does not depend on immunity to the infectious agent

In certain infections such as tetanus and diphtheria, disease is entirely due to the action of toxins as discussed in Ch. 8. Immunity to the disease requires only immunity (antibody) to the toxin. For the production of vaccine, therefore, a toxin is modified by chemical or physical treatment (alcohol, phenol, UV irradiation) so that it is no longer toxic, but maintains its antigenic character. The resulting toxoid is a very effective vaccine when combined with an adjuvant (see below).

5. There are important differences in principle between killed and live vaccines

The primary response to an antigen is classically distinguished from the secondary response. After the first injection of an antigen the immune response begins and at the same time the antigen itself is generally degraded and disposed of in the body. The second injection of antigen now induces a greatly enhanced response, and subsequent injections give further boosts (see Fig. 39). Each killed vaccine must therefore be given in repeated doses if an adequate immune response and resistance is to be induced. The microorganisms in live vaccines, on the other hand, multiply in the host after administration. The antigenic mass contained in the vaccine itself is small but it is increased many thousand times following growth of the microorganism in the body. The effective dose is greatly amplified in this way, and

Table 35. Comparison of live and killed vaccines

Live	Killed
Must be attenuated by passage in cell culture or bacteriological media	Can be produced from fully virulent microorganisms e.g. polio virus (Salk), typhoid vaccines
Given as a single dose[a]	Given in multiple doses
Smaller number of microorganisms needed	Large number of microorganisms needed
Tend to be less stable	Tend to be more stable
Possibility of spread of infection to unvaccinated individuals	Spread is not possible

[a] Live polio (Sabin) vaccine is an exception. Each dose contains the three types of polio virus that interfere with each other's replication in the intestine, and it must be given on three occasions to ensure an adequate response to each type.

the primary merges into the secondary immune response giving a high level of immunity (Fig. 39). Only one dose of vaccine is therefore needed to produce satisfactory immunity. Nearly all the successful viral vaccines, both medical and veterinary, consist of living attenuated virus. Examples of different types of vaccine are given in Table 36, and differences between live and killed vaccines are summarized in Table 35.

Table 36. Types of vaccines

Vaccine	Live vaccines	Killed vaccines
Viral	Smallpox[a]	Poliomyelitis (Salk)[a]
	Rubella[a]	Influenza
	Measles[a]	Rabies (human diploid cell)[a]
	Poliomyelitis (Sabin)[a]	Hepatitis B
	Yellow fever[a]	
	Mumps[a]	
	Varicella-zoster	
	Also 10–20 commonly used veterinary vaccines (dog, cat, cattle, horse, chicken, pig, sheep)	
Bacterial	BCG[a]	Cholera
	Brucella (veterinary use)	Typhoid
		Whooping-cough
Bacterial polysaccharide vaccines		Pneumococcus[b]—14 antigenically distinct polysaccharides
		Meningococcus—serogroups A and C[c]
Rickettsial		Typhus
Bacterial toxoid vaccines	Diphtheria,[a] tetanus[a]	
	Clostridium welchii (veterinary use)	
Helminths	Cattle lung worm	
	No effective vaccines for human helminth infestations	
Important diseases with no effective vaccine available	Trachoma, chlamydial urethritis,[f] malaria Syphilis, gonorrhoea, trypanosomiasis, leprosy, schistosomiasis Human herpes viruses (H. simplex,[d] EB virus, cytomegalovirus,[d] Hepatitis A, HIV (AIDS) Rheumatic fever[e]	

[a] Highly effective.
[b] There are 84 pneumococcal serotypes but most serious illnesses are due to the 14 more common types. Children less than two years old generally give poor antibody responses to polysaccharide vaccines. Capsular polysaccharides are being used to produce vaccines to other bacteria, such as *Haemophilus influenzae*. Polysaccharides are T-independent antigens (see footnote p. 124) and their immunogenicity in infants can be enhanced when they are converted to T-dependent antigens by conjugation with protein "carriers".

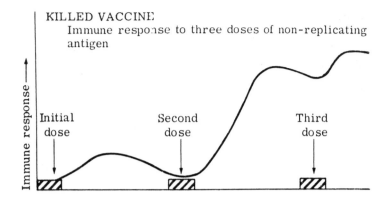

KILLED VACCINE
Immune response to three doses of non-replicating antigen

Immune response ⟶

Initial
dose

Second
dose

Third
dose

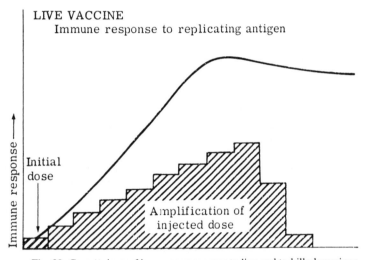

LIVE VACCINE
Immune response to replicating antigen

Immune response ⟶

Initial
dose

Amplification of
injected dose

Fig. 39. Comparison of immune responses to live and to killed vaccines.

Notes to Table 36 continued

[c] Unfortunately most cases of meningitis in the UK and USA are due to serogroup b, but this particular polysaccharide is poorly immunogenic in man.

[d] New vaccines undergoing clinical trials.

[e] Still an important disease in three-quarters of the world's population. A vaccine would induce immune responses to M proteins from the relevant streptococcal types (see p. 206), but there is the possibility that these responses could lead to heart damage, as in the disease itself. The M proteins, however, have type specific determinants localized to 20 amino acid residues, which are highly immunogenic when coupled to polylysine.

[f] The chlamydia responsible for trachoma, urethritis, salpingitis, conjunctivitis and lympho-granuloma inguinale (see Table 3, p. 44) exist as at least 15 serotypes. In diseases such as trachoma, promoted by flies, crowding and shortage of water, and where re-infection is probably important, improvements in hygiene may in the end be as important as vaccines. In one study in Mexico, a daily face wash reduced the incidence of trachoma in children from 48% to 10%.

6. The disease should be serious enough to justify vaccination

Rubella, for instance, is a very mild disease, and vaccination would not be worthwhile were it not for the fact that infection during pregnancy can lead to serious damage to the foetus. This incidentally is the only vaccine that is used to protect an as yet nonexistent individual. Many coxsackie and echo virus infections cause little or no illness and vaccines are not therefore required. Vaccines are sometimes given particularly to certain groups of individuals. This is generally because they are susceptible to some complication of the infection, as in the case of rubella infection of the foetus in pregnant women. Similarly, older people and those with chronic respiratory diseases are often given influenza virus vaccines because they are susceptible to influenzal pneumonia. Children with leukaemia have been given the live varicella-zoster vaccines that are being developed because varicella is often fatal in these children. Again the new 14-valent pneumococcal polysaccharide vaccine can be given to children with sickle cell disease, who are very susceptible to pneumococcal infection. Restricted vaccination is sometimes based on the likelihood of exposure to the disease as with vets or workers in quarantine kennels who receive rabies virus vaccine.

7. Factors determining the duration of resistance

Clearly the longer protection lasts the better; no vaccine would prove popular if an injection were required every six months throughout life. The duration of resistance to disease depends to some extent on the type of infection. In the case of systemic infections with an incubation period of a week or two, a low residual level of immunity gives resistance to disease, because even if re-infection does occur, the immune response is boosted during the incubation period and the infection is terminated before the onset of disease. Repeated subclinical booster infections may be important in maintaining immunity to diseases such as measles and rubella. Infections of the body surfaces, in contrast, have incubation periods of only a few days, and if there is a low residual level of immunity * re-infection can occur and cause disease before there has been time for the immune response to be boosted and the infectious process controlled. Thus it is difficult to induce long lasting immunity to parainfluenza virus infections or to gonorrhoea, but easier for measles or mumps.

We have little understanding of the factors responsible for the long lasting immune responses to microorganisms that are seen in the absence of

---

* Secretory IgA responses tend to be short lived compared with IgG responses. Accelerated secondary IgA responses are seen, but are weaker than with IgG (see p. 133).

persistent infection or re-infection. Immunity to live yellow fever virus vaccine, for instance, is probably life-long, although the infection is not a persistent one, and viable virus is apparently completely eliminated from the body. Perhaps small amounts of viral antigen remain sequestered in some site in the body (see p. 133). Live vaccines give longer lasting protection than killed ones, if the infectious agent persists in the body and produces antigens, to give continuous stimulation of immune responses (BCG, Marek's disease vaccine for poultry).

8. The concept of attenuation

It would seem ridiculous to use the naturally occurring disease agent as the vaccine, because it would tend to cause the disease that one wishes to prevent. In the early days of smallpox vaccination, however, living virus from the scabs of smallpox patients was used as a vaccine. Lady Montague, wife of the British Ambassador to Turkey, brought this type of vaccination ("variolation") to England 250 years ago. It was effective, but could be fatal, and was made illegal in 1840 * when Jenner developed his calf lymph vaccine. Usually it is necessary to reduce the pathogenicity of the microorganism by growth in artificial media such as cell culture (measles, Sabin polio) or bacterial growth media (BCG). This is an empirical procedure, depending on the fact that prolonged passage of a microorganism in an artificial system tends to select mutants better suited to growth in that system than in the original host. Unless the microorganism can be conveniently cultivated artificially such attenuation is impossible, and this is why a live vaccine for a given virus soon follows its successful cultivation *in vitro*. Attenuation has usually been a "blind" procedure, and the microorganism has to be tested for virulence during its continued cultivation in the laboratory. The yellow fever vaccine strain of virus (17D) arose in this way, and only arose once, by what amounts to sheer good fortune. Nowadays attenuation can sometimes be carried out more rationally. For instance, influenza and respiratory syncytial virus mutants have been produced that grow poorly at 37°C, the temperature of the lower respiratory tract, but well at the temperature of the nose, 33°C. These temperature sensitive (ts) mutants multiply after instillation into the nose and induce immunity, but are unable to spread to the lower respiratory tract.

---

* Variolation had a mortality of about 1%, as compared with a mortality of 15–20% for smallpox itself (the milder form of smallpox, variola minor, did not arise until around 1900). Variolation was carried out a good deal in England, especially in the 1760s, someone called Daniel Sutton having variolated 300 000 people, and Jenner himself was variolated as a boy in 1756.

The process of attenuation must be taken far enough so that the vaccine does not cause disease. An early live measles vaccine (Edmonston strain) caused fever and a rash, and human gammaglobulin was administered at the same time to decrease the severity of the vaccine disease. Attenuation, however, must not be taken too far, because the microorganism may then fail to replicate fully enough to induce a good immune response.

9. The concept of monotypic microbes

Certain microorganisms are antigenically much the same, wherever and whenever they occur, so that resistance to disease, once established, is secure. This is so for measles, yellow fever or tuberculosis. Sometimes a given disease is caused by a number of microorganisms which differ antigenically, and resistance to only one of them will not provide resistance to the disease. There are dozens of antigenically distinct types of streptococci, for instance, and resistance to streptococcal infection is not complete until there have been immune responses to them all. The same is true for the common cold, which can be caused by more than 100 antigenically distinct viruses belonging to at least five different groups. Some microorganisms are undergoing repeated antigenic changes during the course of their circulation in the community. Respiratory viruses in particular are evolving rapidly in this way. Vaccination against today's strains may give no protection against tomorrow's variant. This is true of influenza viruses in man, which always tend to be one step ahead of the vaccinators, and of foot and mouth disease virus in animals.

10. Adjuvants

Adjuvants are materials that increase the immune response to a given antigen without being antigenically related to it. Aluminium salts act in this way, and in diphtheria and tetanus vaccines the toxoids are combined with aluminium hydroxide or phosphate. The aluminium salt converts the soluble toxoid into a particulate precipitate and thus increases immunogenicity. Killed *Bordetella pertussis* bacteria, as used in the pertussis vaccine, have a slight adjuvant action, and increase the immune response to vaccines that are given at the same time.

Various oils are effective as adjuvants. The vaccine material is generally administered with the oil as a water-in-oil emulsion, and the mechanism of action is partly because of the very slow breakdown of the mass of oil and consequently slow release of antigen. However, mineral oils, at least, are potentially carcinogenic, and oils tend to cause local sterile abscesses after injection. Finally, mycobacterial products act as adjuvants, and Freund's original complete adjuvant consists of killed, dried mycobacteria (usually *Mycobacterium tuberculosis*) suspended in mineral oil. Mycobacterial adjuvants are given to experimental animals, but can cause granulomas and are not acceptable for human use. Fame and riches await the discoverer of a safe and potent adjuvant for human use. A more lasting immunity could then be induced, and antigens that were poor immunogens could be used. In the past materials as varied as lecithin, starch, tapioca and breadcrumbs have been tried out, but modern immunology gives a more logical basis for the development of a good adjuvant. Muramyl dipeptide, for instance, a synthetic product that is also a component of the cell wall of various bacteria and responsible for the adjuvant activity of mycobacteria shows great promise. The enclosure of antigens in synthetic lipid vesicles (liposomes), from which they are released very slowly after injection, is also being tried out.

11. Interference

The ultimate objective of vaccination programmes might be to administer all vaccines at the same time, thus giving a once and for all protection against everything that matters. There is evidence, however, that when too many antigens are combined they sometimes interfere with each other, so that the immune response to each is not so great as if they had been given separately. More importantly, live viruses occasionally interfere with each other. Live measles virus vaccine, for instance, could inhibit the growth of other live virus vaccines given at the same time, perhaps by inducing interferon. Live poliovirus vaccine (Sabin) given at the same time as other vaccines is unlikely to interfere with them because it grows in a different part of the body, establishing an exclusively intestinal infection. Sabin vaccine, however, contains the three distinct strains of poliovirus, and these tend to interfere with each other during their multiplication in the intestine. They can also be interfered with by any naturally acquired enteroviruses that happen to be multiplying in the intestine at the same time. After the first dose there is often a response to only one of the strains. The same Sabin vaccine is therefore given three times, to ensure that a satisfactory response to each of the virus strains takes place. This is the reason for this apparent exception to the principle about single doses of live vaccines being adequate (see above). But the theoretical problem of interference seems less important in practice and there are immense advantages (cost, organization) in using combined vaccines. For instance, there is increasing and successful use of MMR vaccine (a mixture of live measles, mumps and rubella virus vaccines) given to children aged one year or older, sometimes together with live oral poliovirus vaccine.

12. The age at which vaccines should be given

Human infants are born with a supply of maternal IgG antibody derived from the placental route, and they thus acquire resistance to all infections to which the mother had antibody-mediated immunity. They also receive secretory IgA antibodies in colostrum and milk, and these provide some protection against intestinal infections. Live poliovaccine (Sabin) is less likely to immunize in the first few months of life because secretory IgA antibodies from maternal milk inhibit the growth of the vaccine virus.

The first encounter with many microorganisms thus takes place under an umbrella of maternal immunity, and when infection takes place it is likely to be mild yet at the same time significant enough to generate some immunity in the infant. Maternal antibody persists for up to six months after birth and vaccines, particularly live vaccines, are likely to be less effective if given before this time. Diphtheria, tetanus and whooping cough vaccines are not given until the infant is three to six months old. Certain infections, however, such as measles and whooping cough are particularly severe in infants and very young children (two-thirds of deaths from whooping cough occur during the first year of life) and there is a need to give protection as soon as possible after maternal immunity has faded. Pertussis vaccination, therefore, is commenced at three months to give protection during the first year of life, and live measles vaccine is given at one year. The complications of diphtheria and pertussis vaccination are commoner in older individuals, and this is another reason for giving these vaccines early in life. The contra-indications for smallpox vaccination (congenital immunological deficiencies) are not easily recognized early in life, and this vaccine therefore used to be given at one to two years. Rubella is designed to protect the foetus, and in the UK at present live rubella vaccine is given to girls aged 10–13 years, who are old enough to develop a good immune response, but presumably too young to be pregnant. Finally, it may be worthwhile vaccinating elderly people against infections to which they are particularly susceptible, such as influenza or pneumococcal pneumonia.

13. Problems of testing

All vaccines have to be tested, and their safety and effectiveness evaluated. This may take many years. Human vaccines must be tested on human beings. Preliminary trials in experimental animals are useful, but do not always give results applicable to man. The effectiveness of a vaccine cannot be reliably assessed merely by measuring the immune responses induced; it must be tested in those exposed to natural infection. Trials of this sort are difficult when the disease is an uncommon or serious one (e.g. rabies). Trials must, of course, be large enough and well planned; large numbers may be needed for the proper evaluation of safety. Many vaccines are still of uncertain status because trials have been too small, or because of differences in the potency or composition of a given type of vaccine.

14. Problems of vaccine production

Even when a vaccine of known potency has been developed, its large-scale use depends on efficient methods of mass production. For instance, there would be problems with a leprosy vaccine derived from whole bacteria because these bacteria cannot be grown in culture but must be obtained from artificially infected armadillos. There are not enough armadillos in the world to give an adequate supply of bacteria. A similar problem would have arisen with the hepatitis B virus vaccine derived from the blood of human carriers. Genetic engineering (see below) has solved this problem, and doubtless the key immunogen(s) for protection against leprosy will be produced in a similar way.

15. Problems with immunological unresponsiveness

Failure to give an adequate response to a vaccine may be due not only to immaturity (see p. 314) or immunosuppression, but also to the following factors.

(1) Malnutrition (see Ch. 11).
(2) Interference. Very frequent enterovirus infections in children in developing countries can interfere with the "take" of live poliovirus vaccine. There are suggestions that failures of BCG vaccination in India are due to previous infection with related mycobacteria which induced immune tolerance to cross-reactive but protective antigens in the BCG vaccine.
(3) Unknown factors. For instance, infants develop poor antibody responses to the polysaccharides of type b meningococci, and it is precisely this type that causes serious infection in this age group. The cause for this is not known, but one solution is to couple covalently a protein (e.g. outer membrane protein of the meningococcus) to the polysaccharide, which then induces a good (and now T-dependent)

response. Again, there are reports that hepatitis B vaccine fails to induce protective antibodies in certain individuals. It is not known why, but there is the possibility that the unresponsiveness is genetically controlled.

Complications and Side-effects of Vaccines

Virulent infectious material in vaccine

Virulent microorganisms are inactivated to make killed vaccine. If inactivation has been incompletely carried out, vaccination introduces infection. On one occasion, incomplete inactivation of virulent poliomyelitis virus by formaldehyde in the killed (Salk) vaccine caused paralytic poliomyelitis in large numbers of vaccinated children. There have also been injurious effects because of the presence of additional unsuspected microorganisms in a vaccine. Live yellow fever virus vaccine was at one time stabilized by the addition of human serum, and during the last war thousands of US servicemen vaccinated against yellow fever became jaundiced because of the presence of hepatitis B virus in the "normal" serum. Poliomyelitis virus for the killed (Salk) vaccine was produced in normal monkey kidney cells and then inactivated by formaldehyde. Subsequently, however, the normal monkey kidney cell cultures were shown to contain a papovavirus, SV40 (simian virus 40), which was present in the vaccine and was not inactivated by the formaldehyde treatment. This virus transforms cells and causes tumours experimentally. The thousands of children who had been injected with live SV40 virus were therefore followed with some anxiety, but fortunately there were no harmful effects.

Allergic effects of vaccines

First, nonmicrobial antigens in vaccines can cause allergic responses, especially in vaccines that are given more than once. Vaccines containing penicillin and egg proteins, for instance, have given trouble. Even the microbial components in a vaccine may sometimes give allergic responses (local swelling, rash etc.) in hypersensitive individuals. Second, certain vaccines induce autoimmune type responses in the host. The post-vaccinial encephalitis, or the peripheral neuritis (Guillain-Barre syndrome) that very occasionally occurs a week or two after administration of various killed or live virus vaccines (as well as after natural infection) appears to arise in this way. For instance 10 per million Americans developed the Guillain-Barre syndrome after being given inactivated influenza virus vaccine in 1976 in a nationwide attempt to protect against swine influenza. Possible autoimmune side effects must be considered, especially with vaccines for infectious diseases where there is a significant amount of immunopathology. Microbial components in the vaccine might induce cross-reactive autoimmune responses that could be harmful (e.g. trachoma, rheumatic fever).

Toxicity of vaccines

Large numbers of killed salmonellas are given in the vaccine for typhoid, and this vaccine therefore contains large amounts of endotoxin (see Ch. 8). Accordingly, fever and malaise are not uncommon sequels to vaccination, although these side effects are reduced by injection of the vaccine by the intradermal route.*

Influenza virus vaccines containing inactivated whole virus particles often give troublesome febrile and local reactions in children. This is not seen with vaccines containing disrupted virus material, nor of course with live virus vaccines. The current pertussis (whooping cough) vaccines cause a variable incidence of neurological sequelae. Up to 1 in 5000 vaccinated children may be affected with more serious effects in 1 in 100000. The main toxic component in the vaccine is the lymphocytosis promoting factor, which also causes hypoglycaemia and histamine sensitization. It contributes to the illness in the natural infection. New pertussis vaccines in use or undergoing clinical trials consist of purified antigens rather than whole bacteria. They contain the lymphocytosis promoting factor (converted into a toxoid), together with other antigens that protect against bacterial colonization of the respiratory tract. These "cleaner" vaccines will doubtless cause fewer side effects, and it is to be hoped that they give adequate protection.

Harmful effects on the foetus

After vaccination against smallpox, or during the disease smallpox, the foetus was often infected and killed. Live rubella virus can infect the foetus

---

*Typhoid remains a worldwide problem, with an estimated 12.5 million cases per year, and carriers are common in affected areas (for instance nearly 700 carriers per 100000 people in Santiago, Chile). Vaccine trials with an oral live attenuated strain of *S. typhi* are in progress.

but it is not clear whether it causes damage. Live hog cholera and bluetongue vaccines can certainly cause foetal infection and malformations in domestic animals. Because maternal ill health or infection is a risk to the foetus, it is a good general rule not to give vaccines to pregnant women, especially live vaccines, and especially during the first trimester of pregnancy. On the other hand, immunization during pregnancy can give specific protection to the new born (see p. 134). Tetanus vaccine is often given to pregnant women in developing countries to prevent neonatal tetanus (see footnote p. 198), and certain veterinary vaccines can be administered during pregnancy to protect the offspring.

Effects on immunodeficient host

Live vaccines often cause illness in children with immunodeficiencies. Children with agammaglobulinaemia may develop paralytic disease following vaccination with live polio (Sabin) vaccine. Deficiencies in cell-mediated immunity are the most important, and the consequences of giving measles, smallpox or BCG vaccine to children with thymic aplasia have been described in Ch. 9. The infection caused by the live virus or bacterium is readily controlled in the normal individual and induces a good immune response; it is not controlled and may give rise to serious or lethal infection in the immunodeficient child. Live vaccines can also cause disease in those that are immunodeficient as a result of malignant disease of the lymphoreticular system.

Miscellaneous complications

In the days when vaccination against smallpox was common, complications were often seen in children with eczema. The vaccine virus, after spreading through the body in circulating leucocytes, localized in the eczematous areas and caused secondary vaccinial skin lesions which were sometimes serious. The vaccine virus (vaccinia) readily infects the conjunctiva or the traumatized skin of a nonimmune person, and causes a prominent lesion just as at the site of primary vaccination. Residual virus left on the skin after vaccination, or the virus present in the vesicle that appears at the vaccination site, could be mechanically transferred by fingers etc. to other parts of the body or to other individuals. Now that vaccination against smallpox has virtually ceased, the unvaccinated majority become susceptible to cross-infection from the occasional freshly vaccinated individual.

The Development of New Vaccines

Problems

There are four important problems in vaccine development.

(1) A failure to grow satisfactory quantities of the microorganism in the laboratory. Leprosy, hepatitis A and hepatitis B come into this category.

(2) When crude preparations of killed microorganisms are used as a vaccine, they often give poor protection against disease. Only a small number of the microbial antigens that are present induce a protective immune response, and in most cases (gonorrhoea, herpes viruses, typhoid, trachoma etc.) the key antigens have not been identified. As often as not, there is ignorance as to the type of immune response that needs to be induced.

(3) Live vaccines often give effective protection, but the virus vaccines that are most needed are for the herpes virus group (see Table 36). Live vaccines for these viruses are unlikely to be licenced for general use in man because of the possibility of virus reactivation later in life (see pp. 258–260) and because of the remote possibility that they might induce cancer (see p. 268).

(4) Some of the most successful microorganisms induce ineffective immune responses in the host or actually interfere with the development of effective immune responses (see Ch. 7). Examples include gonorrhea, syphilis, and the herpes virus infections. This is likely to be a problem with live vaccines but if a particular microbial component is responsible for this activity it could be eliminated from a killed vaccine.

Many vaccines contain large numbers of irrelevant antigens, derived either from the microorganism itself or from the culture system used to produce it. It would be better to replace these crude soups with cocktails of defined polypeptides. Sometimes it does not matter if the relevant protective antigen or antigens are not known. Certain virus vaccines can be developed as long as relatively clean preparations of virus are available, as in the case of the inactivated rabies vaccine produced from human diploid cells. But for many bacterial and protozoal infections we need to know more about the role of microbial surface components in pathogenesis. The present pertussis vaccine induces satisfactory protection but contains at least 49 different antigens. Only a small number of these act as important toxins or are present on the bacterial surface and likely to be relevant for host protection (see above). Effective vaccines for leprosy, trypanosomiasis, gonorrhoea, and syphilis will come when first the protective antigens are at least partially separated from irrelevant microbial components, and second, when we know what type of immune response is required for protection.

There are a few bacterial diseases where the relevant antigen has been identified. Capsular polysaccharides can be used to induce protection against pneumococcal, meningococcal or *Haemophilus influenzae* infections (see Table 36). Capsular materials are readily obtained by growing bacteria in the laboratory, but it may be noted that many of the genes that code for the enzymes that synthesize capsule have been cloned. The K88 and K99 adhesins (p. 20) that are responsible for the attachment of *E. coli* to the gut wall of piglets and calves can be used to immunize the pregnant mother whose antibodies will then protect the newborn animal against *E. coli* diarrhoea. Also, the diseases due to the action of a toxin can be approached by developing a toxoid vaccine, and promising work is in progress with a cholera toxoid for oral immunization.

The problem of growing the microorganisms can be solved by genetic engineering. If the DNA that codes for the relevant antigen (e.g. hepatitis B surface antigen) can be obtained it is incorporated into a plasmid which is introduced into a bacterium (*E. coli*) or a yeast (*Saccharomyces cerevisiae*). The antigen can then be bulk-produced from cultures. There are innumerable difficulties, but certain vaccines are now being produced in this way.

It is also possible to develop live avirulent vaccines by removing or inactivating the genes that confer virulence. For instance, the gene for the cholera toxin has been cloned in *E. coli*, altered by mutation and then re-introduced into virulent *Vibrio cholerae*. This gives a strain of bacteria that multiplies without producing the toxin when given orally, and induces immunity to cholera.

Synthetic peptides as vaccines

For a given polypeptide only a small proportion of the molecule is important as an immunogen. Once the minimal sized antigenic determinants have been identified, they are often found to be small peptides. For instance, a 14 amino acid peptide of diphtheria toxin, and similar sized peptides from hepatitis B virus surface antigen or from the VP1 polypeptide of foot-and-mouth disease virus are active, in so far as they can induce protective antibodies when covalently linked to a carrier protein. Small peptides like this can be chemically synthesized, by-passing the need to produce the entire polypeptide in *E. coli* or in yeasts. But there are problems with immunogenicity (the need for carriers, adjuvants) and with the level of protection ultimately induced, and the place for synthetic peptides is still not clear.

Attenuated viruses as carriers

Finally, it is possible to introduce the gene for any given viral protein into the genome of an avirulent virus that can then be administered as a live vaccine. The foreign viral protein is produced in infected cells, and induces an immune response. This has been done mostly with vaccinia virus, into which genes from viruses such as hepatitis B, influenza, rabies, herpes simplex and foot-and-mouth disease have been introduced. This has the supreme advantage that genes from up to 10 or more different infectious agents could be introduced into the same strain of vaccinia virus, a single inoculation of which would simultaneously immunize against a wide range of infections. Unfortunately, smallpox-vaccinated people cannot be immunized in this way, and vaccinia virus is not considered safe enough for people by modern standards (see above). But perhaps vaccinia virus can be made less pathogenic by genetic engineering, and in any case such vaccines might be acceptable for veterinary use. In a similar fashion, genes from different pathogenic intestinal bacteria have been introduced into avirulent bacteria. Following oral administration the avirulent bacteria colonize and multiply, the polypeptides from the pathogens are produced, and gut immunity develops against the intestinal pathogen.

New vaccines will certainly be produced and some of them will have a major impact on the health of people in developed and quite possibly in developing countries. But it is unfortunately true that much human illness and death is due to diseases that can be prevented by the effective use of existing vaccines. This is largely a matter of money and organization. The WHO aims to immunize all children in the world against diphtheria, pertussis, tetanus, measles, polio and tuberculosis by the year 1990. These diseases are responsible for five million preventable deaths a year in children (about 10 a minute) together with several million more who are crippled or mentally retarded. This is the expanded programme of immunization (EPI). There can be nothing but praise for such an endeavour, and for the vision and humanity behind it.

References

Fenner, F. (1982). A successful eradication campaign. Global eradication of smallpox. *Rev. Inf. Dis.* **4**, 916.

Kaper, J. B., Lockman, H., Baldini, M. M. and Levine, M. M. (1984). Recombinant nontoxigenic *Vibrio cholerae* strains as attenuated cholera vaccine candidates. *Nature* **308**, 655–658.

Liew, F. Y. (1985). New aspects of vaccine development. *Clin. Exp. Immunology* **62**, 225–241.

Conclusions

One of the most important conclusions from this survey of microbial infection and pathogenicity is that various microorganisms have developed many of the theoretically possible devices that enable them to overcome or by-pass host defences. Microorganisms evolve rapidly compared with their vertebrate host species, and can generally be expected to be one step ahead. They are quick to take advantage of changes in the host's way of life, and the comparatively recent increases in human density, for instance, have been exploited especially by the respiratory viruses. For similar reasons the venereal route of infection has become more and more promising from a microorganism's point of view. Modern syphilis apears to have arisen from an ancestral nonvenereal spirochaete similar to yaws, which infected the skin in warm countries and was spread by contact. The venereal form arose in the towns and cities of temperate countries where people wore clothes and direct mucosal spread was more successful. Contemporary venery appears to have induced a great flowering of chlamydial and other infections of the urinogenital tract.

Transfer of microorganisms via urine, faeces, food and ectoparasites has greatly decreased, at least in developed countries, but aerosol and mucosal (kissing, venereal) transfer continues with ever increasing efficiency (Fig. 7, p. 36). For the forseeable future in our crowded societies respiratory infections will predominate. Infections transmitted by mucosal routes, however, may stay with us for an even longer period. Mucosal contacts are part of loving and caring, at the core of man's humanity, and as long as people are people microorganisms will have the opportunity to spread in this way.

Because microorganisms can evolve so rapidly there is a real possibility that a particularly unpleasant one may emerge at any time. For instance, there have been no influenza A pandemics of very great significance since the 1918 outbreak. If a new strain appeared that spread with great facility and was at the same time highly lethal, say by invading cardiac muscle to produce myocarditis, the human population could be decimated before a more suitable type of virus–host balance emerged (see Ch. 1).

On the other hand, we are learning much more about infectious agents and infectious diseases, as outlined in this book. Vaccines have been of immense importance in the past and hold great promise for the future. The evolution of a microorganism can be decisively terminated by the proper application of knowledge. Smallpox, the most widespread and fatal disease in England in the eighteenth century and a major cause of blindness, has been totally eradicated from the earth.

It is important to contrast the incidence of infectious disease in different parts of the world, as discussed in Ch. 2. Many of the old infections have been eliminated from developed countries, but various latent, persistent and opportunistic infections have taken their place, especially in those who are kept alive by modern medicine and who have serious defects in microbial resistance. We need a greater knowledge of disease processes and pathogenicity not only for its basic biological interest, but also because it helps with the development of vaccines, with the understanding of persistent and latent infections (including certain types of cancer), and with our ability to deal with any strange new pestilences that arise and threaten us.

Reference

Hackett, C. J. (1963). On the origin of the human treponematoses. *Bull. W.H.O.* **29**, 7–41.

Glossary

Active immunity   Immunity acquired actively following infection or immunization by vaccines.

Addison's disease   Disease resulting from destruction of adrenal glands, characterized by weakness, debility and very great susceptibility to the stress of infection, trauma etc. Other features include spontaneous hypoglycaemia and pigmentation.

Adjuvant   A material that enhances the immune response to an antigen.

Agglutination   Clumping together of proteins (in antigen–antibody reactions), or microorganisms, or red blood cells (haemagglutination).

Aleutian disease virus   This virus infects mink and causes a fatal immunopathological disease in the type of mink that are homozygous for a recessive gene conferring the Aleutian coat colour.

Anamnestic response   Secondary immune response (see primed).

Anterior horn cells   The main motor neurons in the anterior horn (as seen in cross-section) of the spinal cord, supplying striated muscle.

Antigen processing   Preparation of antigen in macrophage for delivery to immunologically reactive lymphocyte.

Antigenic determinant   (= epitope) The small site on the antigen to which antibody attaches. Large antigens such as proteins may carry several different antigenic determinants on the molecule, against which several different antibodies are formed.

Arthus response   Inflammatory reaction formed at the site where antigen is given to an animal possessing precipitating antibody to that antigen. Characteristically oedema, haemorrhage and necrosis appear after a few hours ("immediate hypersensitivity"), and complement, polymorphs and platelets are involved in the reaction.

Attenuated   Reduced in virulence for a given host, often as a result of continued growth of a microorganism in an artificial host or culture system.

Autoimmunity   Immunity (humoral or cell mediated) to antigens of the body's own tissues. Can cause tissue damage and disease, but also occurs as a harmless consequence of tissue damage.

Avidity   Refers broadly to the ability of antibodies to bind to antigens. (Affinity is a more precisely used term referring to activity per antibody-combining site.)

Bacterial cell wall   Comprises up to 20% dry weight of cell. Basically peptidoglycan (= mucopeptide = polymer of aminosugars cross-linked by peptide chains) containing components unique to microorganisms (e.g. muramic acid). Peptidoglycan may constitute nearly all of wall (certain Gram-positive bacteria), sometimes with additional polysaccharides and teichoic acids. Gram-negative bacterial cell walls are mostly lipopolysaccharides and lipoproteins, with little mucopeptide (p. 70).

Bacteriocin   Complex bacteriocidal substance released by certain bacteria, active against related bacteria, e.g. colicins produced by *E. coli*; pyocins produced by *Pseudomonas aeruginosa*.

Basement membrane   A sheet of material up to 0.2 μm thick lying immediately below epithelial (and endothelial) cells and supporting them. Contains glycoproteins and collagen and to some extent acts as a diffusion barrier for microorganisms. Thickness and structure varies in different parts of the body.

B cells Population of lymphoid cells derived from bone marrow developing without the need for the thymus. Differentiate to form antibody-producing cells. Comprise 10–20% circulating lymphocytes in man.

Capsid Protein coat enclosing the nucleic acid core of a virus.

Cell-mediated immunity (CMI) Specific immunity mediated by and transferrable to other individuals by cells (T cells), not by serum.

Challenge Administration of antigen or pathogen to provoke an immune reaction, usually in a primed individual.

Coccus Spherical or ovoid bacterium.

Colicins see Bacteriocin.

Commensal ("table-companion") Associated with a host, often deriving nourishment from host, but neither beneficial nor harmful.

Complement An enzymic system of serum proteins, made up of nine components (C1–C9) that are sequentially activated in many antigen–antibody reactions. Complement is involved in immune lysis of bacteria and of some viruses and other microorganisms. It plays a part in phagocytosis, opsonization, chemotaxis and the inflammatory response.

Connective tissue Forms an all-pervading matrix, connecting and supporting muscles, nerves, blood vessels etc. Consists of a mucopolysaccharide "ground substance" containing cells (fibroblasts, histiocytes etc.), collagen and elastic fibres.

C-reactive protein A protein with subunits of molecular weight 24 300 that happens to react with the C carbohydrate of the pneumococcus. It is synthesized in the liver and is detectable in the serum when inflammation or tissue necrosis has taken place. It binds to substances from microorganisms and damaged tissues, activating the complement system.

Cryptococcus neoformans A yeast-like fungus found universally in soil, occasionally causing local or generalized infection in man.

Cushing's syndrome A disease resulting from excessive secretion of hormones from the adrenal cortex. Patients show wasting of muscle and bone, fat deposits on face, neck and back, and small blood vessels are easily ruptured.

Cutaneous anaphylaxis Antigen injected intradermally into an actively or passively immunized individual causes a local inflammatory response following the interaction of antigen with antibody. This is visible as a weal and flare response, or by the local leakage of dyed plasma protein from blood vessels into tissues. Plasma proteins are dyed blue by the intravenous injection of Evan's blue. A similar response takes place when antigen in the skin reacts with IgE (reaginic) antibodies bound to mast cells, but injected antibodies need a few days to bind to cells before the response is seen.

Cytophilic antibody Antibody that combines with Fc receptors on macrophages, enabling these cells to carry out immunologically specific phagocytosis.

Defective virus replication Incomplete virus replication, with production only of viral nucleic acid, proteins or noninfectious virus particles.

Delayed type hypersensitivity (dth) Hypersensitivity reaction visible 1–2 days after introduction (usually intradermally) of antigen into a sensitized individual. An expression of cell-mediated immunity (c.f. Arthus reaction).

Dendritic cell A large cell with long tree-like (dendritic) processes, present in lymphoid tissues. Concerned with presentation of antigens; not phagocytic and does not bear Fc receptors.

Dorsal root ganglia A series of ganglia lying dorsal to the spinal cord (as seen in cross-section). Contain cell bodies of principal sensory neurons, each receiving impulses along fibres from skin etc., and sending impulses along shorter fibres to spinal cord.

Enathem Lesions on mucosae (e.g. mouth, intestines) in virus infections (c.f. exanthem).

Endocytosis The uptake of material by the cell into membrane-lined vacuoles in the cytoplasm. The term includes pinocytosis (uptake of fluids) and phagocytosis (uptake of particles).

Endogenous pyrogen (= Interleukin-1) Substance released from leucocytes (in man) acting on hypothalamus to produce fever. Endotoxin (q.v.) causes fever by liberating endogenous pyrogen.

Endotoxin Toxic component associated with cell wall of microorganism. Generally refers to lipopolysaccharide of Gram-negative bacilli, the toxic activity being due to lipid A (see Fig. 14).

Enterotoxin Toxin acting on intestinal tract.

Envelope Limiting membrane of virus derived from infected host cell membrane.

Exanthem Skin rash in virus infections (c.f. enanthem).

Exotoxin Toxin released from living microorganism (e.g. tetanus toxin).

Fimbriae (pili) Thread-like processes (not flagella) attached to cell walls of certain bacteria, often mediating attachment to host epithelial cell.

Fomites Comprehensive word for patients' bedding, clothes, towels, and other personal possessions that may transmit infections.

Germinal centre A rounded aggregation of lymphocytes, lymphoblasts, dendritic cells and macrophages. Germinal centres develop in primary nodules (follicles) of lymphoid tissue in response to antigenic stimuli.

Gram negative Losing the primary violet or blue during decolorization in Gram's staining method. The method, developed by Hans Gram, a Danish physician, in 1884, gives a simple and convenient distinction between groups of bacteria (see p. 296). The staining reaction reflects differences in cell wall composition (see Fig. 14), but the mechanism is not clear.

Gram positive Retaining the primary violet or blue stain in Gram's method.

Granuloma A local accumulation of densely packed macrophages, often fusing to form giant cells, together with lymphocytes and plasma cells. Seen in chronic infections such as tuberculosis and syphilis.

Haemolysis Destruction of red blood cells. Caused by bacterial toxins, or by the action of complement on red cells coated with specific antibody.

Hapten A small molecule which is antigenic (combines with antibody) but is not immunogenic, i.e. does not induce an immune response *in vivo* unless attached to a larger ("carrier") molecule.

Heterophile antibody Antibody to heterophile antigens which are present on the surface of cells of many different animal species.

HLA see MHC.

Horizontal transmission The transmission of infection from individual to individual in a population rather than from parent to offspring.

Humoral immunity Specific immunity mediated by antibodies.

Immune complex A complex of antigen with its specific antibody. Immune complexes may be soluble or insoluble, and may be formed in antibody excess, antigen excess, or with equivalent proportions of antibody and antigen. They may contain complement components.

Immune tolerance   An immunologically specific reduction in immune responsiveness to a given antigen.

Immunopathology   Pathological changes partly or completely caused by the immune response.

Infarction   Obstruction of blood supply to a tissue or organ.

Interleukins   A group of proteins, all of them cloned and sequenced, that carry vital signals between different immune cells.

    Interleukin 1   produced by macrophages, promotes activation and mitosis of T and B cells. Causes fever (identical with endogenous pyrogen) as well as a variety of effects on muscle cells, fibroblasts and osteoblasts.

    Interleukin 2   produced by T (especially Th) cells, is essential for the continued proliferation (clonal expansion) of activated T cells.

    Interleukin 3   multicolony stimulating factor; stimulates precursor cells (e.g. in bone marrow) to divide and form colonies of polymorphs, monocytes etc.

In vitro   "In glass", that is to say not in a living animal or person.

In vivo   In a living animal or person.

Kinins   Low molecular weight peptides generated from percursors in plasma or tissues and functioning as important mediators of inflammatory responses. C2 kinin is derived from complement, and other kinins from α_2-globulins.

Lactic dehydrogenase virus   A virus that commonly infects mice, and multiplies only in macrophages. The macrophages fail to remove certain endogenous enzymes from the blood and an infected mouse is identified because there is a rise in the level of plasma lactic dehydrogenase. Infection is life long, and there are no pathological lesions or harmful effects.

Latency   Stage of persistent infection in which microorganism causes no disease, but remains capable of activation and disease production.

Legionellosis   Infection with *Legionella pneumophila*. The bacteria colonize cooling towers, creeks, showerheads, air conditioning units etc., and are inhaled after becoming airborne. Some patients develop pneumonia.

Leishmaniasis   Disease caused by protozoa of genus *Leishmania*, e.g. cutaneous leishmaniasis (Delhi boil etc.) or generalized leishmaniasis (kala-azar).

Leucocytes   Circulating white blood cells. There are about 9000 mm^{-3} in human blood, divided into granulocytes (polymorphs 68–70%, eosinophils 3%, basophils 0.5%) and mononuclear cells (monocytes 4%, lymphocytes 23–25%).

LCM   Lymphocytic choriomeningitis virus. Naturally occurring virus infection of mice displaying many phenomena of great biological interest, e.g. vertical transmission, immunopathology, noncytopathic infection of cells.

Lymphokine   Soluble factor released by primed lymphocyte on contact with specific antigen. Important in CMI.

Lysosome   Cytoplasmic sac present in many cells, bounded by a lipoprotein membrane and containing various enzymes. Plays an important part in intracellular digestion.

Lysozyme   An enzyme present in the granules of polymorphs, in macrophages, in tears, mucus, saliva and semen. It lyses certain bacteria, especially Gram-positive cocci, splitting the muramic acid–β-(1→4)-N-acetylglucosamine linkage in the bacterial cell wall. It potentiates the action of complement on these bacteria. Presumably lysozyme is not exclusively an antibacterial substance because large amounts are present in cartilage. It is present in glandular cells in the small intestine, especially in the Brazilian ant bear, where it's chitinase-like activity may help with the digestion of insect skeletons.

Macrophage processing   Uptake of antigens by macrophages, especially in the form of large particles or microorganisms, and preparation of antigen or antigens for delivery to adjacent immunocompetent lymphocytes.

Marek's disease virus   A herpes virus, commonly infecting chickens, and causing lymphocyte infiltration of nerves with demyelination and paralysis, and lymphoid tumours. Infectious virus present in oral secretions and feather follicles. Controlled successfully by a live virus vaccine.

Memory cells   Sensitized cells generated during an immune response, and surviving in large enough numbers to give an accelerated immune response on challenge.

MHC = Major Histocompatibility Complex   A region of the genome coding for immunologically important molecules.

Class I MHC molecules are HLA (human leucocyte antigen A, B, C in man and H2 k-d in mice). They are associated with β_2 microglobulin and expressed on the surface of nearly all cells. They confer uniqueness on the cells of each individual and ideally the Class I characteristics of donor and recipient should be matched for successful organ transplantation.

Class 2 MHC molecules (HLA-D, DR etc. in man; Ia or Immune-associated in mice) are present on antigen-presenting cells (some macrophages, dendritic cells, Langerhan's cells).

Class 3 MHC molecules are complement components.

Monoclonal antibody   A given B cell makes antibody of a certain class, avidity and specificity. Serum antibody consists of the separate contributions from tens of thousands of B cells. Dr Caesar Milstein discovered how to induce an individual B cell to divide and form a large enough population (clone) of cells to give bulk quantities of the unique antibody. This is a monoclonal antibody.

Natural antibodies   Antibodies present in normal serum, reacting with a wide range of organisms. To a large extent they reflect specific responses to previous subclinical infections, e.g. normal sera lyse many Gram-negative bacteria because of antibodies induced by the normal intestinal flora.

Nucleocapsid   Viral nucleic acid enclosed in a capsid consisting of repeating protein subunits.

Opsonin   (Gk *opson*, a seasoning or sauce). Serum component that combines with antigen or the surface of a microorganism and promotes its phagocytosis by polymorphs or macrophages.

Otitis media   Infection and inflammation of middle ear.

Passive immunity   Transfer of preformed antibodies to nonimmune individual by means of blood, serum components etc., e.g. maternal antibodies transferred to foetus via placenta or milk, or immunoglobulins injected to prevent or modify infections.

Pathogenic   Producing disease or pathological changes.

Persistent infection   An infection in which the microorganism persists in the body, not necessarily in a fully infectious form, but often for long periods or throughout life.

p.f.c.   Plaque forming cells. Refers to lymphocytes that form areas of lysis in a layer of erythrocytes to which the lymphocytes are immunologically sensitized.

p.f.u.   Plaque forming units. Refers to virus that forms plaques (holes) in cell sheets.

Phage typing   Different strains of *Salmonella typhi*, *Staphylococcus aureus*, or *Mycobacterium tuberculosis* can be distinguished on the basis of their different susceptibility to a battery of bacteriophages.

Pili   See Fimbriae.

Pleural and peritoneal cavities   Potential cavities surrounding organs of thorax and abdomen. Lined by "mesothelial" membrane and containing macrophages and other cells.

Plasma cell   B cell which has differentiated to form rough surfaced (ribosome studded) endoplasmic reticulum, with basophilic cytoplasm. It is the major antibody producing cell.

Pneumocystis carini   Exceedingly common protozoan parasite of respiratory tract of man and various animals; normally of zero pathogenicity. Little is known of its structure, life cycle or epidemiology. It attaches to host cells *in vitro* by means of a tubular projection but does not enter the cell except when phagocytosed, e.g. by an alveolar macrophage.

Polyclonal activator   Something that activates many clones of lymphocytes. Infections that activate B cells in this way cause the formation of large amounts of circulating antibody directed against unknown antigens as well as against the infectious agent, and often against host tissue antigens.

Primary infection   The first infection with a given microorganism.

Primed   Exposed to antigen for the first time to give a primary immune response. Further contact with the same antigen leads to a secondary immune response.

Properdin system   Consists of Factor A (a serum protein), Factor B (a β-glycoprotein) and properdin. Not completely defined and role not understood, but may have antibacterial and antiviral action. It is an alternative pathway for the activation of complement, in which C1, C2 and C4 are short-circuited.

Pyogenic   Causing production of pus.

Pyrogen   A substance causing fever.

Reservoir   Animal (bird, mammal, mosquito etc.) or animals in which microorganism maintains itself independently of human infection.

Reticulocytosis   Presence in blood of increased numbers of early form of red cell (reticulocyte), due to increased rate of production in bone marrow.

Reticuloendothelial system   A system of cells that take up particles and certain dyes injected into the body. Comprises Kupffer cells of liver, tissue histocytes, monocytes, and the lymph node, splenic, alveolar, peritoneal and pleural macrophages.

Schistosomiasis   (=bilharzia) Disease with urinary symptoms common in many parts of Africa. Caused by the fluke (trematode) *Schistosoma haematobium*; larvae from infected snails enter water and penetrate human skin.

Shedding   The liberation of microorganisms from the infected host.

Streptococci   Classified into groups A–H by antigenic properties of carbohydrate extracted from cell wall. Important human pathogens belong mostly to Group A (=*Streptococcus pyogenes*), which is divided into 47 types according to antigenic properties of M protein present on outermost surface of bacteria.

Streptolysin O   Exotoxin produced by *Streptococcus pyogenes*. Oxygen-labile, haemolytic and a powerful antigen.

Streptolysin S   Exotoxin produced by *Streptococcus pyogenes*. Oxygen-stable, causing β haemolysis on blood agar plates, but not demonstrably antigenic.

Stress   Physical or mental disturbance severe enough to initiate a coordinated response originating in the cortex and hypothalamus and involving either the autonomic nervous system or pituitary–adrenal axis. Catecholamines and corticosteroids are released in an attempt to counter the harmful systemic effects of the disturbance (or often the threatened disturbance in the case of mental stress).

Symbiotic   Living in a mutually beneficial association with the host.

Systemic infection   Infection that spreads throughout the body.

Teleology   Doctrine that biological phenomena generally have a purpose, serving some function.

T cells (T lymphocytes)   Population of lymphoid cells whose development depends on the presence of the thymus. Responsible for cell-mediated immunity. Comprise 75% circulating lymphocytes in man.

Titre   (1) A measure of units of antibody per unit volume of serum, usually quoted as reciprocal of last serum dilution giving antibody-mediated reaction, e.g. 120. (2) Measure of units of virus per unit volume of fluid or tissue. Usually given in $\log_{10}$ units per ml or g, e.g. $10^{5.5}$ p.f.u. ml^{-1}.

Toxoid   Toxin rendered harmless but still capable of acting as antigen.

Toxoplasma gondii   A protozoan parasite of the intestine of cats, which also infects mice, humans, sheep and other animals. Humans ingest oocysts originating from cat faeces or cysts from infected meat, and about half of the inhabitants of the UK eventually develop antibodies. It is generally asymptomatic, but disease (toxoplasmosis) sometimes occurs, and infection during pregnancy can result in congenital abnormalities involving the brain and eyes.

Transfer factor   A preparation derived from disrupted human leucocytes which on transfer to other individuals can supply certain missing CMI responses. The active constituent is unidentified, but it has been successfully used to treat chronic mucocutaneous candidiasis.

Transformation   A change in the behaviour of a cell, for instance after infection with an oncogenic virus, so that it acquires the properties of a cancer cell. Transformed cells undergo continued mitosis so that the cells in a monolayer are not inhibited from growth by contact with neighbouring cells, and continue to multiply and form a heap of cells. The word also refers to changes in a lymphocyte associated with onset of division.

Tuberculin test   A skin test for delayed hypersensitivity to antigens from *Mycobacterium tuberculosis*. In man the antigen is introduced into the skin by intradermal injections (Mantoux test) or by multiple puncture (Heaf test and tine test).

Vector   As used in this book the word refers to an arthropod that carries and transfers an infectious agent. Quite separately a vector means a replicating genetic unit such as a virus or a plasmid, which will carry and replicate a segment of foreign DNA that has been introduced (spliced) into it.

Vertical transmission   The transmission of infection directly from parent to offspring. This can take place *in utero* via egg, sperm, placenta, or postnatally via milk, blood, contact etc.

Viraemia   Presence of virus in blood stream. Virus may be associated with leucocytes (leucocyte viraemia), or free in the plasma (plasma viraemia), or occasionally associated with erythrocytes or platelets.

Virion   The complete virus particle.

Index